Primary Hypertension

Basic Mechanisms and Therapeutic Implications

Edited by
W. Kaufmann G. Bönner R. Lang
K. A. Meurer

With 72 Figures and 52 Tables

Springer-Verlag
Berlin Heidelberg New York Tokyo

Professor Dr. Werner Kaufmann
Dr. Gerd Bönner
Professor Dr. Robert Lang
Professor Dr. Karl August Meurer

Department of Internal Medicine II
Merheim Hospital and Policlinic of the
University of Cologne
Ostmerheimer Str. 200, D-5000 Köln 91

ISBN-13:978-3-540-16390-0 e-ISBN-13:978-3-642-71125-1
DOI: 10.1007/978-3-642-71125-1

Library of Congress Cataloging in Publication Data.
Primary hypertension. Papers from an international symposium on primary hypertension, held in Cologne, Mar. 1985. Includes index. 1. Hypertension – Congresses. I. Kaufmann, W. (Werner), 1924– . RC 685.H8P75 1986 616.1'32 86-3792 ISBN-13:978-3-540-16390-0 (U.S.)

2125/3130-543210

Preface

Some of the leading scientists in the field of hypertension accepted an invitation to actively participate in an international symposium on primary hypertension. Scientists from 13 countries – from western, southern, and eastern Europe, Australia, and the United States – were present. The meeting was held in Cologne in March 1985. After previous meetings and workshops at Titisee in the Black Forest and several symposia on the renin-angiotensin-aldosterone system here in Cologne, this symposium on primary hypertension was organized in order to induce and to stimulate critical discussion on the basic pathogenetic mechanisms involved and the recently established therapeutic implications.

Numerous studies have been based on the concept that the elevation in blood pressure is mediated by several vasopressor substances. For this reason the renin-angiotensin system has been considered to be the essential endocrine mechanism involved in developing and sustaining arterial hypertension. Other vasopressor factors, such as catecholamines, vasopressin, and serotonin, have been studied extensively and were assumed to play additional parts in blood pressure regulation. However, several other approaches have been initiated in recent years.

One approach is based upon the assumption that blood pressure elevation is not necessarily due only to overactive pressure substances, but may be a consequence of a deficiency in vasodilating agents. It has been shown by several authors that kinins and prostaglandins are such substances, generated in the kidney, vascular beds, and other organs. From data obtained in recent years it can be derived that the kallikrein-kinin and the prostaglandin systems seem to contribute to blood pressure regulation by counteracting the vasoconstricting and sodium-retaining action of the renin-angiotensin-aldosterone mechanism.

Another rapidly emerging scientific approach concerns extensive studies on the significance of the central and peripheral nervous system in the control of arterial blood pressure. Evidence on the probability that the central nervous system is involved in blood pressure control has resulted from studies demonstrating that the brain is a principal site of action of several potent hypotensive agents and that hypotension can be induced and/or prevented experimentally by direct chemical and surgical manipulations at defined brain structures. The hypothalamic area seems to integrate somatic, endocrine, and autonomic functions in response to a wide variety of ambient as well as endogenous stimuli. Those responses are apparently mediated by increased sympathic outflow and release of catecholamines from the adrenal medulla with concomitant increase of peripheral vasomotor tone and peripheral resistance. In view of the experimental significance of the endocrine and neurogenic mechanisms, a coupling between humoral factors and the nervous system must be considered a logical consequence in explaining the development of high blood pressure in primary hypertension. We were forced to realize, however, that it is not possible at the moment to combine endocrine and neural mechanisms in such a way that a generally accepted concept explaining the development and maintenance of primary hypertension can be established.

Irrespective of its pathogenesis, hypertension is one of the main risk factors of the vascular system. Epidemiological follow-up studies have demonstrated clearly that the risk of developing either fatal or nonfatal complications of hypertension is directly proportional to the level of arterial pressure. The main objectives of hypotensive treatment are thus consecutively defined as:

(1) Prevention or possibly even regression of vascular damage.
(2) Reduction of the increased workload on the heart and, hence, reversal of cardiac hypertrophy.

In view of these objectives, a critical evaluation of the established drug therapy of arterial hypertension seems mandatory. The effects of drugs must be related as closely as possible to the pathogenetic mechanisms involved in blood pressure control. Alpha- and beta-blocking agents as well as angiotensin I converting-enzyme (ACE) inhibitors are definite examples of this, and serotonin antagonists are possible examples.

In addition, there is another group of hypotensive compounds, the calcium antagonists, which deserve special interest for at least two reasons:

(1) By blocking the calcium channels of vascular muscle membranes, they interfere with the pathogenetic mechanism, which has until recently been almost neglected with respect to blood pressure control, in contrast to all the other possible factors already mentioned.
(2) Calcium channel blockers have been shown experimentally to have a vascular effect that might be classified as angioprotective.

If this concept could be proved, not only for animals but also for humans, a new era of hypotensive treatment would begin.

In summary, then, the symposium had the following objectives:

(1) To critically evaluate the basic endocrine and neural mechanisms involved in developing and sustaining primary hypertension.
(2) To define the objectives of hypotensive treatment as preventing progression of arteriosclerosis, thus protecting organ function and inhibiting or even reversing cardiac hypertrophy.
(3) To critically discuss and evaluate recently introduced hypotensive agents, especially calcium antagonists, ACE inhibitors, and serotonin-blocking compounds.

The meeting was stimulating, and there were numerous critical and constructive discussions, with results and ideas exchanged in a free and open atmosphere of friendship and cooperation.

This meeting was made possible by a fund from Bayer Pharmaceutical, whom we would like to thank for all the financial and administrative help.

Cologne, March 1986

W. Kaufmann
G. Bönner
R. Lang
K. A. Meurer

Table of Contents

List of Contributors

You will find the addresses at the beginning of the respective contribution

Critical Review of Pathogenesis of Primary Hypertension

Sodium Chloride and Blood Pressure

G. A. MacGregor[1]

Introduction

The balance between salt intake and excretion of sodium chloride plays an important role in determining the volume of extracellular fluid. When mammals moved away from the sea, particularly herbivorous mammals, they had some difficulty in obtaining enough sodium chloride and this could account for their salt appetite and the powerful mechanisms that conserve both sodium and chloride in urine and sweat. In early civilisations man found that sodium chloride was able to preserve food and this allowed the preservation of food during the winter. Salt, therefore, became of economic importance. Large amounts of salt are now consumed in most societies in the world (100–400 mmol/day) compared with what was eaten during man's evolution (approximately 1–10 mmol/day) [1].

Animal Studies

Normal Animals. In the early 1950s Meneely and colleagues showed that in ordinary laboratory rats fed on different amounts of salt for 9 months blood pressure during this time was related to the amount of salt in the diet [2]. An increase in salt intake has also been shown to cause a rise in blood pressure in normal baboons [3] and sheep [4]. Grollman has also shown that feeding pregnant rats additional sodium chloride resulted in their offspring having a higher blood pressure than rats born to mothers who were given less sodium [5].

Inherited Hypertension in Rats. Dahl, by selective inbreeding of rats over 5–7 generations, produced strains which were sensitive (S) or resistant (R) to salt [6]. He showed that in the S-rats that developed high blood pressure there was a critical phase, when they were young, when they were much more susceptible to the effects of salt. Parabiotic experiments between S-rats that developed high blood pressure and R-rats that did not, demonstrated that the rise in blood pressure in the S-rats was at least in part due to a blood-borne factor which could cause a rise in pressure in the R-rat when parabiosed with the S-rat [7]. Furthermore, kidney cross-transplantations between the two strains of rats before high blood pressure had developed demonstrated that the kidney was responsible for the development of the high blood pressure [6]. Studies in spontaneously hypertensive rats (SHR) have also shown that

[1] Blood Pressure Unit, Department of Medicine, Charing Cross & Westminster Medical School, London W6 8RF, Great Britain.

Primary Hypertension
Ed. by W. Kaufmann et al.

increasing salt intake causes a rise in blood pressure [8]. Furthermore, increasing salt intake in all forms of experimental hypertension causes a rise in blood pressure [9].

Studies in Man

For obvious reasons, studies that have been done in man are much less clear-cut and rely mainly on epidemiological and intervention studies. The strongest epidemiological evidence is the comparison between different communities where sodium intake has been shown to relate to both systolic and diastolic blood pressure [10]. Simpson has recently reanalysed several of these studies and added some more recent ones. He was able to confirm separately in both men and women that for an increase in sodium intake of 100 mmol/day, there was an increase in systolic pressure of 12 mmHg and of diastolic pressure of 7 mmHg, although, as he points out, it is not clear whether there is a linear relationship between salt intake and blood pressure between different communities [11] (Fig. 1). Most studies, however, within one community have shown no relationship between individuals' sodium intake and blood pressure. The finding may not be unexpected. Day-to-day variation in salt intake in one individual is almost as large as the variation between individuals, so that the measurement of 24-h urinary sodium excretion will reflect quite accurately the average intake for the population, but will not characterise accurately the salt intake for one individual. The Framingham survey (F in Fig. 1) in the United States illustrates this point in that when subjects were divided into four groups according to increasing sodium excretion, there was an increase in the prevalence of high blood pressure in each group as sodium excretion increased [12]. However, overall, there was no relationship between individuals' sodium excretion and blood pressure. In other communities where there is a wider range of salt intake and intake in one individual tends to be more consistent, for instance, in Korea [13] and Japan [14, 15], direct relationships have been shown between sodium intake and blood pressure.

Overall, therefore, taking the animal and epidemiological evidence, there is quite substantial circumstantial evidence to suggest that as salt intake increases in different communities of the world, so does the prevalence of high blood pressure. Indeed, in Japan where there is a wide variation in sodium intake from one region to another, the amount of sodium in the diet has been directly related to the number of strokes that occur [16]. Nevertheless, some sceptics remain unconvinced and point out that

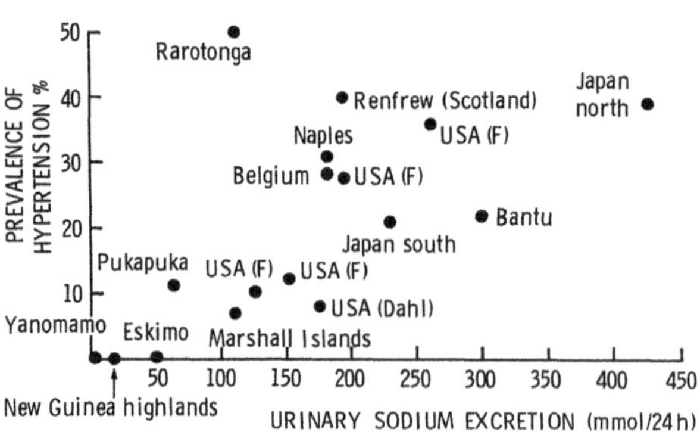

Fig. 1. The geographical distribution of relationship between the prevalence of hypertension and 24-h urinary sodium excretion. *F*, Framingham study

it could be some other factor other than salt in the diet that could account for these differences although this would seem unlikely in the controlled animal experiments.

Intervention Studies. There are now several studies in which salt intake has been altered in a community. In Kenya, soldiers were given a daily 16-g salt ration, and with this increase in salt intake, blood pressure rose [17]. A study of an African rural tribe, some of whom have migrated to the city, has shown that in the urban environment sodium excretion rises and potassium excretion falls [18]. Part of the rise in blood pressure that occurred with this migration was attributed to the increase in salt intake and reduction in potassium intake. Government campaigns in Japan [19, 20] and Belgium [21] have resulted in a reduction in salt intake and during this time there was a fall in the prevalence of high blood pressure and a decrease in cerebrovascular mortality.

However, by far the best intervention study has been performed in Holland by Hoffman et al. [22] who randomly allocated 476 newborn babies into two groups, one of which had a normal sodium intake and the other, a low sodium intake. The mothers were provided with all the nutrients and did not know in which group their child had been placed. There was a progressive increasing difference in systolic blood pressure between the two groups so that at 6 months of age, the babies on the normal sodium intake had a mean systolic pressure 2.1 mm Hg higher than those on the low sodium intake. At 6 months of age the difference in diet was discontinued, nevertheless, this carefully controlled study does illustrate the important role of salt intake in determining blood pressure levels in early infancy. Clearly, this type of study should be continued for longer, but there are obvious practical difficulties in maintaining differences in sodium intake for the 20 or 30 years that would be needed to prove beyond doubt that salt does cause or predispose to essential hypertension in man. It is unlikely that such studies will ever be done. Careful observation of the communities in which intake of sodium is being reduced, for instance, as is now happening in Japan, Belgium and the United States may, perhaps, retrospectively provide the evidence to justify the reduction in salt intake in the world.

How Does Salt Cause a Rise in Blood Pressure?

Kidney cross-transplantation experiments in three forms of inherited hypertension in rats have shown that the kidney carries the underlying abnormality for the high blood pressure [6, 23, 24]. In the Dahl S-rat, Tobian et al. [25] have shown that the kidney is less able to excrete sodium even before high blood pressure has developed, suggesting that at least in this form of inherited hypertension, the abnormality in the kidney is a difficulty in excreting sodium. Two studies in man of renal transplant recipients now suggest that the kidney may also be important in human essential hypertension. In Milan it has been shown that in renal transplant recipients, the donor's family history of hypertension plays an important role in determining subsequent blood pressure in the transplanted patient [26]. In other words, kidneys that come from donors with a family history tend to result in a higher blood pressure in the recipient when they are matched for all of the other factors that may also influence blood pressure in transplanted patients. In the United States, it has been shown that

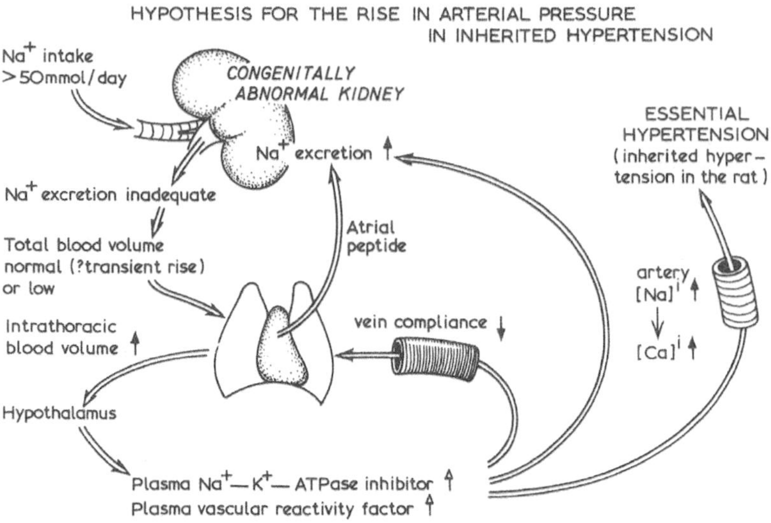

Fig. 2. Sequence of events to explain a postulated inherited defect in the kidney's ability to excrete sodium. The observed rise in a concentration of a circulating sodium transport inhibitor, salt intake and the rise in peripheral resistance in essential hypertension

in patients who develop renal failure secondary to essential hypertension without malignant hypertension kidney transplantation cured their high blood pressure [27]. Based on experiments in parabiotic rats, Dahl was the first to suggest the idea that the rise in blood pressure in Dahl S-rat might be caused by an increase in a sodium-excreting hormone [7]. Subsequently, this idea was developed by Haddy and Overbeck [28] and Blaustein [29] in volume-expanded hypertension and man with essential hypertension. Blaustein pointed out that a rise in intracellular sodium could, through inhibition of sodium-calcium exchange, cause a rise in intracellular calcium and, thereby, increase vascular reactivity of arteriolar smooth muscle. Following these ideas and the kidney cross-transplantation experiments in inherited hypertension in rats, de Wardener and MacGregor [30] suggested that most forms of hypertension whether primary or secondary, could be due to normal volume control mechanisms correcting a persistent inherited or acquired renal difficulty in excreting sodium. In other words, the demonstrated rise in the level of a sodium transport inhibitor might be secondary to an inherited difficulty in the kidney's ability to excrete sodium. The rise in the level of this inhibitor and with time, the severity of the blood pressure, could depend on the extent of the kidney's defect to excrete sodium and the salt intake. At the same time these suggestions could also account for many other related abnormalities that are known to occur in human essential hypertension (Fig. 2).

Abnormalities of Sodium Transport in Human Essential Hypertension

Several different abnormalities of sodium transport have been described in the red cells of patients with essential hypertension [30]. More consistent, however, have been the findings in white cells. Subjects with high blood pressure have been shown to have an increase in white cell sodium concentration which appears to be related to a reduction in the ouabain-sensitive component of the sodium pump [31–34]. This latter finding is consistent with either an inborn abnormality of the cell membrane or an increase in the levels of a circulating inhibitor of the sodium pump. Cross-incubation experiments where normotensive leucocytes have been incubated in the plasma have shown that hypertensive plasma induces the same change in normotensive white cells as found in the hypertensives' own white cells [35] and the degree of inhibition of the sodium pump achieved is related to the height of the subjects from which the plasma was obtained [36]. Other studies using cytochemical bioassays for the ability of plasma to inhibit Na^+-K^+-ATPase and glucose-6-phosphate-dehydrogenase [37] and biochemical assays of Na^+-K^+-ATPase [38] and ouabain displacement of plasma binding to red cells [39] have all suggested there may be a raised level of a circulating inhibitor of the sodium pump in patients with essential hypertension. Whether this increased level of a circulating sodium transport inhibitor is in any way responsible for the increase in peripheral resistance in high blood pressure is not known. Furthermore, its exact identity, unlike the atrial peptides, is not known. However, ouabain is known to increase reactivity of arterioles to agonists such as noradrenaline [40], and digoxin given orally to normotensive subjects for 5 days increased their blood pressure response to infused angiotensin II and noradrenaline [41].

Salt Restriction in Established Hypertension

Restriction of sodium intake can cause substantial falls in blood pressure when it is raised. The first report of this was in patients with renal disease and the reduction in blood pressure was attributed to a reduction in chloride intake [42]. Careful work by Allen and Sherill [43] in the 1920s confirmed these earlier findings. This work was largely forgotten until Kempner [44] revived the idea in the 1940s with his rice and fruit diet. He and others clearly demonstrated a major fall in blood pressure in subjects with severe hypertension and malignant hypertension with clearing of papilloedema and heart failure [45]. These findings are, in some ways, all the more impressive as we now know that patients with malignant hypertension tend not to have much of a fall in blood pressure with salt restriction because of the increase in renin secretion that occurs. Some evidence also suggested that increasing sodium intake from around 10 mmol/day to 25–35 mmol/day caused a rise in blood pressure, although blood pressure did not return to pretreatment levels [45]. Many physicians took this evidence to mean that less severe sodium restriction would not lower blood pressure. However, more recent evidence has shown that less severe restriction of sodium intake to around 80 mmol sodium/day causes a fall in blood pressure even in patients with less severe essential hypertensions [46–48]. Two recent studies have been claimed to show no effect of salt restriction in patients with mild essential hypertension. However, blood pressure in one study during the control phase when patients were on a normal sodium intake was in the normal range [49]. The second study in which there were only 12 patients did show a fall in blood pressure with salt restriction which just failed to reach statistical significance [50]. When all the 20 or

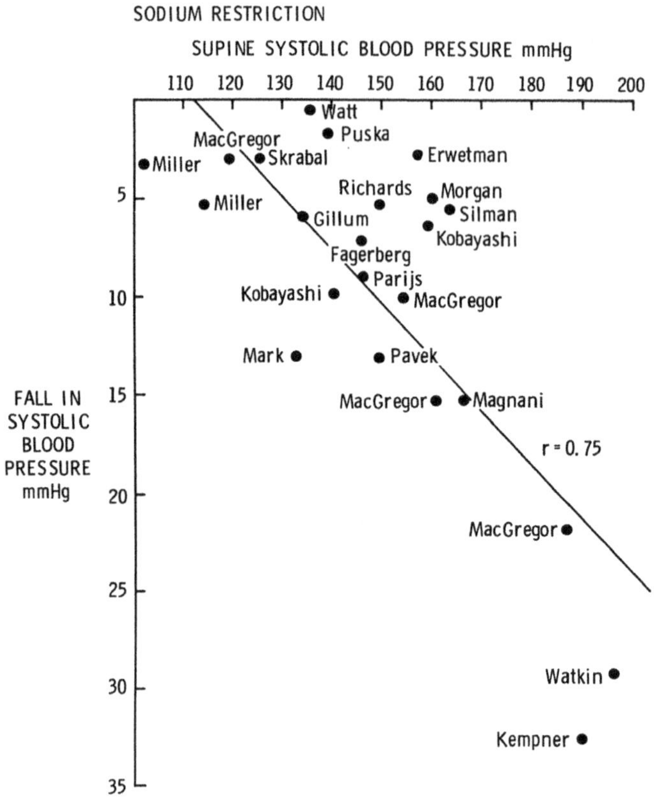

Fig. 3. Fall in supine systolic blood pressure with sodium restriction against pretreatment supine systolic blood pressure

so published studies that we have been able to find where pretreatment or control blood pressure and the fall in blood pressure with sodium restriction alone are given, it can be seen that the higher the initial blood pressure, the greater the effect of salt restriction (Fig. 3). In our own double-blind study of moderate sodium restriction in patients with mild to moderate essential hypertension, there was overall a highly significant fall in blood pressure of 6%, and of the 19 patients studied, 16 had a fall in blood pressure with salt restriction. The fall in blood pressure that was seen was equivalent to that seen in double-blind studies of a beta-blocker alone or a diuretic alone [48]. Several studies have now shown that the effect of salt restriction, as would be expected, is additive to that of blood-pressure–lowering drugs [49, 50] (Fig. 4).

Several studies have suggested that as with diuretics the blood pressure fall with sodium restriction is mediated by a diminished renin response in the hypertensives [51, 52]. In other words, normotensives with salt restriction have a much greater increase in renin release and thereby angiotensin II and less of a fall in blood pressure, whereas patients with lower initial levels of renin have the same loss of sodium and water with sodium restriction, but much less of a rise in renin and angiotensin II and,

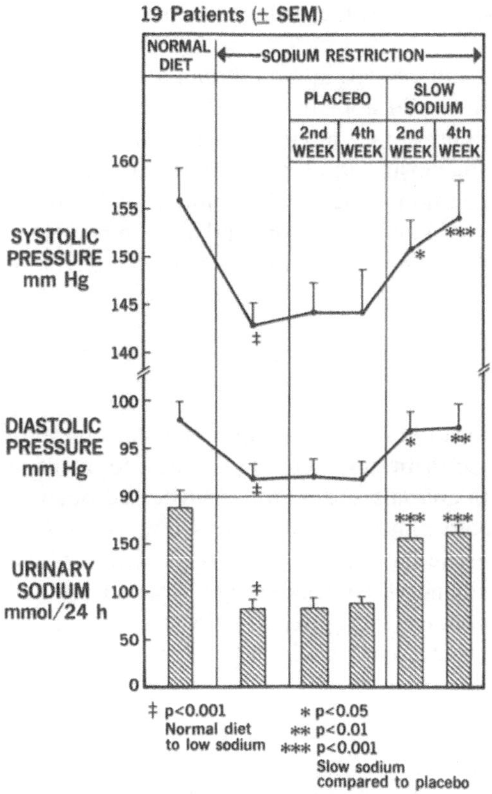

Fig. 4. Average systolic and diastolic blood pressure and urinary sodium excretion on normal diet 2 weeks after dietary sodium excretion, at 2-week intervals during a randomised crossover trial of Slow sodium vs placebo in 19 patients with mild to moderate essential hypertension on no drug treatment. ***, $P<0.001$; **, $P<0.01$; *, $P<0.05$ comparing equivalent measurement on Slow sodium to placebo. ‡, $P<0.001$ for comparison of normal diet and 2 weeks of dietary sodium restriction

therefore, a bigger fall in blood pressure. We examined this relationship directly with the use of saralasin, a competitive inhibitor of angiotensin II, and found that in patients on a low salt diet, the fall in blood pressure with saralasin was inversely correlated with the fall in blood pressure that had occurred with the salt restriction, directly implicating the importance of the renin-angiotensin system to the salt restriction in the fall in blood pressure that occurred [53].

Is It Practical to Reduce Salt Intake?

Clearly, there is no point in instructing patients to change their habits when, in fact, they are not going to be able to do this. A good example is weight loss and alcohol reduction which are extremely difficult to achieve in patients with high blood pressure. Many physicians who had experience of the Kempner rice and fruit diet felt the same way about salt restriction. However, more moderate salt restriction is quite easily achieved in patients who eat predominantly at home. Five percent of the sodium that we currently eat naturally occurs in food; the rest is added to processed foods or during cooking or at the table [54]. Our experience and that of others is that after 1 or 2 months of moderate sodium restriction, most patients prefer the diet [11] and find that the previous high salt foods that they used to eat have become distasteful as the taste receptors become much more sensitive to lower concentrations of sodium chloride.

Several other dietary factors may also be important in modulating blood pressure such as potassium, fat and fibre intake. It would appear reasonable, therefore, to combine moderate salt restriction with other dietary advice that is currently being given by nutritionists, i.e. to reduce total fat consumption, particularly saturated fat, to increase fresh fruit and vegetable consumption as well as fibre intake. All of these will help with compliance to moderate sodium restriction and may have other benefits apart from their blood-pressure–lowering effect in preventing the development of premature vascular disease.

Summary

Evidence from animal and epidemiological studies suggests that a high consumption of sodium chloride may be an important contributing factor to the development of high blood pressure. Recent work on both animals and man has suggested possible mechanisms whereby a high salt intake could cause high blood pressure. When high blood pressure has already developed, restricting salt intake causes a fall in blood pressure in many patients but not necessarily into the normal range. The fall in blood pressure is greater the higher the blood pressure and appears, at least in part, to be related to suppression of the renin system that occurs as blood pressure rises.

References

1. MacGregor GA (1983) Dietary sodium and potassium intake and blood pressure. Lancet 1:750–753
2. Ball OT, Meneely GR (1957) Observations on dietary sodium chloride. J Am Diet Assoc 33:366
3. Cherchovichg M, Capek K, Jaefremova Z, Pohlava I, Jelink J (1976) High salt intake and blood pressure in lower primates. J Appl Physiol 40:601
4. Whitworth JA, Coghlan JP, Denton DA, Hardy K, Scoggins BA (1979) Effect of sodium loading and ACTH on blood pressure of sheep with reduced renal mass. Cardiovasc Res 13:92
5. Grollman A, Grollman EF (1962) The teratonenic induction of hypertension. J Clin Invest 41:710–714
6. Dahl LK, Heine N (1975) Primary role of renal homographs in setting chronic blood pressure levels in rats. Circ Res 36:692–696
7. Dahl LK, Knudsen D, Iwai J (1980) Humoral transmission of hypertension. Am J Med 69:746–758
8. Aoki K, Yamori Y, Ooshim A (1972) Effects of high or low sodium intake in spontaneously hypertensive rats. Jpn Circ J 36:539
9. Haddy FJ (1980) Mechanism, prevention and therapy of sodium dependent hypertension. Am J Med 69:746–758
10. Gleibermann L (1973) Blood pressure and dietary salt in human populations. Ecol Food Nutr 2:143–155
11. Simpson FO (1984) Salt and hypertension: current data, attitudes and policies. J Cardiovasc Pharmacol 6:S4–S9
12. Dawber TR, Kannel WB, Kaga ANA, Donabedian RK, McNamara PM (1967) Environmental factors in hypertension. In: Stamler I, Stamler R, Pullman TN (eds) Epidemiology of hypertension. Grune and Stratton, New York, pp 255–288
13. Kesteloot H, Park BC, Lee CS, Brems-Heyns E, Joossens JV (1980) A comparative study of blood pressure and sodium intake in Belgium and in Korea. In: Kesteloot H, Joossens JV (eds) Epidemiology of arterial blood pressure. Nijhoff, The Hague, pp 453–470

14. Shibarta H, Hatano S (1979) A salt restriction trial in Japan. In: Gross F, Strasser T (eds) Mild hypertension: Natural history and management. Pitman, Bath, pp 147–158
15. Yamori Y, Kihara M, Nara Y, Ohtaka M, Horje R, Tusunematsu T, Note S (1981) Hypertension and diet, multiple regression analysis in a Japanese farming community. Lancet 1:120
16. Sasaki N (1962) High blood pressure and salt intake of the Japanese. Jpn Heart J 3:313
17. Shaper AG, Leonard PJ, Jones KW, Jones M (1969) Environmental effects on the body build, blood pressure and blood chemistry of nomadic warriers serving in the army of Kenya. East Afr Med 46:262–289
18. Poulter N, Kahw KT, Hopwood BEC, Mugambi M, Peart WS, Sever PS (1984) Salt and blood pressure in various populations. J Cardiovasc Pharmacol 6:S197–S203
19. Ministry of Health and Welfare (1981) National Nutritional Survey. Koseisho
20. Ministry of Health and Welfare (1980) National Survey on Circyulatory Disorders. Koseisho.
21. Joossens JV, Geboers J (1983) Salt and hypertension. Prev Med 12:53
22. Hoffman A, Hazebroek A, Valenburg HA (1983) A randomised trial of sodium intake and blood pressure in newborn infants. JAMA 250:370–373
23. Bianchi G, Fox U, di Francesco GF, Giovanetti AM, Pagetti D (1974) Blood pressure changes by kidney cross-transplantation between spontaneously hypertensive rats and normotensive rats. Clin Sci Mol Med 47:435–438
24. Kawabe K, Watanebe TX, Shiono K, Sokabe H (1979) Influence of blood pressure on renal isographs between spontaneously hypertensive and normotensive rats utilising the Fl hybrids. JPN Heart J 20:886–894
25. Tobian L, Lange J, Azei S, Iwai J, Koop E, Coffee J, Johnson MA (1978) Reduction of natriuretic capacity in renin release in isolated blood perfused kidneys of Dahl hypertension-prone rats. Circ Res 43:I 92–97
26. Guidi C, Avanzi C, Bianchi G (1984) Familial factors in hypertension after renal transplantation. Proceedings of 9th International Congress of Nephrology , Los Angeles, 209A
27. Curtis JJ, Luke RG, Dusten HP, et al. (1983) Remission of essential hypertension after renal transplantation. N Engl J Med 309:1009–1015
28. Haddy FJ, Overbeck JW (1976) The role of humoral agents in volume expanded hypertension. Life Sci 19:935–948
29. Blaustein MP (1977) Sodium ions, calcium ions, blood pressure regulation and hypertension: a reassessment and a hypothesis. Am J Physiol 232(3):C165–C173
30. De Wardener HE, MacGregor GA (1983) The relation of a circulating sodium transport inhibitor (the natriuretic hormone?) to hypertension. Medicine (Baltimore) 62:310–326
31. Edmondson RPS, Thomas RD, Hilton PJ, Patrick J (1975) Abnormal leucocyte concentration and sodium transport in essential hypertension. Lancet 1:1003–1005
32. Ambrosioni E, Costa FV, Montebugnoli L, Tartagni F, Magnani B (1981) Increased intralymphocytic sodium content in essential hypertension: an index of an impaired sodium cellular metabolism. Clin Sci 61:181–186
33. Araoye MA, Khatri IM, Yao LL, Freis ED (1978) Leucocyte intracellular cations in hypertension: effective antihypertensive drugs. Am Heart J 96(6):731–738
34. Heagerty AM, Bing RF, Milner M, Thurston H, Swales JD (1982) Leucocyte membranes, sodium transport in normotensive populations, the association of abnormalities of sodium efflux from raised blood pressure. Lancet 2:894–896
35. Poston L, Sewell RB, Wilkinson SP, Richardson PJ, Williams R, Clarkson EM, MacGregor GA, de Wardener HE (1981) Evidence for a circulating sodium transport inhibitor in essential hypertension. Br Med J 282:847–849
36. Kuske R, Renner D, Schoner W (1984) Demonstration of an inhibitor of the Na pump of human lymphocytes in the serum of patients with essential hypertension. Biomed Biochim Acta 43:S21
37. MacGregor GA, Fenton S, Alaghband-Zadeh J, Markandu ND, Roulston JE, de Wardener HE (1981) Evidence for a raised concentration of a circulating sodium transport inhibitor in essential hypertension. Br Med J 283:1355–1357
38. Hamlyn JM, Ringel R, Schaeffer J, Levinson PD, Hamilton BP, Kowarski AA, Blaustein MP (1982) A circulating inhibitor of ($^{+}$-K^{+}) ATPase associated with essential hypertension. Nature 100:650
39. Devynck MA, Pernollet MG, Rosenfeld JB, Meyer P (1983) Measurement of digitalis-like compound in plasma: application in studies of essential hypertension. Br Med J 287:631–634

40. Gebert G, Piechowiak H (1974) Effect of potassium and norepinephrine on the tone of the isolated artery: changes by ouabain pretreatment. Experientia 30:46–47
41. Guthrie TP Jr (1984) Effects of digoxin on the responsiveness to the pressor action of angiotensin and norepinephrine. J Clin Endocrinol Metab 58:76–80
42. Ambard L, Beaujard E (1904) Causes de l'hypertension artérielle. Arch Gen Med 1:520–533
43. Allen FM, Sherril JW (1922) The treatment of arterial hypertension. J Metab Res 2:429–545
44. Kempner W (1948) Treatment of hypertensive vascular disease with rice diet. Am J Med 4:545–577
45. Watkin DM, Froeb HF, Hatch FT, Gutman AB (1950) Effects of diet in essential hypertension. Am J Med 9:441– 493
46. Parijs J, Joossens JV, van der Linden L, Verstreken G, Amery AKIC (1973) Moderate sodium restriction and diuretics in the treatment of hypertension. Am Heart J 855:22–34
47. Morgan T, Gillies A, Morgan G, Adams W, Wilson M, Carney S (1978) Hypertension treated by salt restriction. Lancet 1:227–230
48. MacGregor GA, Markandu ND, Best FE, Elder DM, Cam JM, Sagnella GA, Squires M (1982) Double-blind randomised crossover trial of moderate sodium restriction in essential hypertension. Lancet 1:351–356
49. Watt GCM, Edwards C, Hart JT, Hart M, Walton P, Foy CJW (1983) Dietary sodium restriction for mild hypertension in general practice. Br Med J 286:432–436
50. Richards AM, Espiner EA, Maslowski AH, Nicolls NG, Ikram, H., Hamilton, EJ, Wells, J Blood pressure response to moderate sodium restriction and potassium supplementation in mild essential hypertension. Lancet 1:757–761
51. Parfrey PS, Markandu ND, Roulston JE, Jones BE, Jones JC, MacGregor GA (1981) Relations between arterial pressure, dietary sodium and renin system in essential hypertension. Br Med J 283:94–97
52. Longworth BL, Dreyer JIM, Lieber MA, Laragh J (1980) Divergent blood pressure responses during short-term sodium restriction in hypertension. Clin Pharmacol Ther 27:544–546
53. Cappuccio FP, Markandu ND, Sagnella GA, MacGregor GA (to be published) Sodium restriction lowers high blood pressure through a decreased response of the renin system – direct evidence using saralasin. J Hypertens
54. MacGregor GA (1984) The salt-free diet book. Dunitz, London

Non-Modulating Essential Hypertension: A Subset with Sodium Sensitivity

G. H. Williams[1] and N. K. Hollenberg[1]

Introduction

Multiple lines of evidence suggest a role for sodium intake in the pathogenesis of hypertension, although it appears that only some hypertensives have a special sensitivity to sodium [7, 13, 25]. The frequency of "sodium-sensitive" hypertension has been estimated to be around 60% based on the efficacy of sodium restriction [4] or diuretic agents [6] in lowering blood pressure. There is also evidence to indicate that diuretics are efficacious in the same patients as respond to a reduced sodium intake [17]. A pressor response to a sodium load also occurs in about 50% of unselected, but small groups of patients [7, 13].

It is unlikely that sodium-sensitive hypertension is a homogeneous group. For example, in patients with bilateral renal artery stenosis, primary aldosteronism, or mild renal failure – all forms of sodium-sensitive hypertension, the mechanisms underlying their volume dependency are different [14]. The attempt to subclassify patients with essential hypertension on the basis of a renin-sodium profile has been partially successful in this regard. Patients with "low renin essential hypertension" show a more striking and consistent response to diuretics than does any other subgroup of patients with essential hypertension [14]. However, even low renin hypertension is unlikely to be homogeneous.

Two questions arise from this analysis: First, can the known forms of volume-dependent hypertension account for all sodium-sensitive hypertension? Second, is there a common mechanism underlying each? The answer to both questions is clearly: No. Not only is the cumulative frequency of bilateral renal artery stenosis, primary aldosteronism, chronic renal failure, and low renin essential hypertension too low, it is clear that some patients with normal renin essential hypertension also have a pressor response to sodium loading [7, 13]. Furthermore, none of the hypotheses proposed to explain sodium-sensitive hypertension can account for the known sodium sensitivity of these normal renin essential hypertensives – potentially the largest subgroup.

The purposes of this essay are threefold: to review (a) the normal factors involved in sodium homeostasis, (b) the ways in which abnormalities in these normal regulatory systems may lead to altered sodium homeostasis, and (c) the potential therapeutic implications of such findings.

[1] Harvard Medical School and Brigham and Women's Hospital, 75 Francis Street, Boston, MA 02115, USA.

Primary Hypertension
Ed. by W. Kaufmann et al.

The Renin-Angiotensin-Aldosterone System

Several studies on the role of the renin-angiotensin-aldosterone system have primarily addressed its involvement in regulating blood pressure, ignoring the evidence that this system exerts its primary influence on extracellular fluid volume. This fact can be appreciated best by reviewing how this system evolved.

The simplistic interpretation of several [2, 20, 22, 26] reports is that the renin-angiotensin-aldosterone system initially evolved to control extracellular fluid volume, primarily by modifying renal plasma flow and thereby regulating glomerular filtration rate [23]. With an increasingly complex environment, aldosterone also came under the control of renin, further potentiating the ability of this system to respond appropriately to swings in sodium intake. A final modification which has occurred with these systems is the ability of sodium intake to modify vascular (particularly) renovascular and adrenal response to angiotensin II. The effect is reciprocal: sodium restriction enhances adrenal and reduces vascular responses while dietary sodium loading produces the opposite effect [11, 16].

Altered Renal and Adrenal Responsiveness to Angiotensin II in Essential Hypertension

During the 1970s, it became clear that normal control of both the renal vasculature and adrenal responses with changes in sodium intake were dominated by angiotensin II and that there were abnormalities in these relationships in hypertensive subjects. For example, in a subset of patients with essential hypertension, renal circulation was not modified by sodium restriction [10, 12]. A second set of studies reported that some patients with essential hypertension had alterations in the adrenal response to volume depletion [28]. These studies also suggested that the underlying problem was a defect in the interaction of angiotensin II with the adrenal responses – a hypothesis later confirmed [15].

Thus, a substantial body of evidence has accumulated suggesting that in some patients with essential hypertension changes in sodium intake do not produce changes in the sensitivity of the adrenal and renal vasculature to angiotensin II. Uncertain until recently was whether these abnormalities coexist in the same patient. However, two recent studies, one using both acute volume depletion to determine whether an adrenal defect was present and xenon washout to assess renal blood flow [29] and the other administering angiotensin II infusions in patients on a high and low sodium intake [21], have verified that there is a subgroup of patients with essential hypertension who fail to modulate their renal blood flow and aldosterone responses to angiotensin II with changes in dietary sodium intake. We have termed these individuals "non-modulators".

Relationship Between Non-Modulation and Hypertension

One of the major recent conceptual advances in hypertension research has been the recognition that with changing conditions, even in a simple model, the factors responsible for the elevated blood pressure also may vary. For example, angiotensin II is certainly the prime factor mediating the hypertensive process in early renovascular hypertension and even in later stages, if sodium intake is restricted. However, it is equally apparent that other mechanisms are important in maintaining the elevated blood pressure when these patients are salt loaded with suppression of the renin-angiotensin system [1, 3, 8]. How does this apply to the pathogenesis of essential hypertension? Again, it is likely to be relevant where sodium handling is deranged, as seems to be the case in non-modulators. For example, angiotensin II dominates the control of both the adrenal and renal vasculature, and in normal subjects both show reciprocal changes in responsiveness as sodium intake changes. Therefore, the adrenal defect is most apparent with sodium restriction, while the renal abnormality becomes most evident with sodium loading. Thus, the expression of this abnormality at any moment is likely to be a reflection of the amount of sodium ingested.

How could these abnormalities produce an elevated blood pressure? To answer this question, one needs to assess the impact of each in the situation where its function is most important. In normal subjects with sodium restriction, the adrenal responses to angiotensin II are enhanced, thus facilitating sodium retention. In the non-modulators, this is defective. As a result, aldosterone secretion is reduced, which leads to an increased renin release and angiotensin II formation as the obligatory response of this negative feedback loop. Thus, the non-modulator's blood pressure will be more angiotensin dependent.

What happens with sodium loading? Several mechanisms in which the renal vasculature participates contribute to an appropriate renal response to a sodium load. First, the sodium load presented to the renal tubule is determined by the glomerular filtration rate, which is dependent up on renal blood flow. Second, renal hemodynamics also determine peritubular oncotic and hydrostatic pressure, which in turn are determinants of proximal tubular sodium reabsorption. Thus, to the extent that the renal perfusion is fixed in these patients [5, 21, 24] these factors cannot modify renal sodium handling, requiring the recruitment of alternative mechanisms. Thus, non-modulation may provide an explanation for why some normal and high renin hypertensive patients are salt sensitive.

What is the role of non-modulation in the altered sodium handling of some hypertensive subjects? Recently in 28 patients divided into modulators and non-modulators, according to the criteria noted above, the time necessary to achieve low sodium balance was assessed. The half-time of disappearance of sodium from the urine for the non-modulators was 36 h, nearly 50% longer than in modulators or normotensive subjects (24 h), theoretically leading to an increased sodium retention. These individuals also would require longer to achieve sodium balance.

A second study has documented the validity of these theoretical calculations [19]. Twenty-five patients in balance on a low sodium intake were given 200 mEq of sodium per day for 5 days. In the modulators, which comprised almost half of these patients, sodium balance was achieved in approximately 2 days with a net sodium accumulation of approximately 100 mEq. In contrast in the non-modulators, balance had not been achieved even by the end of the 5th day at a time when the cumulative sodium balance was nearly double (200 mEq) that observed in the modulators. What was the effect of this difference in sodium handling on blood pressure? Again in this same study, only the non-modulators had a pressor response to sodium loading.

Thus, it appears likely that non-modulators are "salt-sensitive" and that the salt sensitivity results from their failure to excrete a sodium load appropriately, presumably secondary to the defect in their renal blood supply. Since in over 400 patients [27] in whom modulation or non-modulation could be determined, approximately 50% of the normal and high renin essential hypertensive patients were non-modulators, this abnormality could account for nearly all normal and high renin essential hypertensives with salt sensitivity.

Future Directions and Relationship to Other Abnormalities in Essential Hypertension

In this essay we have reviewed the potential role that target tissue resistance to angiotensin II may play in raising blood pressure. Presently available data would suggest that nearly half of white normal and high renin essential hypertensive subjects are non-modulators, i.e., sodium intake fails to modulate adrenal and renal vascular responsiveness to angiotensin II. As a consequence of this abnormality these individuals fail to excrete a sodium load appropriately, and thus have sodium-sensitive hypertension.

Does this evolving hypothesis account for other abnormalities described in hypertensive patients? Theoretically, one would assume that if the major system used to respond to various sodium loads is defective, then secondary systems will be activated in an attempt to maintain normal sodium homeostasis. Thus, with sodium loading and the failure of renal blood flow to increase, presumably most of the sodium is finally excreted by the recruitment of other factors including dopamine, the atrial natriuretic peptide and the ouabain-like inhibitor of sodium potassium ATPase. While this would presumably facilitate sodium excretion, a price would be paid, in that tissue responsiveness to vasoconstrictor agents would be increased [9, 18]. Furthermore, abnormalities in sodium transport across red blood cell membranes have been reported in some hypertensives. Theoretically, this abnormality may be occurring in those hypertensive patients who are non-modulators, again because of their abnormality in sodium homeostasis [30]. If true, then assessment of red cell sodium transport may be an effective screening procedure to determine which hypertensives are non-modulators. Such an approach is necessary because, at the present time, the only reliable way non-modulators are detected is complex and time consuming – either by assessing the adrenal response to angiotensin II on a low sodium intake or the renal vascular response on a high sodium intake. This complexity precludes their application for general screening.

References

1. Barger AC 1979 The Goldblatt Memorial Lecture, Part 1. Experimental renovascular hypertension. Hypertension 1:447–455
2. Berne HA (1967) Hormones and endocrine glands of fishes. Science 158:455–462
3. Brunner HR, Kirshman JD, Sealey JE, Laragh JH (1971) Hypertension of renal origin: Evidence for two different mechanisms. Science 174:1344

4. Chapman B (1951) Some effects of the rice-fruit diet in patients with essential hypertension. In: Bell ET (ed) Hypertension. A symposium. University of Minnesota, Minneapolis, p 516
5. Dluhy RG, Bavli SZ, Leung FK, Solomon HS, Moore TJ, Hollenberg NK, Williams GH (1979) Abnormal adrenal responsiveness and angiotensin II dependency in high renin essential hypertension. J Clin Invest 64:1270–1276
6. Freis E (1979) Comparative effects of ticrynafen and hydrochlorothiazide in the treatment of hypertension (Veterans Administration Cooperative Study Group on Antihypertensive Agents). New Engl J Med 301:293
7. Fujita T, Henry WL, Bartter FC, Lake CR, Delea CS (1980) Factors influencing blood pressure in salt-sensitive patients with hypertension. Am J Med 69:334–344
8. Gavras H. Brunner HR, Vaughan ED Jr, Laragh JH (1973) Angiotensin-sodium interaction in blood pressure maintenance of renal hypertensive and normotensive rats. Sciene 180:1369
9. Gruber KA, Whitaker JM, Buckalew VM Jr (1980) Endogenous digitalis-like substance in plasma of volume-expanded dogs. Nature 287:743–745
10. Hollenberg NK, Merrill JP (1970) Intrarenal perfusion in the young 'essential' hypertensive: A subpopulation resistant to sodium restriction. Trans Assoc Am Physicians 83:93–101
11. Hollenberg NK, Chenitz WR, Adams DF, Williams GH (1974) Reciprocal influence of salt intake on adrenal glomerulosa and renal vascular responses to angiotensin II in normal man. J Clin Invest 54:34–42
12. Hollenberg NK, Borucki LJ, Adams DF (1978) The renal vasculature in early essential hypertension: Evidence for pathogenetic role. Medicine (Baltimore) 57:167–178
13. Kawasaki T, Delea CS, Bartter FC, Smith H (1978) The effect of high-sodium and low-sodium intakes on blood pressure and other related variables in human subjects with idiopathic hypertension. Am J Med 64:193–198
14. Laragh JH (1973) Vasoconstriction-volume analysis for understanding and treating hypertension. The use of renin and aldosterone profiles. Am J Med 55:261–273
15. Moore TJ, Williams GH, Dluhy RG, Bavli SZ, Himathongkam T, Greenfield M (1977) Altered renin-angiotensin-aldosterone relationships in normal renin essential hypertension. Circ Res 41:167–171
16. Oelkers W, Brown JJ, Fraser R, Lever AF, Morton JJ, Robertson JIS (1974) Sensitization of the adrenal cortex to angiotensin II in sodium-deplete man. Circ Res 34:69–77
17. Parijs J, Joossens JV, van der Linden L, Verstreken G, Amery AKPC (1973) Moderate sodium restriction and diuretics in the treatment of hypertension. Am Heart J 85:22
18. Poston L, Sewell RB, Wilkinson SP, Richardson PJ, Williams R, Clarkson EM, MacGregor GK, de Wardener HE (1981) Evidence for a circulating sodium transport inhibitor in essential hypertension. Br Med J 282:847–849
19. Redgrave JE, Rabinowe SL, Hollenberg NK, Williams GH to be published Correction of abnormal renal blood flow response to angiotensin II by converting enzyme inhibition in essential hypertensives. J Clin Invest
20. Sawyer WH, Blair-West JR, Simpson PA, Sawyer MK, (1976) Renal responses of Australian lungfish to vasotoxin, angiotensin II and NaCl infustion. Am J Physiol 231:593–602
21. Shoback DM, Williams GH, Moore TJ, Dluhy, RG, Podolsky S, Hollenberg NK (1983) Defect in the sodium-modulated tissue responsiveness to angiotensin II in essential hypertension. J Clin Invest 72:2115–2124
22. Sokabe H (1974) Physiology of the renal effects of angiotensin. Kidney Int 6:263–277
23. Sokabe H, Mizogame S, Sato A (1968) Role of renin in adaptation to sea water in eruyhaline fishes. Jpn J Pharmacol 18:332–343
24. Taylor TT, Moore TJ, Hollenberg NK, Williams GH (1984) Converting enzyme inhibition corrects the altered adrenal response to angiotensin II in essential hypertension. Hypertension 6:92–99
25. Tuck ML, Williams GH, Dluhy RG, Greenfield M, Moore TJ (1976) A delayed suppression of the renin-aldosterone axis following saline infusion in human hypertension. Circ Res 39:711–716
26. Vinson GP, Whitehouse BJ, Goddard C, Sibley CP (1979) Comparative and evolutionary aspects of aldosterone secretion and zona glomerulosa function. J Endocrinol 81:5P–24P
27. Williams GH, Hollenberg NK (to be published) Defect in sodium mediated adrenal and renal responsiveness to angiotensin II in essential hypertension: Implications for pathogenesis. In: Carey RM (ed) Is essential hypertension an endocrine disease? Butterworth, London

28. Williams GH, Rose LI, Dluhy RG, McCaughn D, Jagger PI, Hickler RB, Lauler DP (1970) Abnormal responsiveness of the renin-aldosterone system to acute stimulation in patients with essential hypertension. Ann Intern Med 72:317–326
29. Williams GH, Tuck ML, Sullivan JM, Dluhy RG, Hollenberg NK (1982) Parallel adrenal and renal abnormalities in the young patient with essential hypertension. Am J Med 72:907–914
30. Woods JW, Parker JC, Watson BS (1983) Perturbation of sodium-lithium countertransport in red cells. Engl J Med 308:1258–1261

Vasodepressor Hormones (Kinins) in Blood Pressure Regulation*

O. A. CARRETERO[1] and S. F. RABITO[1]

Introduction

There are many mechanisms by which blood pressure can be regulated. These mechanisms interact in a complex fashion with each other to maintain blood pressure homeostasis.

Vasopressor systems such as the renal renin-angiotensin system have been clearly shown to have a major role in the control of blood pressure and in the pathogenesis of certain types of hypertension [86]. The role of vasodepressor systems in the control of blood pressure and in the pathogenesis of hypertension is less well defined. However, the hypothesis that a balance among vasopressor and vasodepressor systems contributes to the maintenance of normal blood pressure and that an alteration of this balance could cause hypertension or hypotension is reasonable (Fig. 1). Kinins are one of the most potent vasodilator substances known. These peptides are released from precursor proteins known as kininogens (substrate) by a group of enzymes known as kininogenases. The best known and most potent kininogenases are plasma and glandular kallikreins. Plasma kallikrein (EC 3.4.21.33) circulates as a

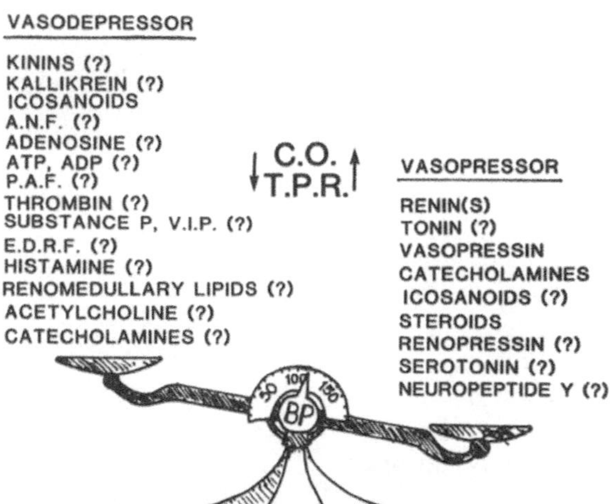

Fig. 1. Hypothetical role of vasoactive substances in hypertension

* This study was supported in part by NIH grant HL 28982.

[1] Hypertension Research Division, Henry Ford Hospital, 2799 W. Grand Boulevard, Detroit, MI 48202, USA.

Primary Hypertension
Ed. by W. Kaufmann et al.

proenzyme complexed to its substrate, high molecular weight kininogen (HMWK). Plasma prekallikrein is activated by and in turn activates Hageman factor (coagulation factor XII). This system, in addition to its kinin generating and procoagulant activity, has fibrinolytic activity (through the activation of plasminogen to plasmin) and complement activating capability [19]. Glandular kallikrein(s) (EC 3.4.21.34) are serine proteases with 60%–75% homology with tonin, γ-subunit of nerve growth factor and epidermal growth factor-binding protein, [3, 32, 51, 56] and 35%–50% homology with trypsin, chymotrypsin, and elastase [7, 25, 56, 91]. Kallikrein(s) appear to originate from the expression of 25–30 different genes located in chromosome 7 [56]. Kallikreins are found in the salivary and sweat glands, pancreas, intestines, kidney, prostate, spleen, arteries and veins, and brain (Fig. 2). This ubiquitous location

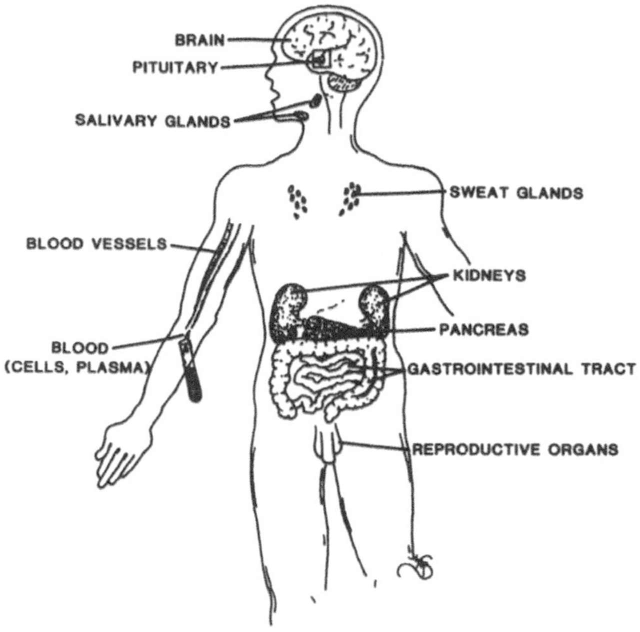

Fig. 2. Localization of kallikrein

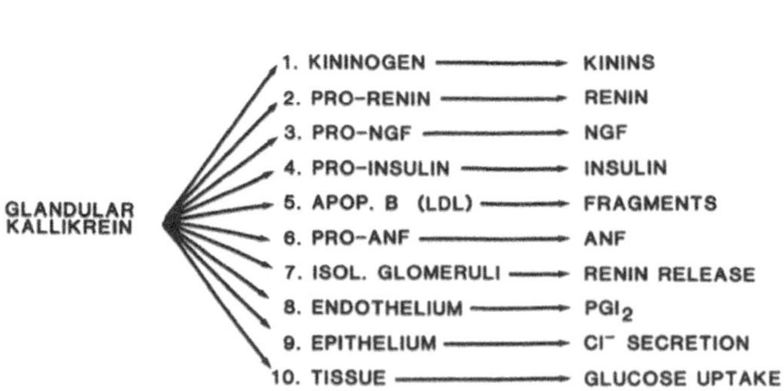

Fig. 3. Proposed functions of glandular kallikrein

and the presence of multiple kallikrein genes suggest multiple functions for this enzyme(s).

Although glandular kallikrein has a much narrower range of substrate specificity than trypsin, it can hydrolyze many other substrates. In addition to its kininogenase activity (kinin generating capacity), glandular kallikrein has the capability to process pro-hormone to hormone (proinsulin [64], pro-renin [28, 80], pro-atrial natriuretic factor [26]), to activate growth factors [10, 12, 34], to generate angiotensin from plasma [57], to break down apoprotein B from LDL [13], to stimulate the release of renin and PGI_2 [6, 14, 61, 90, 92], and to produce contraction of the uterus [8, 9, 16] and ureter [53] (Fig. 3). These in vitro and pharmacological effects of the enzyme are not mediated by the release of kinins. Although, at the present time, it is not known whether these events also occur in physiological and pathological situations, they open the possibility that kallikrein participates in multiple biological regulatory functions.

The kininogenase activity of kallikrein is an important one although kininogen is not the exclusive substrate for this enzyme. Glandular kallikrein can release kinins from both HMWK and low molecular weight kininogen (LMWK). When released into the circulation, glandular kallikrein is rapidly inactivated by plasma inhibitors, while generated kinins are destroyed by a group of peptidases known as kininases. Thus, both the rapid inactivation of glandular kallikrein and the rapid degradation of kinins in normal circumstances suggest that if this vasodepressor system plays a role in blood pressure regulation, it is not as a systemic but as a local hormone (autacoid).

Salgado et al. [79] in our laboratory have shown that during the infusion of bradykinin, the arterial blood kinin concentration required to decrease blood pressure in normotensive and hypertensive rats was 40 to 100 times higher than that found in non-infused normal rats. This finding makes it unlikely that circulating kinins play a role in blood pressure regulation. As autacoids, the glandular kallikrein-kinin system could regulate vascular resistance, particularly in tissues rich in glandular kallikrein. Furthermore, in the kidney, the renal kallikrein-kinin system could participate in the control of sodium and water excretion and, consequently, in blood pressure regulation.

The Brain Kallikrein-Kinin System

All the components of the kallikrein-kinin system are present in the central nervous system (CNS) where they may participate in the modulation of nervous, neuroendocrine, and cardiovascular functions. Kininogenase activity has been found in brain homogenates [41], in the anterior pituitary gland [72, 74, 84], pituitary pars intermedia [73, 84], hypothalamus, pineal gland, and cerebrospinal fluid (CSF) [84]. Bradykinin-like substances have been extracted from brain, and using an immunofluorescence method, bradykinin was localized in hypothalamic neurons and in nerve fibers [23]. In addition, functional bradykinin receptors have been identified in a cultured nerve cell population derived from neuroblasts [88]. Kinins and kininogen have also been measured in CSF [84, 93]. Kinins may be generated locally, however, the source of CSF kininogen is unknown. Kininases, particularly kininase II and a metalloendopeptidase, are also present in the brain [17, 18, 27, 43, 45].

The cardiovascular effects of kinins given centrally are quite different from the actions of these peptides applied peripherally. Bradykinin, injected intraventricularly, produces a hypertensive response, an effect that is abolished by lateral septal lesions [20, 21, 22, 50]. This central effect of bradykinin is mediated by α-adrenergic mechanisms operating within the lateral septal area [20, 21, 22] and by prostaglandin-related systems of the brain [44]. In the dorsomedial and posterior hypothalamic nuclei, bradykinin increased both heart rate and blood pressure [29]. These effects were blocked by pretreatment with methylatropine, suggesting that the parasympathetic nervous system mediates these actions of bradykinin in these hypothalamic nuclei. The first evidence of an involvement of the endogenous brain kallikrein-kinin system in the central modulation of cardiovascular function was obtained by Thomas et al. [93]. These authors reported that ventriculocisternal perfusion with melittin, an activator of membrane bound kallikrein, caused elevation in the concentration of kinins in CSF accompanied by an increase in blood pressure.

The Glandular Kallikrein-Kinin System in Organs Rich in Glandular Kallikrein

The salivary glands, especially the submandibular gland, have very high concentrations of glandular kallikrein. Glandular kallikrein is found in the cells of convoluted granular tubules and striated ducts of these glands [66]. The exocrine secretions of these glands have significant amounts of glandular kallikrein, although its function is not known.

Studies in our laboratory have demonstrated that under resting conditions the rat submandibular gland releases kallikrein into the vascular compartment [76]. Sympathetic stimulation of the gland produced a 46-fold increase in kallikrein secretion rate into the circulation. This increase was blocked by pretreatment with phentolamine and prazosin, indicating that the sympathetic nervous system, through activation of α_1-adrenoreceptors, controls kallikrein secretion from the submandibular gland into the circulation. Furthermore, we have observed that in 48h nephrectomized rats, the inhibition of converting enzyme or kininase II by captopril significantly increased the blood flow to the unstimulated submandibular gland without changes in blood pressure [68]. In contrast, 10 min after sympathetic stimulation of the gland, captopril produced a marked decrease in blood pressure [67]. Both the changes in blood flow and blood pressure were blocked by antibodies to kinins. Thus, it may be that when glandular kallikrein is released into the circulation in small amounts, it functions as an autacoid regulating local blood flow, and when released in large amounts, such as after sympathetic stimulation of the submandibular gland, it functions as a vasodilator hormone, decreasing systemic blood pressure. However, the results observed in these studies may be unique for the rat since its submandibular gland contains more kallikrein than that of any other species studied, and upon sympathetic stimulation, releases a large amount of kallikrein into the circulation [76]. Therefore, in other organs and species which are not as rich in glandular kallikrein, the kallikrein-kinin system may act only as an autacoid when the tissue is stimulated to release kallikrein into the circulation.

The Renal Kallikrein-Kinin System

The presence of the kallikrein-kinin system in the kidney is especially important since this organ is essential in the long-term regulation of blood pressure. Urinary kallikrein is synthesized by the kidney. Isolated rat kidneys, when perfused with fluids that contain neither prekallikrein nor kallikrein, produce and release active and inactive kallikrein not only in the urine but also in the perfusion fluid [24, 78]. The kallikrein found in the perfusion fluid appears to be secreted directly into the vascular compartment, since it is found in the perfusion fluid of non-filtering kidneys [95]. We found that plasma immunoreactive glandular kallikrein increases three to four times after nephrectomy, and that its concentration was lower in the renal venous than in arterial blood [77]. These data suggest that the kidneys filter and remove plasma immunoreactive glandular kallikrein. In all probability, most of this enzyme is in the inactive form [96]. These studies do not exclude the possibility that in vivo the kidney also releases kallikrein into the vascular compartments as shown in the isolated perfused kidney studies [24, 58, 95]. Furthermore, a simultaneous increase in esterase activity in the renal lymph and urine of dogs during saline infusion has been reported, suggesting that renal kallikrein is released in the interstitial space of the kidney [57]. However, esterolytic methods are highly unspecific, and this study should be interpreted with caution. Renal kallikrein in the interstitial and vascular spaces of the kidney could release kinins from plasma kininogen, thereby possibly playing a role in the regulation of renal blood flow distribution. At the present time, it is not clear whether renal and other glandular kallikreins reach the peripheral circulation in their active form, since there are considerable amounts of protease inhibitors in plasma which very rapidly inactivate this enzyme [40, 94].

Though some of the immunoreactive kallikrein in urine may be filtered from plasma [33], we have evidence that most of the urinary kallikrein is produced by the kidney [81]. It could be that most of the filtered immunoreactive kallikrein is reabsorbed by endocytosis in the proximal tubule [85].

Over 90% of the kallikrein in the kidney is found in the cortex, decreasing from the outer to the inner cortex, with very little kallikrein in the medulla and papilla [63, 82]. Isolated glomeruli have a small amount of kallikrein activity compared with the kallikrein concentration in the total cortex. Using the stop-flow technique, we have shown that kallikrein is secreted in the urine in the distal tubule [81]. In immunohistochemical studies, Ørstavik et al. [69, 70] have shown that in the rat kidney kallikrein is localized in the convoluted distal tubules at a point distal to the juxtaglomerular apparatus, extending along the distal tubule to a point ending in the collecting tubule. In these studies, no kallikrein could be found in the collecting tubule or in the area of the macula densa. We studied the localization of both active and inactive kallikrein in the microdissected rabbit nephron [65]. Active and inactive kallikrein were localized in the granular portion of the distal and cortical collecting tubules. This segment of the nephron contains more than 85% of the active and inactive kallikrein found in the total microdissected nephron. Very little active or inactive kallikrein was found in other segments, including the bright portion of the distal segment which has the macula densa. The granular portions of the distal convoluted and cortical collecting tubules have similar characteristics both morphologically [49] and functionally [42]. They form a single nephron segment called the connecting tubule which has two types of cells, the connecting tubule cells and the intercalated cells. Since the connecting tubule cells and kallikrein localize only in the granular part of the distal and collecting segment, and the intercalated cells are thoroughly distributed from the granular distal tubule to the medullary collecting tubule, it is reasonable to assume that kallikrein is synthesized in the connecting tubule cells. The discrete localization of kallikrein suggests a specific role of renal kallikrein in association with these nephron segments. Recently, we have shown that this segment of the nephron has an anatomical relation with the afferent arteriole which contains renin [5].

Considerable amounts of kinins are present in the urine [1, 39, 59]. They appear to be formed in the kidney and in the urine itself [60]. We found no correlation between kallikrein and kinin excretion in urine collected directly from the ureter of the rat [83]. Further, in this study we found that acidification of the urine by sodium sulfate infusion decreased kinin excretion, while it increased kallikrein excretion. On the other hand, alkalinization of normally acidic urine of the rat by volume expansion or infusion of sodium bicarbonate increased urinary kinin excretion. These data indicate that urinary kallikrein excretion may not reflect the intrarenal formation of kinins. Another possible interpretation is that even when the urine is collected directly from the ureters, urinary kinins do not reflect the activity of the system, since they may, in part, be destroyed before leaving the kidney since renal tissue is very rich in kininases [30, 37].

When bradykinin is infused into the renal artery, 90% is inactivated in one passage through the kidney and less than 0.2% appears in the urine [60]. There are three main types of kininases in the kidney: kininase I [31, 54, 87], kininase II [37, 47, 60], and a neutral metalloendopeptidase (NEP [2, 35]). Kininase II has been studied more extensively than kininase I, partly because kininase II, in addition to hydrolyzing kinins, converts angiotensin I to angiotensin II (angiotensin I-converting enzyme, ACE). Kinins could be considered the preferred substrate for kininase II, since the K_m is lower for this peptide than for angiotensin I. Kininase II has been localized in the brush border of the proximal tubule cells of the kidney using fluorescein-labeled antibody to kininase II, and also by demonstrating a high concentration of this enzyme in brush-border membranes which were separated by differential centrifugation [37, 62]. Small concentrations of kininase II were also found in the distal nephron. An NEP has been recently purified from human kidney that in vitro cleaves bradykinin by releasing the C-terminal dipeptide [2, 35]. Although the K_m of bradykinin is lower with kininase II than with NEP, NEP has a 10-fold higher turnover number [35]. The importance of this NEP in the in vivo degradation of kinins remains to be determined. The presence of these peptidases in the lumen of the proximal tubule prevents filtered kinins from reaching the distal nephron, thus acting as an effective barrier [15].

The origin of the kininogen (substrate) needed for the formation of kinins in the lumen of the nephron is not known. The plasma of different species is very rich in kininogen. The amount is on the order of 4–12 μg/ml when expressed as its capability to release kinins when incubated with trypsin. A small amount of plasma kininogen reaching the distal nephron could account for the kinins found in the urine. In human urine, there is a significant amount of immunoreactive kininogen, however, kininogen is found in small amounts when measured by its capability to generate kinins [71]. It could be that most of the kininogen has already been consumed by the urinary kallikrein. It has been reported that urinary kinins were absent in a subject with a congenital deficiency of HMWK and LMWK [38]. On the other hand, as previously mentioned, in a patient without HMWK, but with normal LMWK (Fitzgerald trait), it was found that the urine contained normal amounts of kinins (unpublished observation). This indicates that kinins in the urine are formed from LMWK and that they are not formed by plasma kallikrein, since this enzyme mainly uses HMWK as substrate [19]. The plasma kininogen appears to be synthesized by the liver [11]. The possibility that kininogen is produced by the kidney itself cannot be completely disregarded, since it has been reported that kidney tissue contains kininogen [97]. However, in this study, the possibility that the kidney extracts were contaminated with blood was not eliminated.

Recently, Proud et al. [75] using antibody to low molecular weight kininogen and immunohistochemical techniques have localized kininogen in cells of distal and collecting tubules. In rabbit renal tissue, we have been unable to demonstrate the presence of kininogen (K. Omata, A. G. Scicli, and O. A. Carretero, unpublished results). The presence of an inhibitor of glandular kallikrein has also been demonstrated in the rat kidney tubules [36]. It is feasible that this inhibitor could play a role in the regulation of intrarenal formation of kinins.

The infusion of kinins into the renal artery results in an increased blood-flow, diuresis, and natriuresis without changes in glomerular filtration rate. Like most vasodilator drugs, kinins produce a greater increase in blood flow in the inner cortex than in the outer. Unlike other vasodilators, kinins do not decrease proximal sodium and water reabsorption in outer cortical nephrons available for micropuncture [89]. Accordingly, the natriuretic effect of kinins is either due to inhibition of sodium reabsorption in the distal part of the nephron or to changes in deep nephron reabsorption. Kinins may affect sodium reabsorption as the result of a direct effect on the transport of sodium in the nephron, a vasodilator effect, changes in the osmotic gradient of the renal medulla, or a combination of all three effects. Changes in the osmotic gradient of the renal medulla could explain the decrease in urinary osmolality and vasopressin-resistant diuresis caused by kinins [98].

Kinins administered into the renal artery probably do not mimic the effects produced by kinins formed intrarenally by endogenous kallikrein, since their sites of action or concentration could be different. Kauker [46] has shown that kinins administered directly into the late proximal tubule increase ^{22}Na excretion, also injected into the tubule. However, he used doses of bradykinin at least 50 times higher than that expected to be found in the distal nephron. The enhancement by kinins of sodium excretion could have occurred proximal to the distal and collecting tubules where kinins are formed in the nephron. Nevertheless, this study suggests that kinins in the lumen of the nephron have natriuretic effects. The role of endogenously generated kinins in the regulation of renal blood flow, and water and electrolyte excretion has been studied by using ACE inhibitors. These inhibitors increase the concentration of endogenous kinins by inhibiting kininase II. After administration of ACE inhibitors, renal blood flow increases in the juxtamedullary cortex with a simultaneous increase in the fractional excretion of sodium [4]. The increase in renal blood flow, sodium excretion, or urinary volume observed after administration of ACE inhibitors correlates positively with both the concentration of kinins in the renal vein and the amount of kinins in the urine [60]. However, the use of ACE inhibitors does not allow for differentiation between the potentiation of kinin activity and the inhibition of the conversion of angiotensin I to angiotensin II. Administration of aprotinin, an inhibitor of kallikrein and other proteases, to volume-expanded rats decreased GFR, renal blood flow, urinary volume, sodium, potassium, and PGE_2 excretion [92]. Furthermore, administration of antibodies against kinins to saline-infused rats resulted in a decrease in sodium excretion [52]. This finding suggests that intrarenally released kinins cause natriuresis, diuresis, and release of prostaglandins.

Summary and Conclusions

Kinins are one of the most potent vasodilator substances known. These peptides are released from substrates called kininogens by a group of serine proteases known as kininogenases. The best known and most potent kininogenases are plasma and glandular kallikreins. Plasma kallikrein circulates as a proenzyme complexed to its substrate, HMWK. This system has kinin generating, procoagulant, fibrinolytic, and complement activating capabilities. Glandular kallikreins are found in the salivary and sweat glands, pancreas, intestines, kidney, prostate, spleen, arteries and veins, brain, and pituitary and pineal glands. Glandular kallikreins can release kinins from both HMWK and LMWK. Because of the rapid inactivation of both kallikrein and kinins in the circulation, this vasodepressor system may play a role in the regulation of blood pressure as a local hormone (autacoids) rather than as a systemic one. As autacoids the glandular kallikrein-kinin system could regulate vascular resistance in tissues rich in glandular kallikrein such as the submandibular gland. In the kidney, the endogenous kallikrein-kinin system could participate in the regulation of sodium and water excretion and, therefore, in the control of blood pressure. The role of the arterial wall and brain kallikrein-kinin systems in the regulation of peripheral vascular resistance needs further investigation.

References

1. Abe K (1965) Urinary excretion of kinin in man with special reference to its origin. Tohoku J Exp Med 87:175–184
2. Almenoff J, Orlowski M (1983) Membrane-bound kidney metalloendopeptidase: interaction with synthetic substrates, neutral peptides, and inhibitors. Biochemistry 22:590–599
3. Ashley PL, MacDonald RJ (1985) Kallikrein-related mRNAS of the rat submaxillary gland: nucleotide sequences of four distinct types including tonin. Biochemistry (In press)
4. Bailie MD, Barbour JA (1975) Effect of inhibition of peptidase activity on distribution of intrarenal blood flow. Am J Physiol 228:850–853
5. Barajas L, Powers K, Carretero OA, Scicli AG, Inagami T (1985) Simultaneous immunocytochemical localization of renin and kallikrein in rat renal cortex. Kidney Int (Submitted)
6. Beierwaltes WH, Prada J, Carretero OA (1985) Effect of glandular kallikrein on renin release in isolated rat glomeruli. Hypertension 7:27–31
7. Bell GI, Quinto C, Quiroga M, Valenzuela P, Craik CS, Rutter WJ (1984) Isolation and sequence of a rat chymotrypsin B gene. J Biol Chem 259:14265–14270
8. Beraldo WT, Araujo RL, Mares-Guia M (1966) Oxytocic esterase in rat urine. Am J Physiol 211:975–980
9. Beraldo WT, Lauar NS, Siqueira G, Heneine IF, Catanzaro OL (1976) Peculiarities of the oxytocic action of rat urinary kallikrein. In: Pisano JJ, Austen KF (eds) Chemistry and biology of the kallikrein-kinin system in health and disease. Fogarty International Center Proceedings, Washington, DC, pp 375–378

10. Berger EA, Shooter EM (1977) Evidence for pro-β-nerve growth factor, a biosynthetic precursor to β-nerve growth factor. Proc Natl Acad Sci USA 74:3647–3651
11. Borges DR, Gordon AH (1976) Kininogen and kininogenase synthesis by the liver of normal and injured rats. J Pharm Pharmacol 28:44–48
12. Bothwell MA, Wilson WH, Shooter EM (1979) The relationship between glandular kallikrein and growth factor-processing proteases of mouse submaxillary gland. J Biol Chem 254:7287–7294
13. Cardin AD, Witt KR, Chao J, Margolius HS, Donaldson VH, Jackson RL (1984) Degradation of apolipoprotein B-100 of human plasma low density lipoproteins by tissue and plasma kallikreins. J Biol Chem 259:8522–8528
14. Carretero OA, Beierwaltes WH (1984) Effect of glandular kallikrein, kinins and aprotinin (a serine protease inhibitor) on renin release. J Hypert 2 (Suppl 1):125–130
15. Carone Fa, Pullmann TN, Oparil S, Nakamura S (1976) Micropuncture evidence of rapid hydrolysis of bradykinin by rat proximal tubule. Am J Physiol 230:1420–1424
16. Chao J, Shimamoto K, Margolius HS (1981) Kallikrein-induced uterine contraction independent of kinin formation. Proc Natl Acad Sci USA 78:6154–6157
17. Checler F, Vincent JP, Kitabgi P (1983) Degradation of neurotensin by rat brain synaptic membranes: involvement of a thermolysin-like metalloendopeptidase (enkephalinase), angiotensin converting enzyme, and other unidentified peptidases. J Neurochem 41:375–384
18. Chevillard C, Saavedra JM (1983) Selective increase of angiotensin-convertying enzyme activity in discrete extrahypothalamic areas of Brattleboro rats. Brain Res 272:283–290
19. Colman RW (1980) Patho-physiology of the kallikrein system. Ann Clin Lab Sci 10:220–226
20. Correa FMA, Graeff FG (1974) Central mechanisms of the hypertensive action of intraventricular bradykinin in the unanesthetized rat. Neuropharmacology 13:65–75
21. Correa FMA, Graeff FG (1975) Central site of the hypertensive action of bradykinin. J Pharmacol Exp Ther 192:670–676
22. Correa FMA, Graeff FG (1976) On the mechanism of the hypertensive action of intraseptal bradykinin in the rat. Neuropharmacology 15:713–717
23. Correa FMA, Innis RB, Uhl GR, Snyder SH (1979) Bradykinin-like immunoreactive neuronal system localized histochemically in rat brain. Proc Natl Acad Sci USA 76:1489–1493
24. Corthorn J, Roblero J (1981) Release of activatable kallikrein by isolated rat kidneys. Hypertension 3 (Suppl II):39–41
25. Craik CS, Choo QL, Swift GH, Quinto C, MacDonald RJ, Rutter WJ (1984) Structure of two related rat pancreatic trypsin genes. J Biol Chem 259:14255–14264
26. Currie MG, Geller DM, Chao J, Margolius HS, Needleman P (1984) Kallikrein activation of a high molecular weight atrial peptide. Biochem Biophys Res Comm 120:461–466
27. Defendini R, Zimmerman EA, Weare JA, Alhenc-Gelas F, Erdös EG (1983) Angiotensin-converting enzyme in epithelial and neuroepithelial cells. Neuroendocrinology 37:32–40
28. Derkx FHM, Tan-Tjiong HL, Man In't Veld AJ, Schalekamp MPA, Schalekamp MAH (1979) Activation of inactive plasma renin by tissue kallikreins. J Clin Endocrinol Metab 49:765–769
29. Diz DI, Jacobowitz DM (1984) Cardiovascular effects of discrete intrahypothalamic and preoptic injections of bradykinin. Brain Res Bull 12:409–417
30. Erdös EG (1979) Kininases. In: Erdös EG, (ed) Bradykinin, Killidin and Kallikrein, Handbook of experimental pharmacology, vol 25 supply. Springer, Berlin Heidelberg New York, pp 427–428
31. Erdös EG, Yang HYT (1967) An enzyme in microsomal fraction of kidney that inactivates bradykinin. Life Sci 6:569–574
32. Evans BA, Richards RI (1985) Genes for the α and γ subunits of mouse nerve growth factor are contiguous. EMBO 4:133–138
33. Fink E, Schleuning M (1982) Studies on the excretion of tissue kallikrein from blood into urine. Hoppe-Seylers Z Physiol Chem 363:1331–1339
34. Frey P, Forand R, Maciag T, Shooter EM (1979) The biosynthetic precursor of epidermal growth factor and the mechanism of its processing. Proc Natl Acad Sci USA 76:6294–6298
35. Gafford JT, Skidgel RA, Erdös EG, Hersh LB (1983) Human kidney "enkephalinase", a neutral metalloendopeptidase that cleaves active peptides. Biochemistry 22:3265–3271
36. Geiger R, Mann K (1976) A kallikrein-specific inhibitor in rat kidney tubules. Hoppe-Seylers Z Physiol Chem 357:553–558

37. Hall ER, Kato J, Erdös EG, Robinson CJG, Oshima G (1976) Angiotensin I-converting enzyme in the nephron. Life Sci 18:1299–1304
38. Hial V, Keiser HR, Pisano JJ (1976) Methionyl-lysyl-bradykinin (MLBK) in human urine and the absence of kinins in subjects with congential deficiency of kininogen. Fed Proc 35:692
39. Hial V, Keiser HR, Pisano JJ (1976) Origin and content of methionyl-lysyl-bradykinin, and bradykinin in human urine. Biochem Pharmacol 25:2499-2503
40. Hojima V, Isobe M, Moriya H (1977) Kallikrein inhibitors in rat plasma. J Biochem 81:37–46
41. Hori S (1968) The presence of bradykinin-like polypeptides, kinin-releasing and destroying activity in brain. Jpn J Physiol 19:772–787
42. Imai M (1979) The connecting tubule: a functional subdivision of the rabbit distal nephron segments. Kidney Int 15:346–356
43. Kariya K, Kawauchi R, Okamoto H (1981) Regional distribution of kininase in rat brain. J Neurochem 36:2086–2088
44. Kariya K, Yamauchi A, Chatani Y (1982) Relationship between central actions of bradykinin and prostaglandins in the conscious rat. Neuropharmacology 21:267–272
45. Kariya K, Yamauchi A, Hattori S, Tsuda Y, Okada Y (1982) The disappearance rate of intraventricular bradykinin in the brain of the conscious rat. Biochem Biophys Res Comm 107:1461–1466
46. Kauker ML (1980) Bradykinin action of the efflux of luminal Na in the rat nephron. J Pharmacol Exp Ther 214:119–123
47. Kokubu T, Kato I, Nishimura K, Hiwada K, Ueda E (1978) Angiotensin I-converting enzyme in human urine. Clin Chim Acta 89:375–379
48. Kramer HJ, Moch T, Von Sicherer L, Dusing R (1979) Effects of aprotinin on renal function and urinary prostaglandin excretion in conscious rats after acute salt loading. Clin Sci 56:547–553
49. Kriz W, Kaissling B (1978) Anatomical and ultrastrucural studies upon heterogeneity of nephrons in the rabbit kidney. In: Proceedings, 7th International Congress of Nephrology, Montreal, Universite de Montreal. Karger, Basel, p 217
50. Lambert GA, Lang WJ (1970) The effect of bradykinin and eledoisin injected into the cerebral ventricles of conscious rats. Eur J Pharmac 9:383–386
51. Lazure C, Leduc R, Seidah NG, Thibault G, Genest J, Chretien M (1984) Amino acid sequence of rat submaxillary tonin reveals similarities to serine proteases. Nature 309:555–558
52. Marin-Grez M (1974) The influence of antiobodies against bradykinin on isotonic saline diuresis in the rat. Pfluegers Arch 350:231–239
53. Marin-Grez M, Bönner G, Gross F (1980) Ureteral contractions induced by rat urine in vitro: probable involvement of renal kallikrein. Experientia 36:865–866
54. Marinkovic DV, Ward P, Erdös EG, Mills IH (1980) Carboxypeptidase-type kininase of human kidney and urine. Proc Soc Exp Biol Med 165:6–12
55. Maruta H, Arakawa K (1983) Confirmation of direct angiotensin formation by kallikrein. Biochem J 213:193–200
56. Mason AJ, Evans BA, Cox DR, Shine J, Richards RI (1983) Structure of mouse kallikrein gene family suggests a role in specific processing of biologically active peptides. Nature 303:300–307
57. Mills IH (1979) Kallikrein, kininogen and kinins in control of blood pressure. Nephron 23:61–71
58. Misumi J, Alhenc-Gelas F, Marre M, Marchetti J, Corvol P, Menard J (1983) Regulation of kallikrein and renin release by the isolated perfused rat kidney. Kidney Int 24:58–65
59. Miwa I, Erdös EG, Seki T (1968) Presence of three peptides in urinary kinin (substance Z) preparations. Life Sci 7:1339–1343
60. Nasjletti A, Colina-Churio J, McGiff JC (1975) Disappearance of bradykinin in the renal circulation of dogs: effects of kininase inhibition. Circ Res 37:59–65
61. Nasjletti A, Malik KU (1979) Relationships between the kallikrein-kinin and prostaglandin system. Life Sci 25:99–110
62. Nishimura K, Erdös EG (1980) Membrane-bound kininase and kallikrein. In: Gross F, Vogel G (eds) Enzymatic release of vasoactive peptides. Raven, New York, pp 225–234
63. Nustad K, Rubin I (1970) Subcellular localization of renin and kininogenase in rat kidney. Br J Pharmacol 39:87–91
64. Ole-Moi Yoi O, Seldin DC, Spragg J, Pinkus GS, Austen FK (1979) Sequential cleavage of proinsulin by human pancreatic kallikrein and a human pancreatic kininase. Proc Natl Acad Sci USA 76:3612–3616

65. Omata K, Carretero OA, Scicli AG, Jackson BA (1982) Localization of active and inactive kallikrein in the isolated tubular segments of the rabbit nephron. Kidney Int 22: 602–607
66. Ørstavik TB (1980) The kallikrein-kinin system in exocrine organs. J Histochem Cytochem 28: 881–889.
67. Ørstavik TB, Carretero OA, Johansen LB, Scicli AG (1982) Role of submandibular gland kallikrein in the hypotensive effect of captopril after sympathetic stimulation of the rat submandibular gland. Circ Res 51: 385–390
68. Ørstavik TB, Carretero OA, Scicli AG (1982) The kallikrein-kinin system in the regulation of submandibular gland blood flow. Am J Physiol 242: H1010–H1014
69. Ørstavik TB, Inagami T (1982) The localization of kallikrein in the rat kidney and its anatomical relationship to renin. J Histochem Cytochem 30: 385–390
70. Ørstavik TB, Nustad K, Brandtzaeg P, Pierce JV (1976) Cellular origin of urinary kallikrein. J Histochem Cytochem 24: 1037–1039
71. Pisano JJ, Corthorn J, Yates K, Pierce JV (1978) The kallikrein-kinin system in the kidney. Contrib Nephrol 12: 116–125
72. Powers CA, Nasjletti A (1982) A novel kinin-generating protease (kininogenase) in the porcine anterior pituitary. J Biol Chem 257: 5594–5600
73. Powers CA, Nasjletti A (1983) A kininogenase resembling glandular kallikrein in the rat pituitary pars intermedia. Endocrinology 112: 1194–1200
74. Powers CA, Nasjletti A (1984) A major sex difference in kallikrein-like activity in the rat anterior pituitary. Endocrinology 114: 1841–1844
75. Proud D, Perkins M, Pierce JV, Yates KN, Highet PF, Herring PL, Mangkornkanok M, Bahu R, Carone F, Pisano JJ (1981) Characterization and localization of human renal kininogen. J Biol Chem 256: 10634–10639
76. Rabito SF, Ørstavik TB, Scicli AG (1983) Role of the autonomic nervous system in the release of rat submandibular gland kallikrein into the circulation. Circ Res 52: 635–641
77. Rabito SF, Scicli AG, Kher V, Carretero OA (1982) Immunoreactive glandular kallikrein in rat plasma: a radioimmunoassay for its determination. Am J Physiol 242: H602–H610
78. Roblero J, Croxatto H, Garcia R, Corthorn J, De Vito E (1976) Kallikrein-like activity in perfusates and urine of isolated rat kidneys. Am J Physiol 231: 1383–1389
79. Salgado MCO, Rabito SF, Carretero OA (1985) Blood kinin in one-kidney, one-clip hypertensive rats. Hypertension (in press)
80. Sealey JE, Atlas SA, Laragh JH, Oza NB, Ryan JW (1978) Human urinary kallikrein converts inactive renin to active renin and is a possible physiological activator of renin. Nature 275: 144–145
81. Scicli AG, Carretero OA, Hampton A, Cortez P, Oza NB (1976) Site of kininogenase secretion in the dog nephron. Am J Physiol 230: 533–536
82. Scicli AG, Carretero OA, Oza NB (1976) Distribution of kidney kininogenases. Proc Soc Exp Biol Med 151: 57–60
83. Scicli AG, Diaz M, Carretero OA (1983) Effects of pH and amiloride in the intrarenal formation kinins. Am J Physiol 245: F198–F203
84. Scicli AG, Forbes G, Nolly H, Dujovny M, Carretero OA (1984) Kallikrein-kinins in the central nervous system. Clin Exper Hypert A6(10&11): 1731–1738
85. Simson JAV, Spicer SS, Chao J, Grimm L, Margolius HS (1979) Kallikrein localization in rodent salivary glands and kidney with the immunoglobulin-enzyme bridge technique. J Histochem Cytochem 27: 1567–1576
86. Skeggs LT, Dorer FE, Kahn JR, Lentz KE, Levine M (1976) The biochemistry of the renin-angiotensin system and its role in hypertension. Am J Med 60: 737–748
87. Skidgel RA, Davis RM, Erdös EG (1984) Purification of a human urinary carboxypeptidase (kininase) distinct from carboxypeptidase A, B or N. Anal Biochem 140: 520–531
88. Snider RM, Richelson E (1984) Bradykinin receptor-mediated cyclic GMP formation in a nerve cell population (murine neuroblastoma clone N1E-115). J Neurochem 43: 1749–1754
89. Stein JH, Congbalay RC, Karsh DL (1972) The effect of bradykinin on proximal tubular sodium reabsorption in the dog: evidence for functional nephron heterogeneity. J Clin Invest 51: 1709–1712
90. Suzuki S, Franco-Saenz R, Tan SY, Mulrow PJ (1980) Direct action of rat urinary kallikrein on rat kidney to release renin. J Clin Invest 66: 757–762

91. Swift GH, Craik CS, Stary SJ, Quinto C, Lahaie RG, Rutter WJ, MacDonald RJ (1984) Structure of the two related elastase genes expressed in the rat pancreas. J Biol Chem 259:14271–14278
92. Terragno NA, Lonigro AJ, Malik KU, McGiff JC (1972) The relationship of the renal vasodilator action of bradykinin to the release of prostaglandin E-like substances. Experientia 28:437–439
93. Thomas GR, Thibodeaux H, Margolius HS, Privitera PJ (1984) Cerebrospinal fluid kinins and cardiovascular function. Effects of cerebroventricular melittin. Hypertension 6 (Suppl I): 46–50
94. Travis J, Salvesen GS (1983) Human plasma proteinase inhibitors. Annu Rev Biochem 52:655–709
95. Vio CP, Churchill L, Rabito SF, Terragno A, Carretero OA, Terragno NA (1983) Renal kallikrein in venous effluent of filtering and non-filtering isolated kidney. Adv Exp Med Biol 156:897–905
96. Vogel R, Werle E (1970) Kallikrein inhibitors. In: Erdös EG (ed) Bradykinin, kallidin and kallikrein. Springer, Berlin Heidelberg New York, pp 213–249 (Handbook of experimental pharmacology, vol 25)
97. Werle E, Busse R, Schmal A (1968) Über die Kallikreinausscheidung im Harn des Menschen nach Nierentransplantation. Klin Wochenschr 46:1315–1317
98. Willis LR (1977) Effects of bradykinin on the renal medullary osmotic gradient in water diuresis. Eur J Pharmacol 45:173–183

Peripheral Adrenergic Mechanisms in Primary Hypertension

S. Z. Langer[1]

Introduction

The general view that neurotransmitters can regulate their own release through presynaptic autoreceptors represents a new concept in the field of neurotransmission which has been demonstrated for noradrenaline, dopamine, serotonin, acetylcholine, and possibly for other transmitters [15, 18, 29].

In the noradrenergic system, the concept of presynaptic modulation of transmitter release developed in parallel with the pharmacological evidence for two subtypes of α-adrenoceptors as defined by a different profile of affinity and relative order of potencies for agonists as well as for antagonists [15, 29].

In blood vessels, both the α_1- and the α_2-adrenoceptor subtypes can be identified postjunctionally where they mediate vasocontriction [10, 12, 19, 22, 23], although the α_1-adrenoceptor predominates in most vascular smooth muscle. Evidently, the predominant presynaptic adrenoceptor which mediates the inhibition of the release of noradrenaline corresponds to the α_2-adrenoceptor subtype [13, 15, 16, 28].

In addition to presynaptic α_2-inhibitory autoreceptors, the noradrenergic varicosity possesses inhibitory dopamine receptors of the D2 subtype [4, 5, 9, 11, 17, 26]. Two types of facilitatory receptors have also been reported to be present on noradrenergic nerve terminals, β-adrenoceptors [1, 13, 24, 27] and angiotensin II receptors [3, 7].

The present article examines the physiological and pharmacological relevance of presynaptic adrenoceptors on peripheral sympathetic nerve terminals in terms of therapeutic potential.

Location and Function of α-Adrenoceptor Subtypes Within the Cardiovascular System

The relative order of selectivities for a range of α_1-adrenoceptor-agonists and antagonists acting on α_1- and α_2-adrenoceptor subtypes are shown in Table 1. For the agonists, methoxamine and amidephrine are the most selective agents for the α_1-adrenoceptor subtype. Noradrenaline and adrenaline stimulate both subtypes of α-adrenoceptors and the α-methyl and 6-fluoro analogs of noradrenaline are preferential α_2-adrenoceptor agonists (Table 1). Among the selective α_2-adrenoceptor agonists which are not phenylethylamines, clonidine, para-aminoclonidine, BHT 920,

[1] Department of Biology, L.E.R.S., 58, rue de la Glacière, F-75013 Paris.

Primary Hypertension
Ed. by W. Kaufmann et al.

Table 1. Pharmacological basis for the subclassification of α-adrenoceptors: α-Adrenoceptor agonists in their order of selectivity for the α_1- and α_2-adrenoceptor subtype

	Order of selectivity for agonists
α_1	Methoxamine
↑	Amidephrine
	Cirazoline
	Phenylephrine
	Noradrenaline
	Adrenaline
	$\alpha - CH_3$-Noradrenaline
	6-F-Noradrenaline
	Clonidine
	Guanfacine
	Paraaminoclonidine
	BHT 933
	M7
	TL 99
↓	BHT 920
α_2	UK 14304

M7 = (2,*N,N*-dimethylamino-5,6-dihydroxy-1,2,3,4-tetrahydronaphthalene); TL 99 = (2,*N,N*-dimethylamino-6,7-dihydroxy-1,2,3,4-tetrahydronaphthalene); BHT 920 = (2-amino-6-allyl-5,6,7,8-tetrahydro-4*H*-thiazolo-[4,5-*d*]azepine); BHT 933 = (2-amino-6-allyl-4,5,7,8-tetrahydro-6*H*-oxazolo-[5,4-*d*] azepine); UK 14304 = (5-bromo-6-[2-imidazolin-2-ylamino]-quinoxaline)

Table 2. Pharmacological basis for the subclassification of α-adrenoceptors: α-Adrenoceptor antagonists in their order of selectivity for the α_1- and α_2-adrenoceptor subtype

	Order of selectivity of antagonists
α_1	Prazosin
↑	Corynanthine
	Labetolol
	Alfuzosin
	WB 4101
	Ifenprodil
	Phentolamine
	Tolazoline
	Piperoxan
	Mianserin
	Yohimbine
	RS – 21361
↓	WY – 26703
α_2	Idazoxan

WB 4101 = (*N*-[2-(2,6-dimethoxyphenoxy)-ethyl]1,4-benzodioxane-2-methylamine); RS 21361 = (±)-2-(1-ethyl-2-imidazolyl)methyl-1,4-benzodioxane; WY 26703 = (*N*-methyl-*N*-1,3,4,6,7,11b α-hexahydro-2H-benzo-[a]-quinolizin-2β-yl)-*i*-butanesulphonamide; Ifenprodil = α-(4-Hydroxyphenyl)-β-methyl-4(phenylmethyl)-1-piperidine-ethanol, Alfuzosin [6]

BHT 933, UK-14304, and the aminotetralines M7 and TL 99 are the most widely used compounds (Table 1). When the α-adrenoceptor antagonists are taken into consideration prazosin is a highly selective α_1-adrenoceptor antagonist, while corynanthine and labetolol, although much less potent than prazosin, are nevertheless selective for the α_1-adrenoceptor. Labetolol, however, is also a β-blocker. Other drugs which block both α_1- as well α_2-adrenoceptor are phentolamine, mianserin, and tolazoline (Table 2). Both yohimbine and rauwolscine are preferential α_2-adrenoceptor antagonists, while idazoxan, WY 26703, and RS 21361 are at present the most selective α_2-adrenoceptor antagonists available (up to 100-fold ratio of selectivity for idazoxan under in vitro conditions). More recently, some analogs of idazoxan have been shown to possess an even greater selectivity ratio for the blockade of the α_2-adrenoceptor subtype [8].

The predominant α-adrenoceptor subtype located presynaptically on noradrenergic nerve terminals corresponds to the α_2-subtype and it is linked to the modulation of transmitter release. Activation of α_2-adrenoceptor by the addition of exogenous agonists reduces transmitter release, while the increase in noradrenaline release ob-

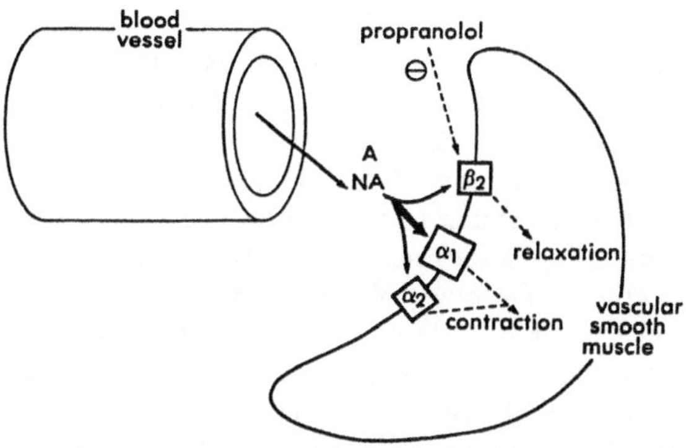

Fig. 1. Schematic representation of the postsynaptic adrenoceptor subtypes located on vascular smooth muscle of certain arteries and veins and which are stimulated by circulating or exogenous catecholamines noradrenaline *(NA)* and adrenaline *(A)* to cause contraction of the smooth muscle cell. The predominant α-adrenoceptor is the α_1-adrenoceptor subtype, and it is also the predominantly innervated α-receptor in vascular smooth muscle. *A* in preference to *NA* can also stimulate vasodilatory β-adrenoceptors in blood vessels, effects which are antagonized ⊖ by propranolol

tained in the presence of α_2-adrenoceptor antagonists depends upon the frequency of nerve impulses and duration of the period of depolarization [28]. These results support the view that there is an operational negative feedback mechanism through which the released transmitter can regulate its own release once a threshold concentration of noradrenaline is achieved in the synaptic cleft [15, 28, 29]. Certain aspects of this concept have, however, recently been challenged [2].

Postsynaptically, in vascular smooth muscle, the α_1-adrenoceptor is the predominant receptor mediating vasoconstriction, but there are also postsynaptic α_2-adrenoceptors which also mediate vasoconstriction in arterial as well as in venous vascular smooth muscle (Fig. 1). The relative proportions of vascular postsynaptic α_1- and α_2-adrenoceptors vary as a function of the vascular bed and also with the diameter of the blood vessel. This latter point may represent an important observation for drug actions in vivo. At the present time, the pharmacology of the pre- and postsynaptic α_2-adrenoceptors appears similar, but it may be possible with future drugs to also discriminate between pre- and postsynaptic α_2-adrenoceptor effects.

In most vascular beds examined so far, the postsynaptic α_1-adrenoceptor appears to be the preferentially innervated subtype [12, 20, 22, 23]. However, in spontaneously hypertensive rats (SHR) [12, 22, 23] and dog saphenous vein [10], there is evidence that postsynaptic α_2-adrenoceptors elicit vasoconstriction in response to both exogenously and endogenously released noradrenaline.

Presynaptic Inhibitory Dopamine Receptors on Peripheral Noradrenergic Nerves

Stimulation of presynaptic dopamine receptors of the D2 subtype by dopamine and other dopamine-receptor agonists can mediate the inhibition of noradrenaline release; effects which have been demonstrated under both in vitro as well as in vivo conditions [4, 5, 9, 11, 17, 26]. The reduction of noradrenaline release, elicited by dopamine-receptor agonists, is accompanied by a decrease in the magnitude of the end-organ responses to sympathetic nerve stimulation [4, 5, 17, 26]. The presynaptic inhibitory dopamine receptors are therefore a target for exogenously applied agonists (e.g., pergolide) which inhibit noradrenaline release and reduce blood pressure and heart rate [4, 5, 17]. In contrast to presynaptic α_2-adrenoceptors, which appear to play a physiological role in modulating noradrenergic neurotransmission, the presynaptic inhibitory dopamine receptors, although pharmacologically relevant, may not be physiologically significant since blockade of presynaptic D2 receptors (e.g., sulpiride) fails to enhance the stimulation-evoked release of noradrenaline, although this D2 receptor antagonist effectively blocks the inhibitory actions of dopamine-receptor agonists [4, 5, 21]. The presynaptic inhibitory D2 receptors on noradrenergic nerve terminals differ pharmacologically from the postsynaptic D1 receptors, which mediate vasodilatation in the mesenteric and renal vascular beds [26].

Presynaptic Facilitatory β-Adrenoceptors on Peripheral Noradrenergic nerves

There is now considerable evidence for the presence of presynaptic facilitatory β-adrenoceptors on peripheral noradrenergic nerve terminals [1, 13, 24, 27]. Exposure to low concentrations of isoproterenol or adrenaline enhances the stimulation-evoked release of noradrenaline and this effect is blocked by propranolol [1, 18], but not by betaxolol [18], indicating that the β-adrenoceptor involved in the facilitation of noradrenergic neurotransmission corresponds to the β_2 subtype.

The fact that adrenaline preferentially stimulates the presynaptic facilitatory β_2-adrenoceptor may be relevant to the pathogenesis of some forms of hypertension [25]. Nevertheless, it remains to be established whether the clinical efficacy of β-adrenoceptor blocking drugs in hypertension relates to some extent to blockade of presynaptic facilitatory β-adrenoceptors [24, 25].

A second facilitatory mechanism at the level of sympathetic nerve endings involves angiotensin II [3, 7, 29] and it is of interest that inhibitors of the angiotensin converting enzyme (ACE) such as captopril, which have antihypertensive properties, can prevent the angiotensin II-mediated facilitation of noradrenergic neurotransmission [3, 7].

Therapeutic Potential of Drugs Acting as Agonists or Antagonists at α_1- and α_2-Adrenoceptors

The characterization of receptor subtypes has often been followed by developments in drug discovery involving novel therapeutic indications.

As discussed in the previous sections, on the whole, the α_1-adrenoceptor appears to be linked to fewer physiological functions than the α_2-adrenoceptor although subclasses of both α-adrenoceptor types may exist. The α_1-adrenoceptor agonists are extensively used as local vasoconstrictors, particularly in the nasal mucosa. Systemic administration of α_1-agonists increases blood pressure through peripheral vasoconstriction and can be used to treat hypotension. Selective blockade of peripheral α_1-adrenoceptor in vascular smooth muscle leads to an effective antihypertensive action with a decrease in peripheral resistance without reflex tachycardia as is the case with prazosin or alfuzosin [6]. A peripheral α_1-adrenoceptor antagonist like prazosin or alfuzosin represents a rational approach in the therapy of essential hypertension. As a result of the blockade of α_1-adrenoceptors in the smooth muscle of the urinary tract, α_1-antagonists may be useful in the treatment of urinary dysfunction at the level of the bladder and the urethra.

Since the α_2-adrenoceptor is more widely distributed, the list of potential therapeutic applications both for agonists as well as for antagonists is more extensive although not always convincingly proven in animals or established in man, mainly because of the limited clinical studies with selective α_2-adrenoceptor antagonists.

Among the well-established therapeutic indications of α_2-adrenoceptor agonists is the antihypertensive and bradycardic action of clonidine, guanfacine and guanabenz which reflect both central and peripheral sites of action. Clonidine has also been used successfully in the withdrawal syndrome from opiate addiction, most likely because of the ability of clonidine to stimulate inhibitory somatodendritic and presynaptic α_2-adrenoceptors on noradrenergic neurons in the central nervous system (CNS). Local administration of α_2-adrenoceptor agonists, such as clonidine, decreases intraocular pressure and they are therefore useful in the treatment of glaucoma.

Since selective α_2-adrenoceptor antagonists have only recently advanced to clinical trials, their therapeutic effectiveness in several indications remains to be proven. One potential use of centrally acting α_2-adrenoceptor antagonists is in the treatment of depression, since blockade of presynaptic inhibitory α_2-adrenoceptors on central noradrenergic neurons will increase the synaptic concentrations of noradrenaline in the CNS. This mechanism of action is clearly different from the inhibition of neuronal uptake of noradrenaline thought to be the mechanism of action of some tricyclic drugs [14]. It remains possible that the combination of α_2-adrenoceptor blockade and neuronal uptake inhibition will provide a most effective antidepressant therapy.

Another potential therapeutic use for α_2-adrenoceptor antagonists preferably not crossing the blood-brain barrier may be in the treatment of diabetes. Blockade of the inhibitory α_2-adrenoceptors in pancreatic islets may increase insulin release, at least in some clinical forms of diabetes.

α_2-adrenoceptor antagonists (perhaps selective for the periphery) may be useful in the treatment of asthma, first because bronchiolar smooth muscle possesses α_2-adrenoceptors which mediate contraction and which can be sensitized by agents such as serotonin or histamine, substances which are released in asthmatic conditions. Second, by increasing noradrenaline release (presynaptic action), these antagonists might stimulate a greater β-adrenoceptor bronchodilatator action in asthmatic conditions.

A more speculative possibility concerns the potential use of peripherally active α_2-adrenoceptor antagonists in peripheral vascular disorders and perhaps in some forms of hypertension. It was recently shown that in the tail artery of SHR, postsynaptic smooth muscle α_2-adrenoceptors mediate vasoconstriction to a larger extent than in normotensive WKY tail arteries [12, 23]. If, as these findings suggest, there is an increased component of vascular smooth muscle α_2-adrenoceptor mediated vasoconstriction in hypertensive states, then a peripherally active α_2-adrenoceptor antagonist may be considered as a drug potentially useful in the treatment of hypertension. All selective α_2-adrenoceptor antagonists currently available penetrate the CNS, and may increase sympathetic discharge to the peripheral vasculature.

Conclusions

It is now well established that prejunctional adrenoceptors (and other receptor types) are located on sympathetic nerve terminals. Stimulation of these receptors can modulate the release of noradrenaline. From a pharmacological standpoint, the stimulation of inhibitory receptor subtypes by agonist drugs, or the blockade of facilitatory receptor subtypes by antagonists offers a new approach to the discovery of novel agents for use in respiratory, endocrine, cardiovascular, and CNS disorders. The design of novel, chemical structures which may be able to discriminate between presynaptic and postsynaptic α_2-adrenoceptors as well as α_1-adrenoceptors will clearly assist in the pharmacological rationale for the treatment of certain clinical disorders.

References

1. Adler-Graschinsky E, Langer SZ (1975) Possible role of a beta adrenoceptor in the regulation of noradrenaline release by nerve stimulation. Br J Pharmacol 53:43–50
2. Angus JA, Bobik A, Jackman GP, Kopin IJ, Korner P (1984) Role of auto-inhibitory feedback in cardiac sympathetic transmission assessed by simultaneous measurements of changes in ^{3}H-efflux and atrial rate in guinea pig atrium. Br J Pharmacol 81:201–214
3. Antonaccio MJ, Kerwin L (1981) Pre- and post-junctional inhibition of vascular sympathetic function by captopril in SHR. Hypertension 3:I54–I62
4. Cavero I, Lefevre-Borg F, Gomeni R (1981) Blood pressure lowering effects of N,N-di-n-propyl-dopamine in rats: evidence for stimulation of peripheral dopamine receptors leading to inhibition of sympathetic vasculature. J Pharmacol Exp Ther 218:515–524
5. Cavero I, Lefevre-Borg F, Lhoste F, Sabatier C, Richer C, Giudicelli JF (1984) Pharmacological haemodynamic and autonomic nervous system mechanisms responsible for the blood pressure and heart rate lowering effects of pergolide in rats. J. Pharmacol Exp Ther 228:779–791
6. Cavero I, Lefevre-Borg F, Manoury P (1984) Alfuzion (SL 77.499), a new antihypertensive agent with a peripheral site of action 1 in vivo pharmacological studies. Br J Pharmacol 81:13
7. Clough DP, Hatton R, Keddie JR, Collis MG (1982) Hypotensive action of captopril in spontaneously hypertensive and normotensive rats. Interference with neurogenic vasoconstriction. Hypertension 4:764–772
8. Doxey JC, Roach AG, Stillings MR, Strachan DA, Virdee NK, Welbourn AP (1984) Potent and selective alpha$_2$-adrenoceptor antagonists in a series of 2-substituted analogues of idazoxan. Br J Pharmacol 81:181
9. Enero MA, Langer SZ (1975) Inhibition by dopamine of ^{3}H-noradrenaline release elicited by nerve stimulation in the isolated cat's nictitating membrane. Naunyn Schmiedebergs Arch Pharmacol 289:179–203
10. Flavahan NA, Rimele TJ, Cooke JP, Vanhoutte PM (1984) Characterization of postjunctional alpha$_1$ and alpha$_2$-adrenoceptors activated by exogenous or nerve released norepinephrine in the canine saphenous vein. J Pharmacol Exp Ther 230:699–705
11. Galzin AM, Dubocovich ML, Langer SZ (1982) Presynaptic inhibition by dopamine receptor agonists of noradrenergic neurotransmission in the rabbit hypothalamus. J Pharmacol Exp Ther 221:461–471

12. Hicks PE, Medgett IC, Langer SZ (1984) Postsynaptic alpha$_2$-adrenoceptors mediated vasoconstriction in SHR tail arteries in vitro. Hypertension 6:12–18
13. Langer SZ (1976) The role of alpha and beta-presynaptic receptors in the regulation of noronrenaline release elicited by nerve stimulation. Clin Sci Mol Med 51:423s–426s
14. Langer SZ (1978) Presynaptic receptors. Nature 275:479–480
15. Langer SZ (1981) Presynaptic regulation of the release of catecholamines. Pharmacol Rev 32:337–362
16. Langer SZ (1981) Presence and physiological role of presynaptic inhibitory alpha$_2$-adrenoceptors in guinea-pig atria. Nature 294:671–672
17. Langer SZ, Armstrong JM (1984) Prejunctional receptors and the cardiovascular system: Pharmacological and therapeutic relevance. In: Antonaccio MJ (ed) Cardiovascular pharmacology. Raven, New York, pp 197–213
18. Langer SZ, Galzin AM (1983) Beta-adrenoceptors and noradrenergic neurotransmission: effects of betaxolol on the stimulation evoked release of ^{3}H-noradrenaline in isolated rat atria and rabbit hypothalamic slices. In: Morselli PL, Kilborn JR, Cavero I, Harrison DC, Langer SZ (eds) Betaxolol: a new β_1-adrenoceptor antagonist, vol 1. Raven, New York, pp 21–30
19. Langer SZ, Shepperson NB (1982) Recent developments in vascular smooth muscle pharmacology – the postsynaptic alpha$_2$-adrenoceptor. Trends Pharmacol Sci 3:440–444
20. Langer SZ, Shepperson NB, Massingham R (1981) Preferential noradrenergic innervation of alpha$_1$-adrenergic receptors in vascular smooth muscle. Hypertension 3:112–118
21. Massingham R, Dubocovich ML, Langer SZ (1980) The role of presynaptic receptors in the cardiovascular actions of N,N-di-n propyldopamine in the cat and dog. Naunyn Schmiedebergs Arch Pharmacol 314:17–28
22. Medgett IC, Langer SZ (1984) Heterogeneity of smooth muscle alpha-adrenoceptors in rat tail artery in vitro. J Pharmacol Exp Ther 229:823–830
23. Medgett IC, Hicks PE, Langer SZ (1984) Smooth muscle alpha$_2$-adrenoceptors mediate vasoconstrictor responses to exogenous norepinephrine and to sympathetic stimulation to a greater extent in SHR than in WKY rat tail arteries. J Pharmacol Exp Ther 231:159–165
24. Misu Y, Kubo T (1983) Presynaptic beta-adrenoceptors. Trends Pharmacol Sci 4:506–508
25. Rand MJ, Majewski H, McCulloch MW, Story DF (1978) An adrenaline mediated positive feedback loop in sympathetic transmission and its possible role in hypertension. In: Langer SZ, Starke K, Dubocovich ML (eds) Presynaptic receptors. Pergamon, Oxford, p 263
26. Shepperson NB, Duval N, Massingham R, Langer SZ (1982) Differential blocking effects of several dopamine receptor antagonists for peripheral pre- and postsynaptic dopamine receptors in the anaesthetized dog. J Pharmacol Exp Ther 221:753–761
27. Stärjne L, Brundin J (1976) β_2-adrenoceptors facilitating noradrenaline secretion from human vasoconstrictor nerves. Acta Physiol Scand 94:88–93
28. Story DF, McCulloch MW, Rand MJ, Stanford Starr CA (1981) Conditions required for the inhibitory feedback loop in noradrenergic transmission. Nature 293:62–65
29. Westfall TC (1977) Local regulation of adrenergic neurotransmission. Physiol Rev 57:659

Neural Transmitters and Central Mechanisms in Primary Hypertension*

P. I. KORNER[1], E. BADOER[1], and G. A. HEAD[1]

Introduction

Much of our current knowledge about the operation of the autonomic nervous system is based on input-output analysis of the mechanisms through which particular disturbances evoke distinctive autonomic response patterns. Most of this work has been based on analysing the responses to stimuli of relatively short duration, of only minutes and hours. However, our focus on circulatory regulation shifts to a longer time frame when considering the pathogenesis of hypertension, or the mechanisms of action of centrally acting antihypertensive drugs. Some of the latter are particularly valuable for probing molecular mechanisms, such as the neurotransmitters and membrane receptors, of cardiovascular neurons.

In human primary hypertension identification of causal mechanisms has turned out so far to be extraordinarily elusive. One of the main reasons for this has been the large contribution made by the amplifier properties of the heart and vessels to the maintenance of the elevated blood pressure in chronic hypertension [26]. Thus, in experimental hypertension due to one-kidney renal artery stenosis the cardiovascular amplifier effects contributed three times more to the maintenance of the elevated blood pressure as did the basic cause. This applies equally to human primary hypertension where the amplification of constrictor and inotropic stimuli will obscure the contribution of the basic cause. We have recently sought a way out of this impasse, by reversing the cardiovascular hypertrophy by a long period of drug treatment, followed by analysis of the factors important in the redevelopment of hypertension when treatment is stopped [22, 36]. Although the number of patients in this programme is still small, our preliminary findings have shown evidence of sympathetic overactivity during redevelopment of hypertension in a higher proportion of patients than in chronic hypertension. This has given a new impetus to identifying the molecular mechanisms important in the central regulation of blood pressure.

In this paper we want to concentrate discussion on the circulatory functions of the central catecholaminergic (CA) and serotonergic (5HT) neurons. This has been somewhat controversial and we want to discuss a new approach, which involves studying the effects of neurotoxin-induced acute endogenous transmitter release. These neurons play an important role in the central actions of clonidine and alphamethyldopa (α-MD), so that analysis of their action helps to identify some of the

* Studies from our laboratory were supported by the Australian National Health and Medical Research Council, the National Heart Foundation of Australia and the Alfred Hospital Research Fund.

[1] Baker Medical Research Institute, Commercial Road, Prahran, Victoria. 3181, Australia.

Primary Hypertension
Ed. by W. Kaufmann et al.

pathways capable of producing long-term alterations in autonomic function. We have examined whether lesions of a number of CA nuclei alter the cardiovascular effects of transmitter release, α-MD and clonidine. Recent studies in animal models of primary hypertension from other laboratories, point to possible developmental "faults" in these systems.

General Organisation of Central Autonomic Pathways

A circulatory disturbance produces changes in the activity of many different sensory receptors, including that of the arterial and cardiac baroreceptors. This information reaches the central nervous system (CNS) through the glossopharyngeal, vagus and many spinal afferent nerves. This is integrated in numerous brain regions, including neurons close to the input in the nucleus tractus solitarii and spinal cord, from which there are polysynaptic projections to many groups of neurons in the bulb, midbrain, hypothalamus, limbic system, neocortex, cerebellum and spinal cord [8, 24, 25]. Thus, integration of information through the many afferent inputs to the CNS, involves "centres" that are widely distributed through the neuraxis. From these sites there is convergence of pathways, to the various groups of autonomic motoneurons, often via a complex polysynaptic route.

One characteristic of the responses of conscious animals is that a reflex response to a particular component of the input profile of the disturbance is often greatly altered by the level of activity of one or more of the other inputs [24, 25]. When the reflex in question is the baroreceptor reflex, changes in its properties (e.g. gain, range) through interactions involving the CNS are sometimes referred to as "central resetting" of this reflex. The underlying mechanisms are identical to the facilitation and occlusion responses, first described by Sherrington [46] in his classic analysis of spinal reflexes.

At present we still have much to learn about the different transmitters released by the central autonomic neurons and about the cardiovascular effects which they subserve. Most likely the same types of transmitters that are released by neurons regulating the different somatic and behavioural functions, will also be released from "cardiovascular" neurons. This includes simple amino acids such as glutamate and gamma-amino butyric acid; amines such as noradrenaline (NA), adrenaline, dopamine (DA) and serotonin (5HT); peptides such as angiotensin, the opioid peptides, oxytocin, vasopressin and substance P. Neurons releasing one transmitter are sometimes in series with those releasing another transmitter [40], much as occurs in the peripheral sympathetic system. Hence, we should guard against too ready labelling of neuron groups as belonging to a particular "system", other than in a molecular sense. Recent work has shown that *several* transmitters are sometimes released simultaneously from particular nerve terminals; what this means in terms of function is still unclear [8].

Catecholaminergic and Serotonergic Neurons

Catecholaminergic and serotonergic neurons were first described by Dahlström and Fuxe [10]. From the distribution of their axons it is likely that they subserve a whole range of somatic, autonomic and behavioural functions [4, 38, 42, 47]. Chalmers and colleagues were the first to show that they played a role in the baroreceptor reflex and that after chemical ablation of their endings by specific neurotoxins the development of hypertension was altered in several experimental models [6, 7, 9]. But there has been much controversy about the cardiovascular effects mediated through CA and 5HT neurons [8, 28, 37].

After intracisternal (i.c.) injection of 6-hydroxydopamine (6-OHDA), we observed large cardiovascular effects over the first few hours [18, 32]. These were due to release of transmitters following the uptake of the neurotoxin into the nerve terminal, as has been described in peripheral sympathetic nerves [16, 32]. The cardiovascular effects that we observed were much greater than the chronic changes after several days or weeks and have provided valuable information about the functions of the CA neurons. One limitation of the method is that the experiment can be performed only once in a given animal. In addition, the effects observed during release of large amounts of transmitter provide information about "potential" pathways, that may not necessarily be involved in moment-to-moment regulation of autonomic function. Subsequently, we found that the neurotoxin 5,6-(or 5,7-)dihydroxytryptamine (DHT) is taken up in a similar manner by the re-uptake pump of the 5HT nerve terminal; many of the acute circulatory effects after i.c. injection are also due to transmitter release. Evidence that after both 6-OHDA and 5,6-DHT the evoked circulatory changes *were* in fact due to transmitter release, included demonstration (a) that they were abolished or attenuated by specific receptor antagonists and (b) that when chronic changes occurred after degeneration of the nerve terminals, they were directionally *opposite* to the acute effects [18–20, 33]. This is because the acute changes are due to enhanced activity in a pathway, whilst chronic changes result from its loss, due to destruction of the specific nerve endings.

Effects of 6-OHDA and 5,6-DHT

In conscious rabbits the effects of transmitter release after i.c. 6-OHDA, consisted of a rise in mean arterial pressure (MAP) after a latency of about 1 h; this became maximal at about 2–3 h and was associated with pronounced cardiac slowing (Fig. 1) [18, 32, 33]. The hypertension was due to systemic vasoconstriction predominantly affecting renal and splanchnic vascular beds [32]. The bradycardia was due to changes in properties of the arterial baroreceptor reflex, with facilitation of vagal efferent activity during rises in blood pressure (Fig. 2) [33].

We also studied the effects of 6-OHDA in pontine rabbits subjected to infracollicular decerebration [32]. Here there was a short latency fall in MAP and heart rate, with time courses similar to the effects of centrally administered clonidine (Fig. 1) [1]. Again the bradycardia was largely due to facilitation of the vagal component of the baroreceptor-heart rate reflex, which was similar to the effects of clonidine and α-MD [1, 31].

Thus, increased activity of different CA neurons does not have uniform effects on blood pressure: the early depressor and heart rate responses observed in pontine rabbits are mediated through bulbo-spinal CA pathways, whilst the late pressor response is mediated through a suprapontine pathway.

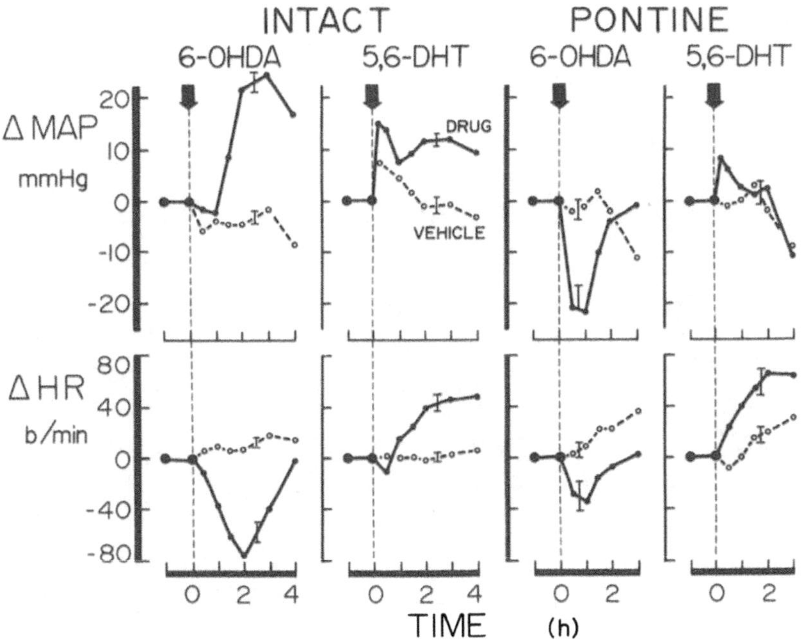

Fig. 1. Average changes in mean arterial pressure *(ΔMAP)* and heart rate *(ΔHR)* produced by i.c. 6-OHDA and 5,6-DHT *(solid lines)* and of vehicle *(interrupted lines)*, injected at *arrow*, in rabbits with intact CNS *(left panels)* and in pontine rabbits *(right panels)*. (From [29])

The chronic effects following 6-OHDA were studied 2 weeks after 6-OHDA, when there is maximal degeneration of nerve terminals [41]. At that time resting MAP and heart rate were completely restored, suggesting that altered activity of other pathways compensated for the loss of CA neurons. Evidence of the importance of CA neurons in normal cardiovascular regulation came from the demonstration of chronic changes in baroreceptor-heart rate reflex properties which were, as expected, opposite to the acute effects (Fig. 2) [33].

Undoubtedly NA neurons are the major group affected by 6-OHDA. But adrenaline neurons may also contribute to the changes observed after 6-OHDA in view of the probable similarity of the re-uptake pumps for NA and adrenaline neurons. Large cardiovascular effects have recently been evoked by stimulating neurons (probably adrenergic) in the ventrolateral medulla, just anterior to the A1 group, electrically or with glutamate [11, 42]. 6-OHDA also reduces brain DA levels, but to a much smaller degree than NA [20]: one group of cells that may participate in the acute effects of 6-OHDA are the A13 group of DA cells, which lie in the dorsal part of the postero-lateral hypothalamus – an area from which large pressor responses can be evoked [2, 13a].

Transmitter release from 5HT neurons, following i.c. administration of 5,6-DHT, produced a biphasic rise in MAP and a rise in heart rate (Fig. 1) [19]. The tachycardia was due to inhibition of the vagal component of the baroreceptor-heart rate reflex (Fig. 2). Transmitter release in pontine rabbits, abolished the late component of the rise in MAP, but the early rise in MAP and the tachycardia responses were similar

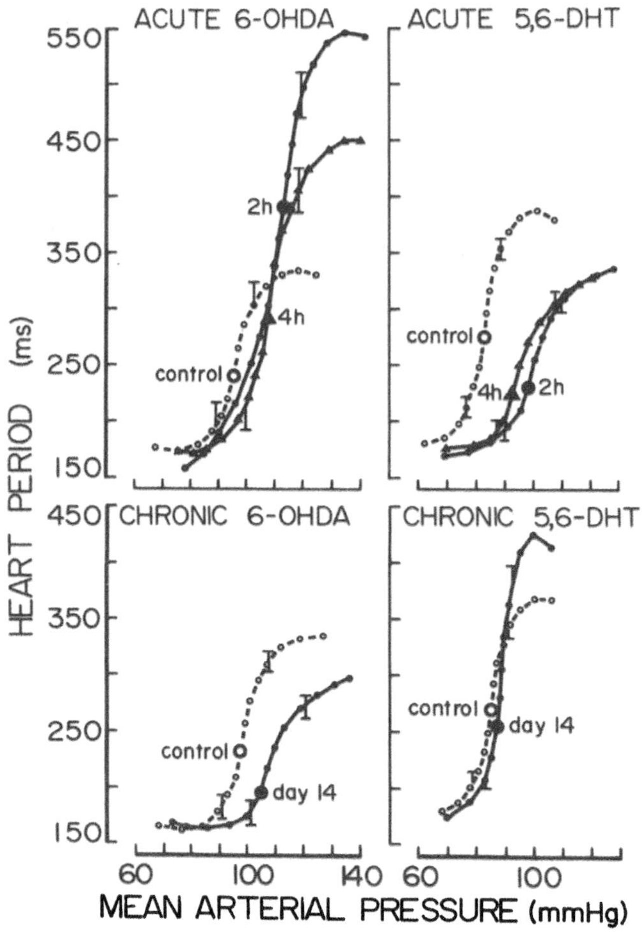

Fig. 2. *Top panels:* Average baroreceptor-heart rate reflex function curves relating mean arterial pressure to heart period (interval between pulses) during control period *(interrupted lines)* and 2 and 4h after injection of 6-OHDA or 5,6-DHT. *Lower panels:* Curves obtained before and 2 weeks after injection of the neurotoxins. (From [29])

to the findings in normal rabbits. Two weeks after 5,6-DHT, resting MAP and heart rate had returned to initial control, but the chronic changes in baroreceptor-heart rate reflex properties were opposite to the changes observed during transmitter release (Fig. 2), indicating that 5HT neurons contribute to the normal regulation of vagal tone.

The interrelationships between CA and 5HT pathways were investigated further, by examining whether the effects of synaptic release of CA or 5HT transmitters produced by i.c. 6-OHDA or 5,6-DHT were altered by giving the other neurotoxin 1 week earlier [29]. From these studies cardiac vagal efferent activity is regulated through independent parallel bulbar pathways of CA and 5HT neurons, with the former facilitating vagal activity and the latter inhibiting it (Fig. 3). There is a similar parallel arrangement of CA and 5HT neurons involved in the direct bulbo-spinal pathways regulating blood pressure, with CA neurons being depressor and 5HT neurons pressor. This is in accord with the effects of iontophoretic injection of NA and 5HT on preganglionic sympathetic motoneuron activity [44].

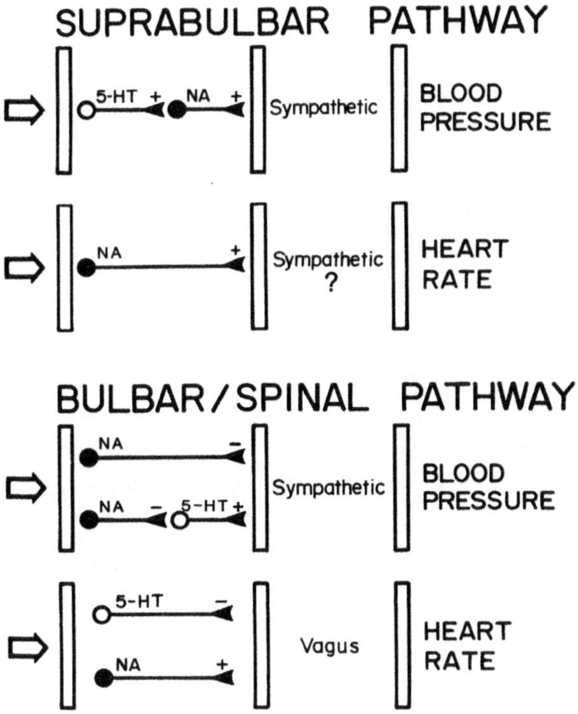

Fig. 3. Schema representing the CA pathways (shown mostly as noradrenergic, *NA*) and *5-HT* pathways regulating blood pressure and heart rate. In the suprapontine pressor pathway a 5HT neuron is in series with a CA neuron. Suprapontine heart rate pathway is based on data obtained in sino-aortically denervated rabbits. Bulbar and spinal CA and 5-HT pathways regulating cardiac vagal activity are arranged in parallel, whilst those regulating blood pressure have a mixed parallel and series arrangement. (Further discussion in text). (From [34])

After 6-OHDA the late pressor effect was not altered by previous administration of 5,6-DHT [29]. By contrast, the 5,6-DHT-induced late component of the pressor response was abolished completely by previous treatment with 6-OHDA. This indicates that the suprapontine pressor pathway includes a 5HT neuron in series with a CA neuron (Fig. 3).

Central and Reflex Components of 6-OHDA Response

The acute effects of 6-OHDA include (a) "true" central effects of transmitter release on the various autonomic outflows discussed above, and (b) reflexly induced changes in autonomic activity as a result of feedback through the arterial and other circulatory baroreceptors. The importance of the reflex component is evident from comparisons of the responses of intact and sino-aortically denervated (SAD) animals (Fig. 4) [35].

In SAD rabbits we observed that early depressor and late pressor components characteristic, respectively, of the responses of pontine and normal rabbits were both present. The heart rate response of SAD rabbits consisted of a short latency bradycardia with a time course similar to that of pontine rabbits, followed by a progressive increase in heart rate above resting that we have not observed in animals with intact sino-aortic nerves.

It follows that feedback through the arterial baroreceptors eliminates the early fall in blood pressure in normal rabbits, but attenuates the late pressor response only

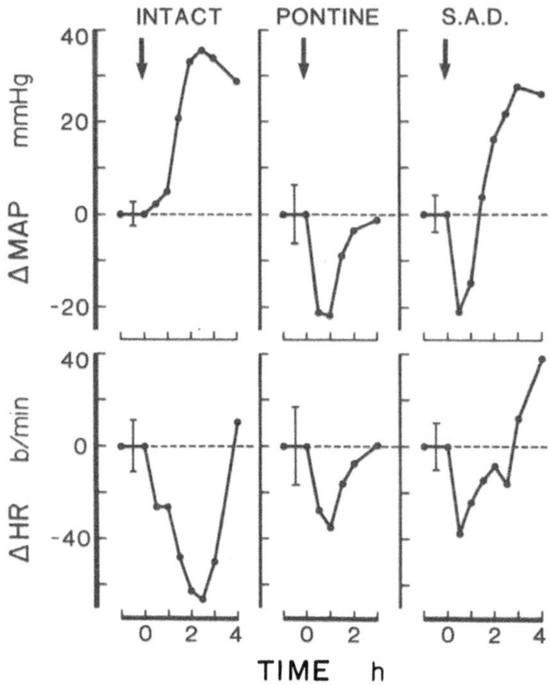

Fig. 4. Time course of changes in mean arterial pressure *(ΔMAP)* and heart rate *(ΔHR)* after i.c. injection of 6-OHDA (at *arrow*) in intact, pontine and sino-aortically denervated *(SAD)* rabbits. (From [34])

slightly. Feedback through the baroreceptors completely masks the late tachycardia response produced by the direct central effects of transmitter release. Hence, the late bradycardia is largely reflex in normal rabbits, secondary to the rise in MAP. We believe that the tachycardia of the SAD rabbit is probably mediated through the cardiac sympathetic, since it occurs at a time when activity in other sympathetic outflows is enhanced [32]. SAD rabbits have low (if any) vagal tone [1, 5, 30, 31] so that their early bradycardia response may be mediated by inhibition of cardiac sympathetic activity through a bulbo-spinal pathway, whilst the late tachycardia may be mediated through sympathetic facilitation through a suprapontine pathway (cf. schema for bulbo-spinal blood pressure pathway in Fig. 3). By contrast, the early bradycardia in pontine (with intact sino-aortic nerves) is largely vagal, with only a small sympatho-inhibitory component [33], which is similar to the effects of clonidine [31].

Thus, in the SAD preparation, feedback through the arterial baroreceptors is eliminated, so that its responses to 6-OHDA are closer to the "true" central effects of transmitter release than those of normal rabbits.

Which CA Nuclei are the Sources of the Central Cardiovascular Effects of 6-OHDA Induced Transmitter Release?

In these experiments bilateral electrolytic lesions were made in the A1, A2, A5 and A6/A7 NA nuclei, together with appropriate sham operations in other rabbits. In most experiments the bilateral lesions involved only one of the above nuclei. We used various landmarks on the surface of the brain or within it to obtain the stereotaxic co-ordinates for each nucleus. For example, we used the obex to map A1 [4] and mapping of the motor nucleus of the trigeminal for obtaining the A6/A7 co-ordinates. The animals were studied 2–3 weeks after making the lesions and on average, we destroyed 85% of NA cells in a given set of nuclei and never less than 73%.

In rabbits with intact sino-aortic nerves resting MAP was significantly lower than in sham-operated rabbits after A6/A7 lesions. Thus, in normal animals the activity of A6/A7 area increased resting blood pressure.

We do not know whether the effects of lesions were due to destruction of cells or of fibres of passage. However, using the residual effects of 6-OHDA-induced transmitter release as a marker, we could determine to what extent a given lesion affected the overall effects of CA release on blood pressure and heart rate in normal and SAD rabbits. Clearly, SAD rabbits were the most appropriate for assessing the changes in the pressor and depressor responses and in the tachycardia response (cardiac sympathetic) which are mediated through the various pathways of Fig. 3. Since SAD rabbits have little vagal tone, the effects on CA pathways affecting the vagus can only be assessed in rabbits with intact sino-aortic nerves.

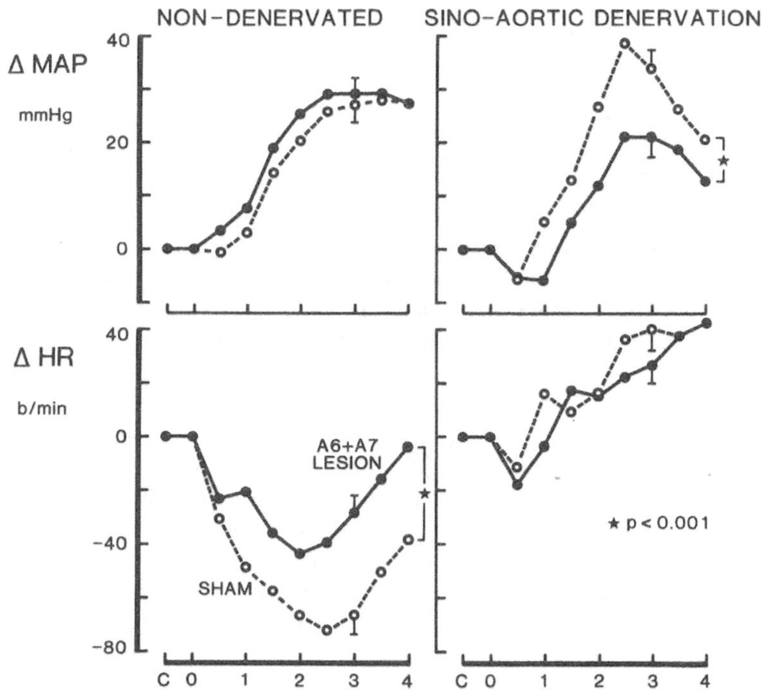

Fig. 5. Changes in mean arterial pressure *(ΔMAP)* and heart rate *(ΔHR)* following injection of 6-OHDA at time zero in intact *(left)* and sino-aortically denervated *(right)* rabbits subjected to either a bilateral lesion of the A6 and A7 nucleus (*solid lines*; $n = 7$) or to sham operation (*interrupted lines*; $n = 10$) 2–3 weeks before experiment. *Asterisk*, $P < 0.01$ for difference between groups; *bar*, 2 SEM from within animals variance in each group

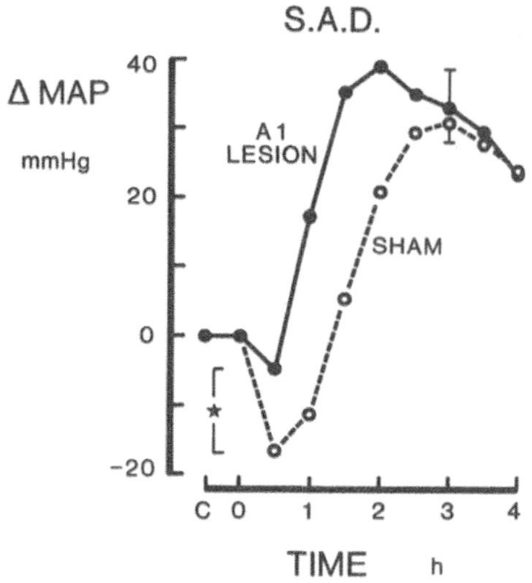

Fig. 6. Changes in mean arterial pressure *(ΔMAP)* in five sino-aortic denervated rabbits subjected to bilateral lesions of A1 nucleus *(solid lines)* or to sham operation *(interrupted lines)*. *Asterisk*, $P<0.025$ for significance of difference between groups; *bar*, 2 SEM from within animal variance in each group

In SAD rabbits, only lesions of A6/A7 (which contains over 40% of all NA neurons) significantly reduced the late pressor response after 6-OHDA, which was attenuated to 58% of the response of sham-operated rabbits ($P<0.01$; Fig. 5). Axons from this nucleus are thus a major contributor to the suprapontine pressor pathway shown in Fig. 3; the most likely integrative sites receiving these fibres are the hypothalamus and/or the amygdala. We also found that A1 nucleus mediated the early depressor effects in SAD rabbits and that these were attenuated by bilateral lesions of this nucleus (Fig. 6). Our findings about a depressor function of this region are in agreement with results of electrical stimulation [3]. It is possible that abolition of the depressor response by A1 lesions was due to destruction of fibres arising from the C1 group of adrenaline-containing neurons, which are just anterior to A1, but some adrenaline neurons mediate rises in blood pressure [11, 42].

The various lesions had only small effects on the tachycardia responses of SAD rabbits. However, the late bradycardia responses of intact rabbits were affected by lesions of A6/A7, A5 and A1 + A2 nuclei (e.g. Fig. 5). Hence, cells or fibres involving these nuclei probably contribute to the vagal pathways in Fig. 3.

In summary, at least some of the pathways in Fig. 3 are influenced by more than one NA nucleus. A1 lesions eliminate the bulbo-spinal depressor response of SAD rabbits given 6-OHDA. We have not completely identified all the sources of the suprapontine pressor pathway, but A6/A7 lesions are one important component of this pathway.

"Faults" in CA Pathways in Experimental Animals with Primary Hypertension

There are still many anatomical gaps in our knowledge of the CA pathways outlined in Fig. 3 and little is known about the role of the various 5HT nuclei. However, the general approach of using neurotoxin-induced transmitter release as a marker for assessing the effects of lesions has proved useful in the analysis of normal function.

The same approach has identified abnormalities of function in the above pathways, in animals with genetic hypertension. Head and de Jong [17] have recently shown significant differences in the relative magnitude of depressor and pressor responses of rats with spontaneous hypertension (SHR), Wistar-Kyoto (WKY), and Wistar rats. In SHR and WKY, the depressor effects were more potent and the late pressor component was virtually absent, whilst in Wistar rats both components were prominent, as in rabbits. Whether or not the observed differences contribute to the development of hypertension in SHR is uncertain; the important point is that genetic factors may produce differences in central autonomic pathways between the different strains. Genetic factors could also influence the distribution and numbers of the α_1- and α_2-adrenoceptors associated with their central autonomic pathways.

Saavedra et al. [45] and more recently Howe et al. [21] observed an increase in activity of the enzyme phenylethanolamine methyl transferase (PNMT), which is important in the synthesis of adrenaline in the young SHR rats. This has also been found in stroke-prone SHR [8]. However, increased PNMT activity was not observed in somewhat older SHR. If these adrenaline neurons play a role in the pathogenesis of primary hypertension in SHR, this may come about during early development.

Central Actions of Clonidine and α-MD in Relation to CA and 5HT Neurons

The actions of clonidine and α-MD are closely similar to the effects obtained during increased activity in the bulbo-spinal CA pathways [1, 20, 31]. Moreover, CA neurons appear to be the major site of biotransformation of α-MD into its active metabolites [14, 20] and the resultant cardiovascular effects are closely similar to those produced by clonidine. Thus, we have found that i.c. administration of α-MD and of clonidine produced similar changes in MAP, cardiac output and total peripheral resistance. In addition, both facilitated the vagal component of the baroreceptor-heart rate reflex and inhibited cardiac sympathetic motoneurons that do not receive baroreceptor projections. The only significant difference relates to those cardiac sympathetic neurons that receive projections from the baroreceptors, which are inhibited by clonidine, but unaffected by α-MD [1]. Thus, clonidine can be regarded as a marker for the neurons on which α-MD metabolites act, distally to the site of central biotransformation.

We studied the effects of the two antihypertensive drugs in rabbits before and 2 weeks after administration of one or other of the two neurotoxins [20]. After 6-OHDA the hypotensive action of i.c. α-MD was completely abolished and the bradycardia response was markedly attenuated (Fig. 7). This indicates the importance of CA neurons in biotransformation of α-MD. By contrast, the hypotensive effect of clonidine was attenuated by only about 50% whilst the attenuation of the heart rate response was slightly greater. After 5,6-DHT the falls in blood pressure and heart rate produced by both clonidine and by α-MD were each attenuated by about 50%.

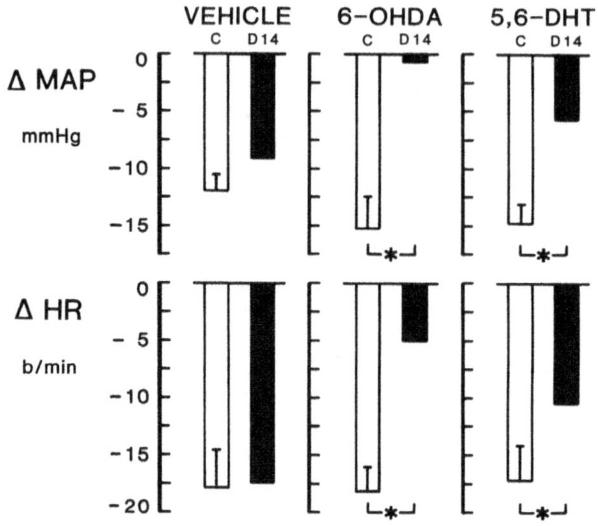

Fig. 7. Changes in mean arterial pressure *(ΔMAP)* and heart rate *(ΔHR)* occurring between 3 and 4 h after i.c. administration of α-methyldopa (0.4 mg/kg). *Open rectangles* are control responses before any treatment; *filled rectangles* are results obtained with α-methyldopa, 2 weeks after giving i.c. vehicle *(left)*, 6-OHDA or 5,6-DHT. *Bar* (in control response rectangle), 1 SEM from ANOVA; *asterisk*, $P<0.05$ for significance of difference within animals. (Based on data of [20])

Thus, CA and 5HT neurons are *both* involved in the central actions of clonidine and α-MD [20, 34, 35]. After destruction of CA neurons the significant residual response to clonidine suggests that α-adrenoceptors are present in other types of neurons (e.g. 5HT), which are inhibited by clonidine. It is unlikely that 5HT neurons are involved in the biotransformation of α-MD so that the presence of residual effects to this drug after destruction of these neurons suggests an arrangement similar to that in Fig. 3, for the bulbo-spinal sympathetic pathway regulating BP: some CA neurons in normal rabbits reach the preganglionic sympathetic motoneurons through a pathway in parallel with 5HT neurons, whilst others are in series with 5HT neurons, which become inhibited during increased CA activity.

We have begun to identify which groups of CA neurons are involved in the actions of α-MD and clonidine. After lesions of the A2 nucleus in the medulla and of combined lesions of the A1 + A2 nucleus the hypotensive effects of α-MD, given by the i.c. route, were not altered in SAD rabbits (Fig. 8, right panels) suggesting that these nuclei do not participate in the central effects on blood pressure or on the sympathetic component of heart rate. However, there was a significant delay in the onset of the hypotensive response to α-MD after A1 + A2 lesions in rabbits with intact sino-aortic nerves, associated with complete abolition of the bradycardia. After A2 lesions alone attenuation of the hypotension and bradycardia were less marked; this also occurred after A1 lesions alone. It follows that cells from both nuclei are essential for the action of α-MD on the vagal component of heart rate. We have found that α-MD lowers blood pressure by about 50% through reduction in cardiac output and by about 50% through reduction in total peripheral resistance [1]. The delayed effect on blood pressure may occur predominantly through the neural effects on cardiac output, accounting for the transient nature of the attenuated response. In these rabbits the bradycardia responses to clonidine were also attenuated. Similarly, after lesions of A6/A7 and A5 nuclei the bradycardia responses to α-MD and to clonidine were attenuated in intact rabbits, suggesting that they also were part of pathways im-

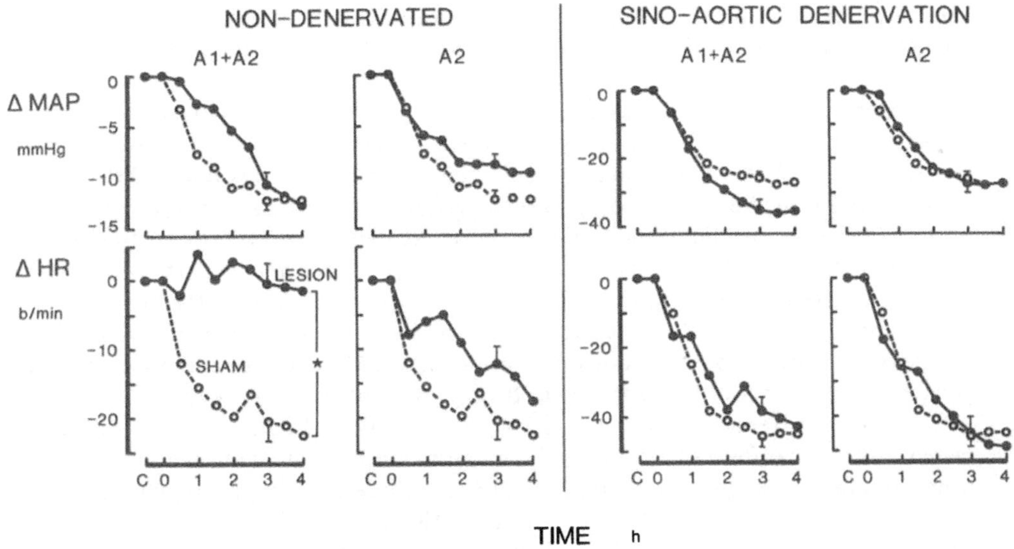

Fig. 8. *ΔMAP* and *ΔHR* in response to i.c. α-methyldopa (0.4 mg/kg) given at time zero to rabbits with intact sino-aortic nerves *(left panels)* subjected to bilateral combined lesions of A1 + A2 nucleus ($n = 8$), to lesions of A2 alone ($n = 6$), or to sham operation ($n = 6$). In the *right panels* responses to α-methyldopa in sino-aortically denervated rabbits subjected to lesions of A1 + A2 ($n = 5$), A2 alone ($n = 5$), or sham operation ($n = 6$). Other symbols as in Fig. 6

portant in the regulation of vagal tone. We have not so far completely abolished the hypotensive effects of these drugs by appropriate lesions. One hypothesis is that both adrenaline neurons of the ventrolateral medulla [42] and the A1 group of cells may be the major groups involved.

In summary, both α-MD and clonidine inhibit sympathetic constrictor tone directly through the effects of CA neurons on sympathetic motoneurons and also by inhibiting 5HT neurons projecting to the motoneurons (Fig. 3). The cardiac sympathetic tone may be inhibited by these drugs through similar pathways. The vagal facilitation could also be mediated through such a more complex arrangement involving both CA and 5HT neurons, rather than through CA neurons alone. The A1 and A2 nuclei are major sites involved in the bradycardia effects of α-MD and of clonidine, with A5 and A6/A7 also contributing to the vagal regulation of heart rate.

How Could Central Autonomic Abnormalities Cause Primary Hypertension?

Although complete removal of CA and 5HT neurons does not alter resting blood pressure, this may not be the case when there is imbalance in the activity of the depressor or pressor pathways, as shown experimentally after A6/A7 lesions. Some of the functional abnormalities in particular pathways are genetically determined, in the light of findings in animal models of primary hypertension. Esler et al. [12] have shown that in a proportion of their subjects there was a fault in the noradrenaline re-uptake pump at peripheral sympathetic nerve terminals. If such an abnormality occurred also in the CNS it could raise blood pressure through some of the pathways that have been discussed.

Recent analysis of noradrenaline kinetics in patients with established primary hypertension has shown that in only about 30% is there evidence of an overall increase in sympathetic neural activity [12]. This low percentage is partly due to the nonuniformity in the activity of different regional sympathetic outflows. For example, elevation of renal sympathetic activity has recently been observed in about 50% of patients with primary hypertension [13]. In chronic hypertension nonautonomic factors are the most important contributors to the maintenance of high blood pressure, notably the amplification by the hypertrophied heart and muscle of all kinds of constrictor and inotropic stimuli [26, 36]. During redevelopment of hypertension after reversal of the hypertrophy, we have recently obtained evidence of sympathetic overactivity affecting a higher proportion of patients than in chronic hypertension. We found that although supine blood pressure returned very slowly when treatment stopped, standing pressure rose more rapidly presumably through enhanced sympathetic activity [22, 36]. Thus there is prima facie evidence of increased sympathetic activity in "early" human hypertension.

One of the characteristics of primary hypertension in both humans and animals is that cardiac and to a lesser extent vascular hypertrophy are present at a very early stage of development [15]. An interesting speculation is whether the sympathetic nervous system plays a role in the early development of hypertrophy. NA released from peripheral nerve endings has been termed the "hypertrophy hormone" [39]; possibly the increased activity of central adrenaline neurons during early development in SHR [8] may exert a trophic role of cardiac and vascular muscle, since the early hypertrophy is proportionately greater than the pressure load.

At present definitive data on causal links between CNS abnormalities and primary hypertension are not available. Sympathetic overactivity does appear to be present in a high proportion of "early" hypertensives. Abnormalities have been demonstrated in the central CA pathways of animals with genetic primary hypertension. CA and 5HT pathways make important contributions to cardiovascular regulation in normal animals and long-term changes in blood pressure can be mediated through these pathways. It remains to be seen whether experimentally induced alterations in their activity can induce chronic hypertension in normal animals.

References

1. Badoer E, Head GA, Korner PI (1983) Effects of intracisternal and intravenous α-methyldopa and clonidine on haemodynamics and baroreceptor-heart rate reflex properties in conscious rabbits. J Cardiovasc Pharmacol 5:760–767
2. Blessing WW, Chalmers JP (1979) Direct projection of catecholamine (presumably dopamine)-containing neurons from hypothalamus to spinal cord. Neurosci Lett 11:35–40
3. Blessing WW, Reis DJ (1982) Inhibitory cardiovascular function of neurons in the caudal ventrolateral medulla of the rabbit: relationship to the area containing A1 noradrenergic cells. Brain Res 253:161–171
4. Blessing WW, Chalmers JP, Howe PRC (1978) Distribution of catecholamine-containing cell bodies in the rabbit central nervous system. J Comp Neurol 179:407–423

5. Blombery PA, Korner PI (1979) Relative contributions of aortic and carotid sinus baroreceptors to the baroreceptor-heart rate reflex of the conscious rabbit. J Auton Nerv Syst 1:161–171
6. Chalmers JP (1975) Brain amines and models of experimental hypertension. Circ Res 36:469–480
7. Chalmers JP, Reid JL (1972) Participation of central noradrenergic neurons in arterial baroreceptor reflexes in the rabbit: a study with intracisternally administered 6-hydroxydopamine. Circ Res 31:789–804
8. Chalmers JP, West MJ (1983) The nervous system in the pathogenesis of essential hypertension. In: Robertson JIS (ed) Clinical aspects of essential hypertension. Elsevier, Amsterdam, pp 64–96 (Handbook of hypertension, vol 1)
9. Chalmers JP, Wurtman RJ (1971) The fate of intracisternally administered norepinephrine-^{3}H in the brain and spinal cord of the rabbit. J Pharmacol Exp Ther 178:8–19
10. Dahlström A, Fuxe K (1964) Evidence for the existence of monoamine-containing neurons in the central nervous system. I. Demonstration of monoamines in the cell bodies of brain stem neurons. Acta Physiol Scand [Suppl 232] 62:1–55
11. Dampney RAL, Goodchild AK, Robertson LG, Montgomery W (1982) Role of ventrolateral medulla in vasomotor regulation: a correlative anatomical and physiological study. Brain Res 249:223–235
12. Esler MD, Jackman G, Bobik A, Leonard P, Kelleher D, Skews H, Jennings G, Korner P (1981) Norepinephrine kinetics in essential hypertension; defective neuronal uptake of norepinephrine in some patients. Hypertension 3:149–156
13. Esler MD, Hasking GJ, Willett IR, Leonard PW, Jennings GL (1985) Noradrenaline release and sympathetic nervous system activity. J Hypertens 3:117–129
13a. Evans MH (1980) Vasoactive sites in the diencephalon of the rabbit. Brain Res 183:329–340
14. Finch L, Haeusler G (1973) Further evidence for a central hypotensive action of α-methyldopa in both the rat and cat. Br J Pharmacol 47:217–228
15. Folkow B (1982) Physiological aspects of primary hypertension. Physiol Rev 62:347–504
16. Haeusler B (1971) Early pre- and postjunctional effects of 6-hydroxydopamine. J Pharmacol Exp Ther 178:49–62
17. Head GA, De Jong W (to be published) Differential blood pressure responses to intracisternal clonidine, α-methyldopa and 6-hydroxydopamine in conscious normotensive and spontaneously hypertensive rats: involvement of a central pressor pathway. J Cardiovasc Pharmacol. In press
18. Head GA, Korner PI (1980) Mechanisms of acute hypertension and bradycardia following intracisternal 6-hydroxydopamine in conscious rabbits. Eur J Pharmacol 66:111–115
19. Head GA, Korner PI (1982) Cardiovascular functions of brain serotonergic neurons in the rabbit as analysed from the acute and chronic effects of 5,6-dihydroxytryptamine. J Cardiovasc Pharmacol 4:398–408
20. Head GA, Korner PI, Lewis SL, Badoer E (1983) Contribution of noradrenergic and serotonergic neurons to the circulatory effects of centrally acting clonidine and α-methyldopa in rabbits. J Cardiovasc Pharmacol 5:945–953
21. Howe PRC, Lovenberg W, Chalmers JP (1981) Increased number of PNMT-immunofluorescent nerve cell bodies in the medulla oblongata of stroke-prone hypertensive rats. Brain Res 205:123–130
22. Jennings G, Korner P, Esler M, Restall R (1984) Redevelopment of essential hypertension after cessation of long-term therapy; preliminary findings. Clin Exp Hypertens [A] 6:493–505
23. Jonsson G, Sachs C (1970) Effects of 6-hydroxydopamine on the uptake and storage of noradrenaline in sympathetic adrenergic neurons. Eur J Pharmacol 9:141–155
24. Korner PI (1971) Integrative neural cardiovascular control. Physiol Rev 51:312–367
25. Korner PI (1979) Central nervous control of autonomic cardiovascular function. In: Berne RM (ed) The heart. American Physiological Society, Bethesda, pp 691–739 (Handbook of physiology, Sect 2: The cardiovascular system, vol 1)
26. Korner PI (1982) Causal and homeostatic factors in hypertension (Sixth Volhard Lecture). Clin Sci [Suppl 8] 63:5s–26s
27. Korner PI (1983) The role of the heart in hypertension. In: Robertson JIS (ed) Clinical aspects of essential hypertension. Elsevier, Amsterdam, pp 97–132 (Handbook of hypertension, vol 1).
28. Korner PI, Angus JA (1981) Central nervous control of blood pressure in relation to antihypertensive drug treatment. Pharmacol Ther 13:321–356

29. Korner PI, Head GA (1981) Effects of noradrenergic and serotonergic neurons on blood pressure, heart rate and baroreceptor-heart rate reflex of the conscious rabbit. J Auton Nerv Syst 3:511–523
30. Korner PI, Shaw J, West MJ, Oliver JR (1972) Central nervous system control of baroreceptor reflexes in the rabbit. Circ Res 31:637–652
31. Korner PI, Oliver JR, Sleight P, Chalmers JP, Robinson JS (1974) Effects of clonidine on the baroreceptor-heart rate reflex and on single aortic baroreceptor fibre discharge. Eur J Pharmacol 28:189–198
32. Korner PI, Oliver JR, Reynoldson JA, Head GA, Carson VJ, Walker MMcD (1978) Cardiovascular and behavioral effects of intracisternal 6-hydroxydopamine in the rabbit. Eur J Pharmacol 53:83–93
33. Korner PI, Reynoldson JA, Head GA, Oliver JR, Carson V (1979) Effect of 6-hydroxydopamine on baroreceptor-heart rate and nasopharyngeal reflexes of the rabbit. J Cardiovasc Pharmacol 1:311–328
34. Korner PI, Head GA, Bobik A, Badoer E, Aberdeen JA (1984) Central and peripheral autonomic mechanisms involved in the circulatory actions of methyldopa. Hypertension [Suppl 2] 6:II-63–II-70
35. Korner PI, Head GA, Badoer E (1984) Effects of sinoaortic denervation on the acute circulatory responses to centrally administered 6-hydroxydopamine and of clonidine in conscious rabbits. J Cardiovasc Pharmacol 6:909–913
36. Korner PI, Jennings GL, Esler MD, Broughton A (1985) Role of cardiac and vascular amplifiers in the maintenance of hypertension and the effect of reversal of cardiovascular hypertrophy. Clin Exp Pharmacol Physiol 12:205–209
37. Kuhn DM, Wolf WA, Lovenberg W (1980) Review of the role of the central serotonergic neuronal system in blood pressure regulation. Hypertension 2:243–255
38. Loewy AD, McKellar S (1980) The neuroanatomical basis of central cardiovascular control. Fed Proc 39:2495–2503
39. Östman-Smith I (1981) Cardiac sympathetic nerves as the final common pathway in the induction of adaptive cardiac hypertrophy. Clin Sci 61:265–272
40. Pickel VM, Joh TH, Reis DJ (1977) A serotonergic innervation of noradrenergic neurons in nucleus locus coeruleus: demonstration by immunocytochemical localization of the transmitter specific enzymes tyrosine and tryptophan hydroxylase. Brain Res 131:197–214
41. Reis DJ, Ross RA, Joh TH (1974) Some aspects of the reaction of central and peripheral noradrenergic neurons to injury. In: Fuxe K, Olsen L, Zotterman Y (eds) Dynamics of degeneration and growth in neurons. Pergamon, Oxford, pp 109–125
42. Reis DJ, Granata AR, Joh TH, Ross CA, Ruggiero DA, Park DH (1984) Brain stem catecholamine mechanisms in tonic and reflex control of blood pressure. Hypertension [Suppl 2] 6:II-7–II-15
43. Ross CA, Ruggiero DA, Joh TH, Park DH, Reis DJ (1983) Adrenaline synthesizing neurons in the rostral ventrolateral medulla: a possible role in tonic vasomotor control. Brain Res 273:356–361
44. Ryall RW (1967) Effect of monoamines upon sympathetic preganglionic neurons. Circ Res [Suppl 3] 20/21:III-83–III-87
45. Saavedra JM, Grobecker H, Axelrod J (1976) Adrenaline-forming enzyme in brainstem: elevation in genetic and experimental hypertension. Science 191:483–484
46. Sherrington CS (1906) The integrative action of the nervous system. Yale University Press, New Haven
47. Ungerstedt U (1971) Stereotaxic mapping of the monoamine pathways in the rat brain. Acta Physiol Scand [Suppl] 367:1–48
48. Wing LMH, Chalmers JP (1974) Participation of central serotonergic neurons in the control of the circulation of the unanesthetized rabbit: a study using 5,6-dihydroxytryptamine in experimental neurogenic and renal hypertension. Circ Res 35:504–513

Brain Peptides in Cardiovascular Regulation

D. GANTEN[1], F. C. LUFT[2], R. E. LANG[1], and TH. UNGER[1]

Introduction

Peptides found within brain tissue, the neuropeptides, number well in excess of 50 [1]. In all likelihood the identification and characterization of these compounds is in its infancy, and many more will subsequently be discovered.

Different modes of action have been described for the neuropeptides. They can, for example, act as neurotransmitters proper, as neuromodulators with positive or negative (presynaptiac) effects on the release of other neurotransmitters, or as neurohormones. The more general term of "chemical messengers" may be more appropriate. At the present time certainly no meaningful generalization about the mode of action can be made for so large a group of molecules which represent the neuropeptides, but there are some special features which merit being pointed out in this context. Neuropeptides frequently coexist with each other or with monoamine transmitters, thereby greatly increasing the number of different chemical signals that a neuron can release and use in communicating with other cells. It is possible that the "synaptic cocktail" consisting of peptides, monoamines, and amino acids is being released simultaneously if these are packaged together in one vesicle of a given nerve ending. They may, however, also be released separately. Peptide actions in general take place over a slower time course and over longer distances ("neurohormonal" action) than is the case for rapid synaptic transmission. A fundamental difference between biogenic amines, amino acids, and peptides is their mode of synthesis and metabolism. Peptides are not as rapidly degraded as classic transmitters and they are probably not recycled. The different speed of synthesis, transport, and replenishment opens up interesting possibilities, e.g., that the same repeated stimulus will in a graded way elicit different postsynaptic patterns in peptidergic and nonpeptidergic neurons. The relevance of this for cardiovascular control remains to be investigated; the functional subdivision of the autonomic nervous system according to the colocalization of peptides has, however, opened new vistas for the understanding and possible treatment of hypertensive desease.

This discussion will be confined to those neuropeptides with known cardiovascular effects.

[1] German Institute for High Blood Pressure Research and Department of Pharmacology, University of Heidelberg, Im Neuenheimer Feld 366, D-6900 Heidelberg.
[2] Indiana University, Indianapolis, IN, USA.

Primary Hypertension
Ed. by W. Kaufmann et al.

Angiotensin

The peripheral actions of renin and angiotensin have been studied since the last century and are well known. The central actions are currently being appreciated. Interestingly, the central effects of angiotensin are complementary to its peripheral effects. Central injection of this peptide is a very potent stimulant for drinking behavior and it also increases salt appetite (for review see [2–4]). Further, administration of angiotensin into the lateral brain ventricle of conscious rats increases blood pressure, in the face of an initial decrease in splanchnic, renal, and adrenal sympathetic tone [5]. The increase in blood pressure is in part mediated through the release of vasopressin into the circulation, since the peripheral administration of vasopressin antagonists substantially diminishes the angiotensin response [5, 6]. Partial attenuation also follows the administration of the alpha-blocking drug prazosin [6] or of other sympatholytic drugs [2]. It is possible that stimulation of brain angiotensin receptors affects sympathetic nervous system activity in a selective, rather than general fashion.

Angiotensin and angiotensin receptors have been localized to various areas of the brain including the median eminence, anterior hypothalamus, the nuclei adjacent to the third ventricle, and the perifornical area. Angiotensin innervation has also been described in the pituitary gland, brain stem areas such as the locus coeruleus, the nucleus ambiguus, and the nucleus tractus solitarii. The material has also been demonstrated in the limbic areas, corpus striatum and the cerebellum (for review see [7–9]). Circulating angiotensin in plasma may also evoke central cardiovascular effects, probably by stimulating the subfornical organ, the organum vasculosum laminae terminalis, and the area postrema [10, 11]. The permeability of the blood-brain barrier is such that circulating angiotensin may have access to these areas. The angiotensin pressor system in the rat forebrain has recently been reviewed [12].

Evidence exists directly implicating angiotensin in the development of hypertension in experimental animal models. For instance, renin was found to be increased in the brains of spontaneously hypertensive rats [13]. Further angiotensin synthesis was also increased, compared with control rats of the same animal model [14]. Finally, renin inhibitors, angiotensin receptor antagonists, and angiotensin converting enzyme (ACE) inhibitors can lower blood pressure when given centrally to this same animal model [15–18]. An additional line of evidence stems from the microiontophoretic application of angiotensin into regions within the blood-brain barrier, such as the septal area, which resulted in a more pronounced neuronal firing response in spontaneously hypertensive rats than control rats [19].

Opioid Peptides

Opioid peptides (endorphins, dynorphins, enkephalins) are widely distributed within the central nervous system (CNS) [20]. The hypothalamus and the brain stem are areas of cardiovascular control which contain substantial amounts of opioid peptides. However, pharmacologic studies involving opioid peptides, their agonists, or their antagonists, have yielded contradictory results with respect to cardiovascular effects depending up on the specific peptide, the site of administration, the species tested, and the state of consciousness of the animals [20]. Prevailing evidence suggests that leu- and met-enkephalin appear to be pressors when administered into the ventricular system of conscious dogs, cats, and rats [21–23]. In anesthetized animals, vasodepressor effects were described [24–27]. Beta-endorphin appears to be primarily a depressor [28, 29]. This opioid peptide may have a direct action on the baroreflex arc [29]; μ receptor agonists have been reported to attenuate the baroreceptor reflex, while antagonists seem to sensitize the baroreceptor mechanism [29]. Injections of beta-endorphin directly into the nucleus tractus solitarii resulted in a bimodal effect with decreases in blood pressure at either low (below 10 ng), or high dosage [30]. Naloxone and beta-endorphin antibody prevented decreases in blood pressure, while antibody to met-enkephalin produced a depressor response. In the nucleus tractus solitarii two opioid pathways were subsequently postulated, one beta-endorphin-like, the other met-enkephalin-like, with depressor and pressor functions, respectively [30]. The presence of a central depressor endorphin pathway is supported by studies examining the effects of naloxone on shock [31–33]. Both intravenous and central administration of naloxone increased blood pressure and improved survival in such models [33]. Evidence supporting a role for opioid peptides in centrally mediated depressor responses also accrues from pharmacologic studies. For instance, naloxone appeared to reverse the antihypertensive action of clonidine and alpha-methyldopa [34]. Moreover, clonidine and alpha-methyl-norepinephrine both released beta-endorphin-like immunoreactivity from brain stem slices of spontaneously hypertensive rats [35]. Finally, beta-endorphin antiserum antagonized the effects of alpha-methyl-norepinephrine, when that compound was injected directly into the nucleus tractus solitarii [36]. A role for maintenance of hypertension in spontaneously hypertensive rats by enkephalins was supported by the results of studies showing that blood pressure in these animals can be lowered by the central administration of diprenorphine [24].

Substance P

A role for substance P in the afferent limb of the baroreceptor reflex arc has already been discussed. In the CNS substance P is found in high concentrations within the hypothalamus [37]. In addition to its central and peripheral role as a mediator of pain, substance P also has cardiovascular effects. When given peripherally, substance P lowers blood pressure [38, 39]. The reverse is true in a dose-dependent fashion, when the peptide is administered centrally [6, 40]. Recent evidence indicates that the effect of substance P on blood pressure and heart rate is the result of sympathetic nervous system stimulation [5, 6]. Interactions between substance P responses and those of opioid peptides are suggested by an enhancing of substance P's effect with naloxone, and an attenuation by morphine [41]. The anterior hypothalamus has been demonstrated to be particularly sensitive to this peptide with respect to its central cardiovascular actions [42]. Substance P has been shown to influence blood flow within the hypothalamus [43], raising the possibility of blood flow control by substance P in certain cardiovascular regulatory centers.

Vasopressin and Oxytocin

Vasopressin, the antidiuretic hormone, and oxytocin, are both peptides synthesized in the hypothalamus and released via the neurohypophysis into the circulation. Vasopressin is recognized for its antidiuretic and vasopressor properties, while oxytocin plays an important role in parturition and lactation. Immunohistochemical techniques demonstrated the presence of vasopressin- and oxytocin-containing neurons in other areas of the CNS including the forebrain, brain stem, hippocampus amygdala, nucleus ambiguus, nucleus tractus solitarii, and the substantia gelatinosa of the spinal cord [44–46]. Quantitative techniques confirmed these histological findings [47, 48]. A role for central vasopressin in the maintenance of behavior and memory has been demonstrated [49]. The presence of both vasopressin and oxytocin within or adjacent to cardiovascular regulatory centers suggests a putative role for these peptides in cardiovascular regulation.

Evidence for a central cardiovascular action of plasma vasopressin stems from experiments comparing infusions of the material either into the inferior vena cava or into the vertebral artery of conscious dogs [50]. Intravertebral vasopressin increased blood pressure less than vena caval administration, even though heart rate decreased to a greater extent. Thus, it is possible that vasopressin may operate to interfere centrally with the baroreceptor reflex, perhaps by augementing its responsiveness. Central (intracerebroventricular) administration of vasopressin increases blood pressure [51, 52] by stimulating the sympathetic nervous system [52], even though the same route of administration appears to attenuate the pressor response evoked by electrical stimulation of the mesencephalic reticular formation [53].

Microinjections of vasopressin into the hippocampal dentate gyrus provided the same effect, suggesting that this area of the brain may play a role in the modulation of depressor functions mediated by vasopressin [53]. On the other hand, microinjections of vasopressin directly into the nucleus tractus solitarii caused dose-related increases in blood pressure, while the vasopressin antagonist $d(CH_2)_5VDAVP$ evoked the opposite (vasodepressor) response [54]. Vasopressin also plays a role in the mediation of pressor responses evoked by central angiotensin II (see above, [5]). The role of vasopressin in hypertension is even less clear. During the developmental phase of hypertension vasopressin was found to be reduced in the brains of spontaneously hypertensive rats [55, 56]. In addition, a strain of rats developed by crossing spontaneously hypertensive rats with the Brattleboro strain of rats, which have diabetes insipidus and no vasopressin, yielded a rat with diabetes insipidus and genetic hypertension [57].

Neurotensin

Neurotensin was identified as a byproduct of substance P isolation [58]. Besides lowering blood pressure by dilating blood vessels, neurotensin alters pituitary hormone release [59], and when injected into the brain, lowers body temperature as well [60]. The material is found in highest concentrations in the hypothalamus and the basal ganglia. The peptide produces selective inhibition of neuronal firing in the locus coeruleus. Neurotensin is distributed in a fashion similar to enkephalin; however, the two peptides are stored in separate neurons and their interaction is as yet unclear [60].

Hypothalamic-Releasing Factors

Releasing factors are contained within the median eminence of the hypothalamus and pass through the portal capillaries to the pituitary gland where they regulate the synthesis and release of pituitary hormones [1]. Thyrotropin-releasing factor was the first to be isolated and was identified to be a tripeptide [61]. Over 80% of thyrotropin-releasing factor occurs outside the hypothalamus. Areas of concentration include motor nuclei of cranial nerves, the ventral spinal cord, the lateral septal nuclei, and the nucleus of the stria terminalis [62]. Its actions seem most concerned with behavioral excitation and anorexia rather than blood pressure regulation per se [63]. On the other hand, corticotropin-releasing factor, a peptide with 41 amino acid residues, clearly increases blood pressure and heart rate when given into the lateral ventricle. This peptide is particularly concentrated in extrahypothalamic nuclei, including those of the limbic system and the medulla. Corticotropin-releasing factor is a potent stimulator of ACTH and beta-endorphin release from the pituitary gland [64]. Its effects on blood pressure following central administration appear to be related to the enhancement of sympathetic tone [65].

Interactions of Neurotransmitters

Information processing in the brain largely involves communication among neurons through release of chemical messengers and neurotransmitters at synapses. Although in theory the brain might make do with one excitatory and one inhibitory neurotransmitter, such is certainly not the case. Until recently, amines such as acetylcholine, nor- and epinephrine, serotonin, glutamic acid, GABA, and histamine were the only well-recognized neurotransmitters. An explosion in the number of possible chemical messengers resulted from the appreciation that various peptides also serve that function [1]. Many of these peptides were first described in the peripheral circulation. The machinery to synthesize these materials has been demonstrated in primitive organisms such as protozoa and bacteria, suggesting that these peptides have served teleologically ancient communicational functions among cells. These compounds regulated energy metabolism, cell hydration, electrolyte transport, and cell growth. With additional cellular differentiation and organization, these same messengers were incorporated into systems which included more direct and rapid neurotransmitters as well. Thus, chemical messengers such as peptides may have evolved to serve hormonal, neurotransmitter, neuromodulator, and neuroregulatory functions simultaneously. Such an arrangement explains the close anatomical relationship between peptide synthesizing cell groups and noradrenergic pathways in the brain [66]. For instance, pathways arising from noradrenergic cells in the dorsal vagal complex, the ventrolateral medulla, and the locus coeruleus were found to terminate in specific subdivisions of the paraventricular and supraoptic hypothalamic nuclei, which are known to be sites of vasopressin and oxytocin synthesis and to be involved in neuroendocrine regulation [66].

An example of interaction and modulation of established amine neurotransmitters by peptides involves the effect of opioid peptides on neuroexcitability. Such an interaction has been reported for cells in the hypothalamus and medulla [67]. The opioids presumably have a presynaptic action, thereby inhibiting release of the excitatory transmitter [68]. Opioids also inhibit the release of substance P from the rat trigeminal nucleus by exerting a postsynaptic effect [69]. The same appears to be the case in the spinal cord, where opioids reduce the depolarization induced by *l*-glutamate. The enkephalins also depress the release of acetylcholine into the spinal fluid [70]. Beta-endorphin is capable of influencing acetylcholine metabolism in several brain nuclei [71]. Opioid peptides also influence the disposition of serotonin within the central nervous system [72], as well as that of GABA [73].

The renin-angiotensin system in the brain and the catecholaminergic system also interact, as suggested by experiments demonstrating the effect of angiotensin on catecholamine turnover in the hypothalamus and medulla [74]. Further, angiotensin participates directly in the release of norepinephrine from brain tissue [75]. In turn, the effects of angiotensin are modulated by endogenous GABA or its agonists [76, 77]. Vasopressin is able to influence the discharges of single neurons in the medulla as well as to excite noradrenergic fibres in the locus coeruleus [78].

The development of drugs with selective effects on peptide disposition awaits clarification of the biosynthesis and inactivation of the peptides. It is likely that further studies of peptide neurotransmitters may well result in important therapeutic applications. Perhaps more important is the likelihood that by obtaining insight into these complex systems and their interactions with more conventionally understood mechanisms, our basic understanding of brain function stands to be substantially enhanced.

References

1. Snyder SH (1980) Brain peptides as neurotransmitters. Science 209:976–983
2. Severs WB, Daniels-Severs AE (1973) Effects of angiotensin on the central nervous system. Pharmacol Rev 25:415–449
3. Fitzsimons JT (1980) Angiotensin stimulation of the central nervous system. Rev Physiol Biochem Pharmacol 87:117–167
4. Lang RE, Unger T, Rascher W, Ganten D (1982) Brain angiotensin. In: Iversen LL (ed) Handbook of psychopharmacology. Plenum, New York, pp 307–361
5. Unger T, Becker H, Petty M, Demmert G, Schneider B, Ganten D, Lang RE (to be published) Differential effects of central angiotensin II and substance P on sympathetic nerve activity in conscious rats: implications for cardiovascular adaptation to behavioral responses. Circ Res
6. Unger T, Rascher W, Schuster C, Pavlovitch R, Schömig A, Dietz R, Ganten D (1981) Central blood pressure effects of substance P and angiotensin II: Role of the sympathetic nervous system. Eur J Pharmacol 71:33–42
7. Schelling P, Speck G, Unger T, Ganten D (1980) The brain renin-angiotensin system: Biochemistry, localization, and functional aspects. In: Parvez H, Parvez S (eds) Advances in experimental medicine: A centenary tribute to Claude Bernard. Elsevier/North-Holland, Amsterdam, pp 243–288
8. Printz MI, Ganten D, Unger T, Phillips MI (1982) Minireview: The brain renin angiotensin system. In: Ganten D, Printz MP, Phillips MI, Schölkens BA (eds) The renin angiotensin system in the brain. Springer, Berlin Heidelberg New York, pp 3–52 (Experimental brain research Supplement, vol 4)

9. Ganten D, Lang RE, Lehmann E, Unger T (1984) Commentary – Brain angiotensin: On the way to becoming a well-studied neuropeptide system. Biochem Pharmacol 33(22):3523–3528
10. Ferrario CM, Gildenberg PL, McCubbin JW (1972) Cardiovascular effects of angiotensin mediated by the central nervous system. Circ Res 30:257–262
11. Phillips MI, Weyhenmeyer D, Felix D, Ganten D, Hoffman WE (1979) Evidence for an endogenous brain-renin angiotensin system. Fed Proc 38:2260–2266
12. Harth DK, Brody M (1984) The angiotensin II pressor system of the rat forebrain. Circ Res 54:355–366
13. Schelling P, Meyer D, Loos HE, Speck G, Phillips MI, Johnson AK, Ganten D (1982) A micromethod for the measurement of renin in brain nuclei: its application in spontaneously hypertensive rats. Neuropharmacology 21:455–463
14. Ganten D, Hermann K, Bayer C, Unger T, Lang RE (1983) Angiotensin synthesis in the brain and increased turnover in hypertensive rats. Science 221:869–871
15. Mann JFE, Phillips MI, Dietz R, Haebara H, Ganten D (1978) Effects of central and peripheral angiotensin blockade in hypertensive rats. Am J Physiol 234:H629–H637
16. McDonald W, Wickre C, Aumann S, Ban D, Moffitt B (1980) The sustained antihypertensive effect of chronic cerebroventricular infusion of angiotensin antagonist in spontaneously hypertensive rats. Endocrinology 107:1305–1308
17. Unger T, Kaufmann-Bühler I, Schölkens B, Ganten D (1981) Brain converting enzyme inhibition: A possible mechanism for the antihypertensive action of captopril in spontaneously hypertensive rats. Eur J Pharmacol 70:467–478
18. Tonnaer JADM, van Put JJ, de Jong W (1981) Intracerebroventricular infusion of n-acetyl-pepstatin attenuates the development of hypertension in the spontaneously hypertensive rat. Eur J Pharmacol 74:113–114
19. Felix D, Schelling P, Haas HL (1982) Angiotensin and single neurons. In: Ganten D, Printz M, Phillips MI, Schölkens BA (eds) The renin angiotensin system in the brain. Springer, Berlin Heidelberg New York, pp 255–269
20. Lang RE, Brückner UB, Kempf B, Rascher W, Sturm V, Unger T, Speck G, Ganten D (1982) Opioid peptides and blood pressure regulation. Clin Exp Hypertens [A] 4 (1–2):249–269
21. Schaz K, Stock G, Simon W, Schlör KH, Unger T, Rockhold R, Ganten D (1980) Enkephalin effects on blood pressure, heart rate and baroreceptor reflex. Hypertension 2:395–407
22. Bellet M, Elghozi JL, Meyer P, Pernollet MW, Schmitt H (1980) Central cardiovascular effects of narcotic analgesics and enkephalins in rats. Br J Pharmacol 71:365–369
23. Yukimura T, Stock G, Stumpf H, Unger T, Ganten D (1981) Effects of (D-Ala-2)-methionine-enkephalin on blood pressure, heart rate, and baroreceptor reflex sensitivity in conscious cats. Hypertension 3:528–533
24. Yukimura T, Unger T, Rascher W, Lang RE, Ganten D (1981) Central peptidergic stimulation in blood pressure control: Role of enkephalins in rats. Clin Sci 61:347s–350s
25. Florez J, Mediavilla A (1977) Respiratory and cardiovascular effects of met-enkephalin applied to the ventral surface of the brain stem. Brain Res 138:585–590
26. Feldberg W, Wei E (1978) Central cardiovascular effects of enkephalins and C-fragment of lipotropin. J Physiol (Lond) 280:18P
27. Laubie M, Schmitt H, Vincent M, Remond G (1977) Central cardiovascular effects of morphinomimetic peptides in dogs. Eur J Pharmacol 46:67–71
28. Bolme P, Fuxe K, Agnati LF, Bradley R, Smythies J (1978) Cardiovascular effects of morphine and opioid peptides following intracisternal administration in chloralose-anaesthetized rats. Eur J Pharmacol 48:319–324
29. Petty MA, Reid JL (1981) Central peptides and baroreflex activity: Studies with opiate analogues, substance P and baroreceptor reflexes in the rabbit. Hypertension [Suppl 1] 3:142–147
30. Petty MA, de Jong W (1982) Cardiovascular effects of ß-endorphin after microinjection into the nucleus tractus solitarii of the anesthetized rat. Eur J Pharmacol 81:449–457
31. Holaday JW, Faden AI (1978) Naloxone reversal of endotoxin hypotension suggest role of endorphins in shock. Nature 275:450–451
32. Faden AI, Holaday JW (1979) Opiate antagonists: a role in the treatment of hypovolemic shock. Science 205:317–318
33. Janssen HF, Lutherer LO (1980) Ventriculo cisternal administration of naloxone protects against severe hypotension during shock. Brain Res 194:608

34. Farsang C, Ramirez-Gonzales MD, Mucci L, Kunos G (1980) Possible role of an endogenous opiate in the cardiovascular effects of central alpha adrenoreceptor stimulation in spontaneous hypertensive rats. J Pharmacol Exp Ther 214:203–208
35. Kunos G, Farsang C (1981) β-Endorphin: Possible involvement in the antihypertensive effect of central alpha-receptor activation. Science 211:82–84
36. Petty MA, de Jong W (1982) Does β-endorphin contribute to the central antihypertensive action of alpha-methyldopa in rats? Clin Sci 63:293S–295S
37. Hökfelt T, Kellerth JO, Nilsson G, Pernow B (1975) Substance P: localization in the central nervous system and some primary sensory neurons. Science 190:889–890
38. Bury RW, Mashford ML (1977) Cardiovascular effects of synthetic substance P in several species. Eur J Pharmacol 45:335–347
39. Pham-Huu-Chanh A, Clavel P, Lehmann-Schad W (1977) Cardiovascular effects of synthetic substance P. Pharmacology 15:341–347
40. Agnati LF, Fuxe K, Bolme P, Lundberg J, Hökfelt T (1979) Evidence for a possible role of substance P and/or its fragments in the central cardiovascular regulation. Neurosci Lett 3:S330
41. Petty MA, Reid JL (1982) The cardiovascular effects of centrally administered substance P in the anaesthetized rabbit. Eur J Pharmacol 82:9–14
42. Unger T, Becker H, Ganten D, König M, Lang RE, Petty M (1983) Central cardiovascular actions of substance P. In: Skrabanek P, Powell D (eds) Substance P. Boole, Dublin, pp 73–74
43. Klugman KP, Lembeck F, Markowitz S, Mitchell G, Rosendorff C (1980) Substance P increases hypothalamic blood flow via an indirect adrenergic cholinergic interaction. Br J Pharmacol 71:623–629
44. Sofroniew MV, Weindl A (1978) Projections from the parvocellular vasopressin- and neurophysin-containing neurons of the suprachiasmatic nucleus. Am J Anat 153:391–430
45. Buijs RM (1978) Intra- and extrahypothalamic vasopressin and oxytocin pathways in the rat. Cell Tissue Res 192:423–435
46. Nilaver G, Zimmerman EA, Wilkins J, Michaels J, Hoffman D, Silverman AJ (1980) Magnocellular hypothalamic projections to the lower brain stem and spinal cord of the rat. Immunocytochemical evidence for predominance of the oxytocin-neurophysin system compared to the vasopressin-neurophysin system. Neuroendocrinology 30:150–158
47. Dogterom J, Snijdewint FGM, Buijs RM (1978) The distribution of vasopressin and oxytocin in the rat brain. Neurosci Lett 9:341–346
48. Glick SM, Brownstein MG (1980) Vasopressin content of rat brain. Life Sci 27:1103–1110
49. Kovacs GL, Bohus B, Versteeg DHG (1979) The effects of vasopressin in memory processes: The role of noradrenergic transmission. Neuroscience 4:1529–1537
50. Liard JF, Deriaz O, Tschopp M, Schoun J (1981) Cardiovascular effects of vasopressin infused into the vertebral circulation of conscious dogs. Clin Sci 61:345–347
51. Pittman QJ, Lawrence D, McLean L (1982) Central effects of arginine vasopressin on blood pressure in rats. Endocrinology 110:1058–1060
52. Unger T, Rohmeiss P, Becker H, Ganten D, Lang RE, Petty M (to be published) Sympathetic activation following central vasopressin receptor stimulation in conscious rats. J Hypertens
53. Bohus B, Versteeg CAM, de Jong W (1982) Vasopressin and central blood pressure control in the rat. In: Rascher W, Clough D, Ganten D (eds) Hypertensive mechanisms. Schattauer, Stuttgart, pp 592–596
54. Matsuguchi H, Sharabi FM, Gordon FJ, Johnson AK, Schmid PG (1982) Blood pressure and heart rate response to vasopressin microinjection into the nucleus tractus solitarius region of the rat. Neuropharmacology 21:687–693
55. Lang RE, Rascher W, Unger T, Ganten D (1981) Reduced content of vasopressin in the brain of spontaneously hypertensive as compared to normotensive rats. Neurosci Lett 23:199–202
56. Rascher W, Lang RE, Unger T, Ganten D, Gross F (1982) Vasopressin in the brain of spontaneously hypertensive rats. Am J Physiol 242:H496–H499
57. Ganten U, Rascher W, Lang RE, Dietz R, Rettig R, Unger T, Taugner R, Ganten D (1983) Development of a new strain of spontaneously hypertensive rats homozygous for hypothalamic diabetes insipidus. Hypertension 5(2):I-119–I-128
58. Carraway RE, Leeman SE (1973) The isolation of a new hypotensive peptide, neurotensin from bovine hypothalami. J Biol Chem 248:6854–6861

59. Nemeroff C, Bissette G, Prange A, Loosen P, Barlow T, Lipton M (1977) Neurotensin: Central nervous system effects of a hypothalamic peptide. Brain Res 128:485–496
60. Uhl Gr, Kuhar MJ, Snyder SH (1977) Neurotensin: Immunohistochemical localization in rat central nervous system. Proc Natl Acad Sci USA 74:4059–4063
61. Burgus R, Dunn TF, Desiderio D, Ward DN, Vale W, Guillemin R (1970) Characterization of bovine hypothalamic hypophysiotropic TSH-releasing factor. Nature 276:321–325
62. Nair RMG, Barrett JF, Bowers CY, Schally AV (1970) Structure of porcine thyrotropin releasing hormone. Biochemistry 9:1103–1106
63. Prange AJ, Wilson IC, Lara PP, Alltop LB, Breese GR (1972) The effects of thyrotropin-releasing hormone in depression. Lancet 2:999–1001
64. Rivier C, Brownstein J, Spiess J, Rivier J, Vale W (1982) In vivo CRF-induced secretion of ACTH, ß-endorphin and corticosterone. Endocrinology 110:272–279
65. Fisher LA, Rivier C, Rivier J, Spiess J, Vale W, Brown MR (1982) Corticotropin releasing factors (CRF): Central effects on mean arterial pressure and heart rate in rats. Endocrinology 110(6):2222–2224
66. Sawchenko PE, Swanson LW (1981) Central noradrenergic pathways for the integration of hypothalamic neuroendocrine and autonomic responses. Science 214:685–687
67. North RA (1979) Opiates, opioid peptides and single neurons. Life Sci 24:1527–1546
68. Zieglgänsberger W, Tulloch IF (1979) The effects of methionine- and leucine-enkephalin on spinal neurons of the cat. Brain Res 167:53–64
69. Jessel T, Iversen LL (1977) Opiate analgesics inhibit substance P release from rat trigeminal nucleus. Nature 268:549–551
70. Jhamandas K, Sawynok J, Sutak M (1977) Enkephalin effects on release of brain acetylcholine. Nature 269:433–434
71. Moroni F, Chency DL, Costa E (1977) β-Endorphin inhibits ACh turnover in nuclei of rat brain. Nature 267267–268
72. Forchetti CM, Marco EJ, Meek JL (1982) Serotonin and gamma-aminobutyric acid turnover after injection into the median raphe of substance P and d-ala-met-enkephalinamide. J Neurochem 38:1336–1341
73. Nistico G, di Giorgio RM, Rotiroti D, Naccari F, Calatroni A (1979) Effects of intraventricular β-endorphin on GABA system in some areas of chick brain. Res Commun Chem Pathol Pharmacol 26:469–478
74. Fuxe K, Andersson K, Ganten D, Hökfelt T, Eneroth P (1980) Evidence for the existence of angiotensin-II-like immunoreactive central neuron system and its interactions with the central catecholamine pathways. In: Gross F, Vogel G (eds) Enzymatic release of vasoactive peptides. Raven, New York, pp 161–170
75. Chevillard G, Duchene N, Pasquier R, Alexandre JM (1979) Relation of the centrally evoked pressor effect of angiotensin II to central noradrenaline in the rabbit. Eur J Pharmacol 58:203–206
76. Brennan TJ, Haywood JR (1983) GABA inhibiton of central angiotensin II and hypertonic CSF pressor responses. Brain Res 267:261–269
77. Unger T, Bles F, Ganten D, Lang RE, Rettig R, Schwab NA (1983) GABA-ergic stimulation inhibited central action of angiotensin II: Pressor responses, drinking and release of vasopressin. Eur J Pharmacol 90:1–9
78. Olpe HR, Baltzer V (1981) Vasopressin activates noradrenergic neurons in the locus coeruleus: A microiontophoretic investigation. Eur J Pharmacol 73:377–378

Critical Evaluation of Basic Mechanisms of Primary Hypertension

K. G. Hofbauer[1] and G. Bönner[2]

Round-Table Discussion with:
O. A. Carretero, Detroit, MI, USA; D. Ganten, Heidelberg, Federal Republic of Germany; P. I. Korner, Victoria, Australia; S. Z. Langer, Paris, France; G. A. MacGregor, London, Great Britain; H. Vetter, Münster, Federal Republic of Germany; G. H. Williams, Boston, MA, USA

Introduction

The round-table discussion was held to evaluate critically the significance of the pathogenetic mechanisms presented during the preceding session. It afforded opportunity to identify areas of consensus or controversy and reflected the progress of current research in hypertension. The fact emerged clearly from the discussion that an understanding of the basic mechansims of cardiovascular control and of the pathogenesis of hypertension is important for the rational application of the available antihypertensive therapies and for the design of new modes of treatment. The following summary covers the main topics dealt with during the last six contributions and the new aspects arising at the round table.

Central and Peripheral Neural Mechanisms

Experimental studies of the central regulation of blood pressure have led to the identification of mechanisms that may be implicated in the pathogenesis of hypertension. In various strains of spontaneously hypertensive rats, genetic differences have been detected in the function of central autonomic pathways (Korner). These findings support the view that central dysregulation may also be a causal factor in human essential hypertension. Overactivity of the sympathetic nervous system, which is observed in patients during the early phase of hypertension, might be an initiating factor in the development of high blood pressure. At a later stage, amplifying factors, such as vascular and cardiac hypertrophy, may obscure the influence of sympathetic overactivity (Korner).

In addition to the "classical" (monoamine) neurotransmitters in the central nervous system, neuropeptides may play an essential part in cardiovascular homoeostasis.

[1] Biological Research Department, CIBA-GEIGY AG, CH-4002 Basel.
[2] Department of Internal Medicine II, Merheim Hospital and Policlinic of the University of Cologne, Ostmerheimer Str. 200, D-5000 Cologne 91.

Primary Hypertension
Ed. by W. Kaufmann et al.

Many peptides, such as angiotensin II, arginine-vasopressin, oxytocin, and substance P, which were originally found in circulating blood or in peripheral organs, have also been detected in the central nervous system, where they may act as neurotransmitters, neuromodulators, or neurohormones. The coexistence of different neuropeptides or of neuropeptides and monoamine transmitters in individual neurons suggests that multiple interactions between these agents may occur (Ganten). It has been demonstrated that central peptidergic mechanisms contribute towards the development and maintenance of high blood pressure in rats with spontaneous hypertension. A better knowledge of the biosynthesis, inactivation, and function of the neuropeptides might lead to the development of drugs capable of interfering selectively with the formation or action of the neuropeptides (Ganten).

The biochemical and biological characterization of central and peripheral adrenoceptors has made it possible to identify subgroups of receptors with different binding properties. Presynaptic receptors modulate transmitter release under physiological conditions; e.g., α_2-adrenoceptors and dopaminergic receptors of the D_2 subtype inhibit the release of noradrenaline, whereas β_2-adrenoceptors have facilitatory effects. These receptors may also be targets for specific new drugs (Langer). Receptor subtypes are coupled to different second-messenger systems; e.g., activation of α_1-adrenoceptors increases the break-down of phosphoinositol and raises intracellular Ca^{2+} concentrations, while activation of α_2-adrenoceptors inhibits adenylate-cyclase activity and lowers intracellular concentrations of cAMP. It has recently been demonstrated that stimulation of α_1-adrenoceptors induces DNA synthesis [1]. These results suggest that α_1-adrenoceptors may play a part in the regulation of cell growth (Langer).

Vasodepressor Hormones

The maintenance of normal blood pressure probably depends on the balance between pressor and depressor factors. Thus, hypertension may be caused either by overactivity of pressor systems, such as the renin-angiotensin and the sympathetic nervous system, or by reduced activity of depressor systems, such as the glandular kallikrein-kinin systems. Although in many recent investigations a reduced activity of the renal kallikrein-kinin system was demonstrated in hypertensive subjects, it is still unclear whether these changes play a role in the pathogenesis of hypertension or are only secondary to the elevated blood pressure. Glandular kallikrein-kinin systems are localized in many organs (salivary glands, sweat glands, pancreas, pituitary, kidney, uterus, gut, chorioid plexus) and are mainly involved in the regulation of secretory function. Thus, it is not easy to imagine what effects on systemic blood pressure regulation all these different kallikrein-kinin systems might exert. Probably all determinations and interpretations of kallikrein activity in vitro or in biological fluids are not valid and do not represent the true activity of the kallikrein-kinin system in the tissues. This is of special importance for the kallikrein-kinin system in arterial walls since at present it is not possible to deduce the activity of glandular kallikrein-kinin systems from measurements on systemic blood (Bönner). The identification of different kinin-receptor subtypes (B_1 and B_2) in the vascular system might help towards a better understanding of the cardiovascular effects of kinins [2]; however, the functional implications of this receptor classification are still controversial (Carretero). Converting-enzyme inhibitors lead to a reduced degradation of kinins, which induce vasodilatation and stimulate the synthesis of prostaglandins. The antihypertensive effects of converting-enzyme inhibition may therefore be partly due to activation of these vasodepressor systems (Romero). However, kinin potentiation has always been reported under pharmacological conditions but not in physiological situations, and the results of direct kinin measurement in the blood after kininase II (angiotensin-converting enzyme) inhibition are equivocal. The absence of kinin potentiation during kininase II inhibition could be due to the plasmatic activity of other kinin degrading enzymes like carboxypeptidase N (kininase I) and an unspecific aminopeptidase, which might compensate for the reduced kininase II activity under physiological conditions. But even if an enhancement of kinins were to occur during acute kininase II inhibition, this increment in kinin levels should be restored to normal during chronic administration of kininase II inhibitors, since these drugs lead to a reduction in the activity of the renin-angiotensin-aldosterone system and thereby effect a marked diminution of glandular kallikrein activity with reduced kinin formation. Thus, the existing experimental and clinical evidence suggests that the main mechanism responsible for the long term antihypertensive action of angiotensin-converting-enzyme inhibitors is blockade of the renin-angiotensin system (Carretero).

Natriuretic Hormones

Diminished capacity of the kidneys to excrete sodium might be the underlying defect in essential hypertension. As a compensatory mechanism, the secretion of a natriuretic hormone that inhibits renal Na^+/K^+-ATPase (ouabain-like factor, endo-ouabain) might be stimulated. This hormone also inhibits Na^+/K^+-ATPase in vascular smooth muscle, which raises the intracellular concentrations of Na^+; this leads via stimulation of Na^+/Ca^{++} exchange to an increase in intracellular Ca^{2+} levels and vasoconstriction. This hypothesis could explain how a defect in renal sodium excretion finally results in an increased systemic vascular resistance and hypertension (MacGregor).

In addition, there is evidence pointing to the existence of a volume-dependent plasma factor that increases vascular sensitivity to pressor agents. It has been observed that in children of hypertensive parents the pressor response to noradrenaline is increased (Weidmann). However, in these normotensive subjects total exchangeable sodium and blood volume are within normal limits. This indicates that changes in central blood volume may be the signal for the release of such a plasma factor, as well as for the secretion of natriuretic hormone (MacGregor).

The identification of natriuretic peptides in the atria of various mammalian species, including man [3], has added a new aspect to the regulation of blood pressure and renal sodium excretion (Hofbauer). These peptides are found in circulating blood, and their release is stimulated by increased atrial stretch (Ganten) [4]. They have not only natriuretic, but also vasorelaxant properties. The blood pressure lowering effect of the atrial natriuretic factor is less prominent than its natriuretic and diuretic effect, since it is possible to stimulate renal sodium and water excretion with doses that do not reduce blood pressure. Pharmacological doses, which are usually needed to lower blood pressure, produce a marked and excessive natriuresis. The exact mechanism of action of atrial natriuretic peptides is unknown, but they have no influence on the activity of Na^+/K^+-ATPase and are therefore not identical with the postulated ouabain-like natriuretic hormone (MacGregor).

The role of atrial natriuretic peptides in the regulation of blood pressure and sodium balance and their pathophysiological significance are not yet clear. In the atria of spontaneously hypertensive rats the concentration of the peptides is reduced, indicating either inadequate synthesis or an increase in atrial secretion rate. Experimental results indicate that the release of atrial natriuretic peptides is stimulated by acute maneuvres, such as volume loading, but not significantly affected by chronic maneuvres, such as high salt intake or mineralocorticoid treatment (Ganten). It therefore appears that the atrial peptides might be important for the acute adaptation of renal function to volume changes, whereas the putative natriuretic hormone (endo-ouabain) may be essential for chronic adaptation (Ganten). However, it has been observed that the ouabain-like factor in the plasma of normal human subjects changed only after an acute sodium load, but not after chronic changes in sodium intake (Carretero). This might indicate that there are still other endogenous natriuretic factors, such as dopamine [5], to be considered (Carretero).

Sodium and Other Ions in Hypertension

The results of epidemiological studies and intervention trials support the concept that a high sodium intake is an important environmental factor in the pathogenesis of essential hypertension (MacGregor). The presence of increased sodium concentrations in red blood cells of hypertensive patients suggests that similar changes might occur in vascular smooth muscle cells, which might lead to increased vascular tone (Vetter) [6]. Recently, ions other than sodium have been implicated in the pathogenesis of hypertension: several experimental studies suggest that chloride [7] might be more important than sodium in the development of salt-sensitive forms of hypertension (Romero). Conversely, decreased K^+ intake has been incriminated as a causative factor in the pathogenesis of essential hypertension (Weidmann).

Epidemiological studies in the United States (Health and Nutrition Examination Survey I, HANES I) [8] revealed certain relations between systolic blood pressure and dietary patterns in the population. In particular, it was found that low Ca^{2+} intake was associated with a high incidence of hypertension. However, the difference in Ca^{2+} intake between hypertensive and normotensive subjects was only about 10% of the total intake (MacGregor). Furthermore, the nutritional habits were assessed by retrospective interviewing and not verified by measurements, which might have distorted the results (Carretero).

Experimental studies in rats with spontaneous hypertension showed an antihypertensive effect of high (4%) Ca^{2+} diets, which could be reversed by the addition of Mg^{2+} (Ganten). However, the Ca^{2+} intake in these studies was equivalent to 30 times the normal dietary intake in humans, which might lead to phosphate depletion. To assess the influence of Ca^{2+} on blood pressure in the population, studies would have to be performed in which its intake is varied within the physiological range (MacGregor).

Subgroups of Patients with Essential Hypertension

Attempts have been made to classify patients with essential hypertension according to various criteria. However, a specific abnormality may show a continuous spectrum of distribution, and the formation of classes may be arbitrary (Ganten). The different criteria applied in defining subdivisions (plasma renin activity, sodium sensitivity, etc.) may give subgroups that overlap considerably (Korner). Moreover, causal factors involved in the development of essential hypertension may be obscured by secondary changes. Such factors will probably only be detectable once methods become available that are much more sensitive than those currently in use (Korner). Studies in normotensive offspring of hypertensive parents are therefore important, but clinical investigations of this nature are restricted by methodological problems, such as the exact documentation of family histories.

The efficacy of a specific pharmacotherapeutic intervention in hypertensive patients should also not be regarded as evidence that a causative factor has been treated (MacGregor). The same applies to dietary measures. Reducing salt intake is a cheap and easy means of lowering blood pressure in a significant proportion of patients with established essential hypertension (MacGregor); however, it is a general measure that concerns all hypertensive patients, yet helps only a minority (Korner). It would be preferable – although not yet practicable – to identify the causes of hypertension in the individual patient and treat it accordingly (Korner).

Non-Modulating Essential Hypertension

A specific example of a subpopulation of essential hypertension might be the group of "non-modulator" hypertensives (Williams). In these patients, renal blood flow fails to increase after sodium loading and the sensitivity of the adrenal angiotensin II receptors does not increase after sodium restriction. The renal response to salt loading shows a unimodal distribution among patients with hypertension, whereas the adrenal response to salt restriction follows a bimodal distribution pattern (Williams). Non-modulation appears to be an inherited defect, which may or may not lead to hypertension, depending upon environmental factors (Oelkers, Williams). Patients with low-renin essential hypertension show exaggerated adrenal sensitivity to angiotensin II after salt intake, i.e., an adrenal abnormality opposite to that seen in non-modulators.

The failure of renal blood flow to increase after sodium loading could make these patients sensitive to an increased sodium intake. However, the response of glomerular filtration rate to salt loading, which is probably even more important than that of renal blood flow (Frohlich), is not known. Experimental studies have shown that marked increases in single nephron perfusion may cause glomerular injury [9]. The question therefore arises whether it is desirable for antihypertensive drugs to increase renal blood flow (MacGregor): most probably a moderate increase is beneficial, whereas a massive increase may be detrimental (Williams).

The problem of identifying a pathogenetic factor by therapeutic interventions is illustrated by the effects of a low salt diet in non-modulators. Theoretically, these patients should show a greater blood pressure reduction after salt restriction than modulators, since compensation for low salt intake is impaired owing to the lack of increased responsiveness of aldosterone secretion to stimulation by angiotensin II. However, this is not the case. Most probably the renin-angiotensin system is overstimulated in non-modulators because their adrenal sensitivity to angiotensin II fails to increase sufficiently. The resultant angiotensin-II-induced vasoconstriction limits the blood pressure lowering effects of sodium restriction in these patients. Consequently, this subgroup of hypertensives responds well to converting-enzyme inhibitors [10]. The efficacy of other agents, such as Ca^{2+} antagonists, in non-modulators is under investigation.

At present, the non-modulator concept has no practical bearing on antihypertensive therapy since it is impossible to identify such patients by means of simple discriminative tests (Williams). Nevertheless, the common functional abnormalities in these patients do suggest that subgroups of patients with essential hypertension may exist. Their identification would not only increase the understanding of pathogenetic mechanisms in essential hypertension, but possibly also provide a rational basis for the choice of antihypertensive treatment.

References

1. Cruise JL, Houck KA, Michalopoulos GK (1985) Induction of DNA synthesis in cultured rat hepatocytes through stimulation of α_1-adrenoceptor by norepinephrine. Science 227:749–751
2. Regoli D, Barabé J (1980) Pharmacology of bradykinin and related kinins. Pharmacol Rev 32:1–46
3. Needleman P, Adams SP, Cole BR, Currie MG, Geller DM, Michener RL, Saper CB, Schwartz D, Standaert DG (1985) Atriopeptins as cardiac hormones. Hypertension 7:469–482
4. Lang RE, Thölken H, Ganten D, Luft FC, Ruskoaho H, Unger T (1985) Atrial natriuretic factor – a circulating hormone stimulated by volume loading. Nature 314:264–266
5. Imbs JL, Schmidt M, Ehrhardt JD, Schwartz J (1984) The sympathetic nervous system and renal sodium excretion: is dopamine involved? J Cardiovasc Pharmacol 6:S171–S175
6. Zidek W, Losse H, Dorst KG, Zumkley H, Vetter H (1982) Intracellular sodium and calcium in essential hypertension. Klin Wschr 60:859–862
7. Whitescarver SA, Ott CE, Jackson BA, Guthrie GP Jr, Kotchen DA (1984) Salt sensitive hypertension: contribution of chloride. Science 223:1430–1432
8. McCarron DA, Morris CD, Henry HJ, Stanton JL (1984) Blood pressure and nutrient intake in the United States. Science 224:1392–1398
9. Dworkin LD, Hostetter TH, Rennke HG, Brenner BM (1984) Hemodynamic basis for glomerular injury in rats with desoxycorticosterone-salt hypertension. J Clin Invest 73:1448–1461
10. Redgrave J, Rabinowe S, Hollenberg NK, Williams GH (1985) Correction of abnormal renal blood flow response to angiotensin II by converting enzyme inhibition in essential hypertensives. J Clin Invest 75:1285-1290

Principal Objectives of Antihypertensive Treatment

Treatment of Vascular Damage in Experimental Malignant Hypertension with Nifedipine and Its Calcium-Antagonistic Dihydropyridine Derivatives

S. Kazda[1], B. Garthoff[1], and G. Luckhaus[2]

Introduction

Calcium antagonists – a new group of antihypertensive drugs – are known to prevent damage of heart muscle due to ischemia, hypoxia, increased sympathetic drive, and other stimuli by preventing the deleterious calcium overload of the cell (for review, see [1, 2]).

In the following it will be shown that some calcium antagonistic dihydropyridine derivatives can also prevent vascular damage associated with malignant hypertension in rats by reducing calcium overload. The tissue protective effect of these drugs is not entirely dependent up on their influence on high blood pressure.

Vascular Damage in Salt-Sensitive Dahl Rats

Dahl rats are a suitable model for studies of malignant hypertension and vascular damage. By systematic breeding, Dahl developed two substrains of Sprague-Dawley rats with different susceptibility to hypertensogenic stimuli including high salt diet [3–5]. Whereas, the sensitive (S) substrain rapidly develops a sustained hypertension when fed a high salt diet, the resistant (R) rats tolerate it without increasing blood pressure. The genetic defect which causes hypertension in S-rats seems to reside in the kidney. In R-rats the sodium excretion increases in parallel with the increased renal perfusion pressure, while a shifted pressure natriuresis curve reduces sodium excretion for a given renal perfusion pressure in S-rats [6].

An increase in blood pressure in S-rats seems to be a compensatory reaction for inducing pressure-natriuresis and corrects the sluggish sodium excretion [7]. However, the fulminantly developed hypertension in S-rats results in a necrotizing vasculopathy with a preferential localization in the kidney [8].

Our extensive investigations of Dahl rats revealed fibrinoid intimal necrosis, medial hyperplasia, and periarteritis in the intrarenal arteries of the hypertensive S-rats on high salt diet. In some nephrons the subendothelial depositions which caused the lumen to be narrower (Fig. 1) in the preglomerular arterioles resulted in a collapse and hyaline degeneration of the glomeruli [9].

[1] Institute of Pharmacology, Bayer AG, Aprather Weg, D-5600 Wuppertal 1.
[2] Institute of Toxicology, Bayer AG, Aprather Weg, D-5600 Wuppertal 1.

Primary Hypertension
Ed. by W. Kaufmann et al.

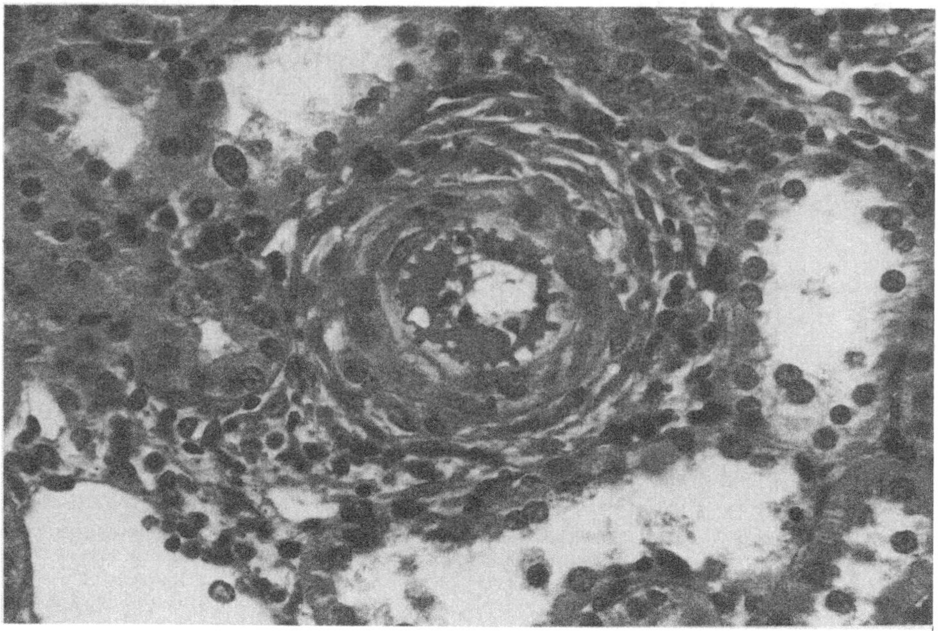

Fig. 1. Interlobular artery of a Dahl sensitive (S) rat with malignant hypertension: marked subendothelial fibrin deposition, endothelial disruption, medial hypertrophy and adventitial inflammatory reaction

The intramural arteries of the right heart of the hypertensive S-rats typically displayed intimal fibrinoid necrosis and periarteritis. Some of these arteries showed occlusive changes which led to necrosis and fibrous replacement of the adjacent myocard [9].

Pronounced hypertensive periarteritis nodosalike changes were seen in the mesenteric arteries of the S-rats. Histologically, these lesions consisted of panarteritis with a medial hyperplasia and intimal fibrinoid necrosis [10].

In salt-loaded R-rats no pathological findings were seen.

Effects of Nifedipine, Nitrendipine, and Nisoldipine

Prevention of Hypertension and Vascular Damage

Treatment of sensitive Dahl rats with nifedipine in addition to high salt diet prevented blood pressure increase, reduced cardiac hypertrophy and mortality (Fig. 2), and improved the impaired renal function [11]. Moreover, the morphological vascular changes in S-rats were completely prevented by the nifedipine treatment. Similar preventive effects were obtained with nisoldipine [12] and nitrendipine [13], but not with captopril [14].

In normotensive Dahl R-rats nifedipine [15], nisoldipine [12], or nitrendipine [13] had no effect on blood pressure.

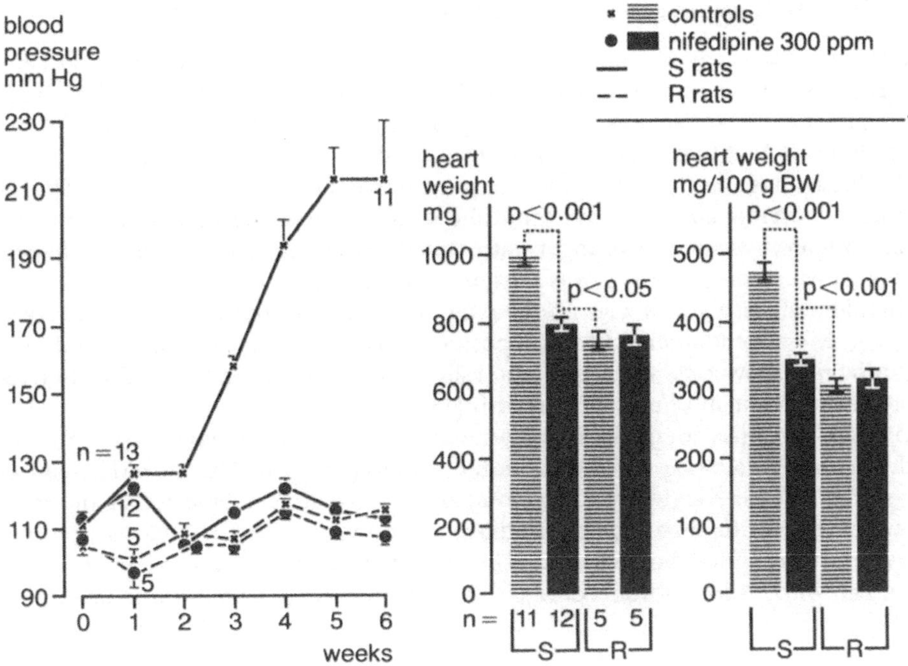

Fig. 2. Prevention of fulminant hypertension, mortality, and cardiac hypertrophy in salt-loaded Dahl S-rats by nifedipine

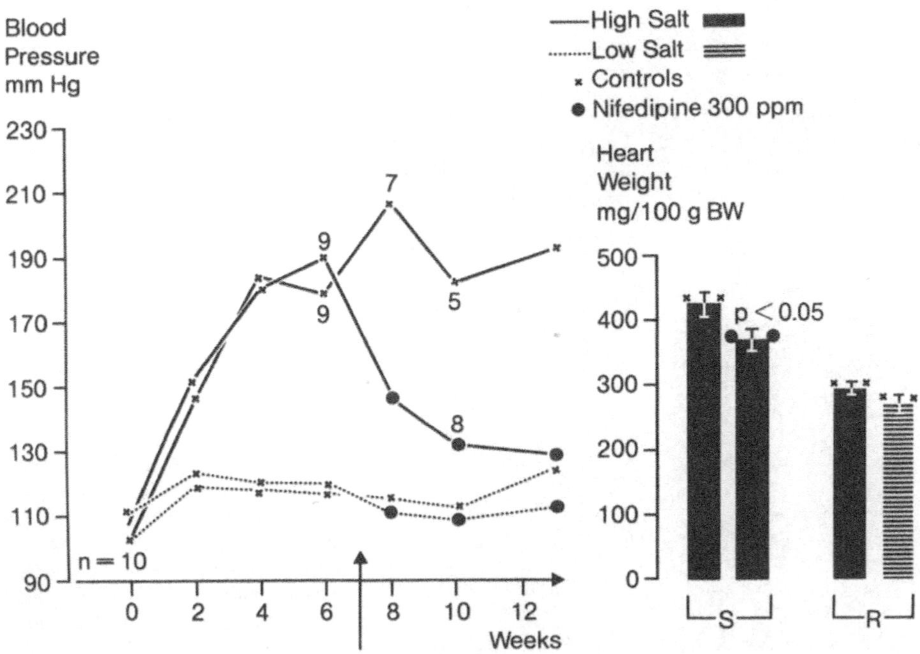

Fig. 3. Therapy of malignant hypertension in salt-loaded Dahl S-rats. Nifedipine normalizes blood pressure and reduces cardiac hypertrophy. In S-rats on low salt diet nifedipine had no effects

Therapy of Malignant Hypertension and Regression of Vascular Lesions

Treatment of salt-loaded Dahl rats with nifedipine, started in the stage of already malignant hypertension, resulted in a rapid normalization of the high blood pressure and regression of cardiac hypertrophy [16] (Fig. 3). Therapy with nisoldipine [12] or nitrendipine [13] at that stage of hypertension had similar beneficial effects.

In the therapeutically treated rats the progressive mortality was reduced. The incidence of vasculopathy was lower and the degree of vascular injury was less pronounced than it was in the younger untreated controls, i.e., at that stage of hypertension at which the treatment was started in this therapeutic trial.

In addition, histological signs of healing of vascular lesions have been observed (Fig. 4). The subendothelial fibrin deposition was no longer present, the internal elastic lamina showed reduplications, and slight adventitial, round cell infiltration reflected some remnant of previous arteritis [17].

The curative effect of nifedipine treatment on the malignant hypertensive arteriopathy in Dahl S-rats was verified in another experiment [18]. The individual course of arterial disease was followed by comparing pretreatment biopsies of the mesenteric arteries with posttreatment findings and necropsy. Within 7 weeks, continuous therapy with nifedipine resulted in healing of early vascular lesions and in a partial repair of the more advanced ones [18] (Figs. 5 and 6). Under normalization of

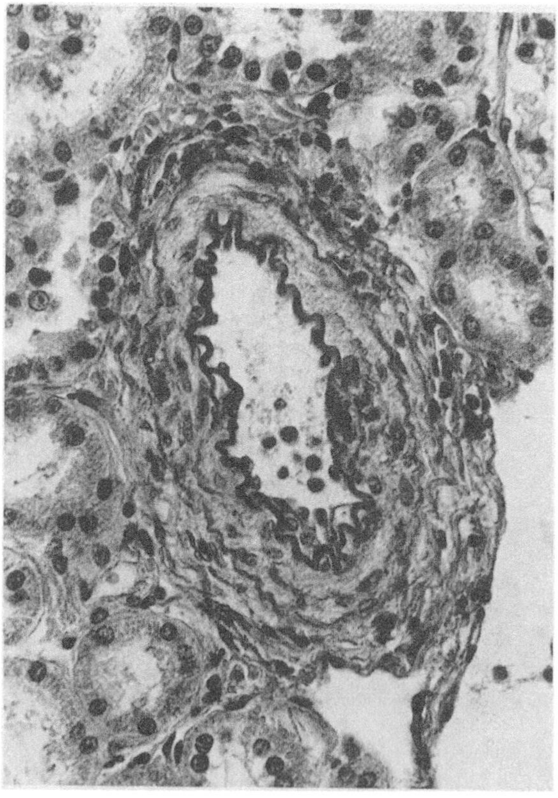

Fig. 4. Healing effect of nifedipine treatment on renovascular lesions in a salt-loaded Dahl S-rat with already established hypertension. Partial reduplication of the internal elastic lamina, focal small alterations of the intima, remnants of previous periarteritis [17]. (With kind permission of The Fellowship of Postgraduate Medicine)

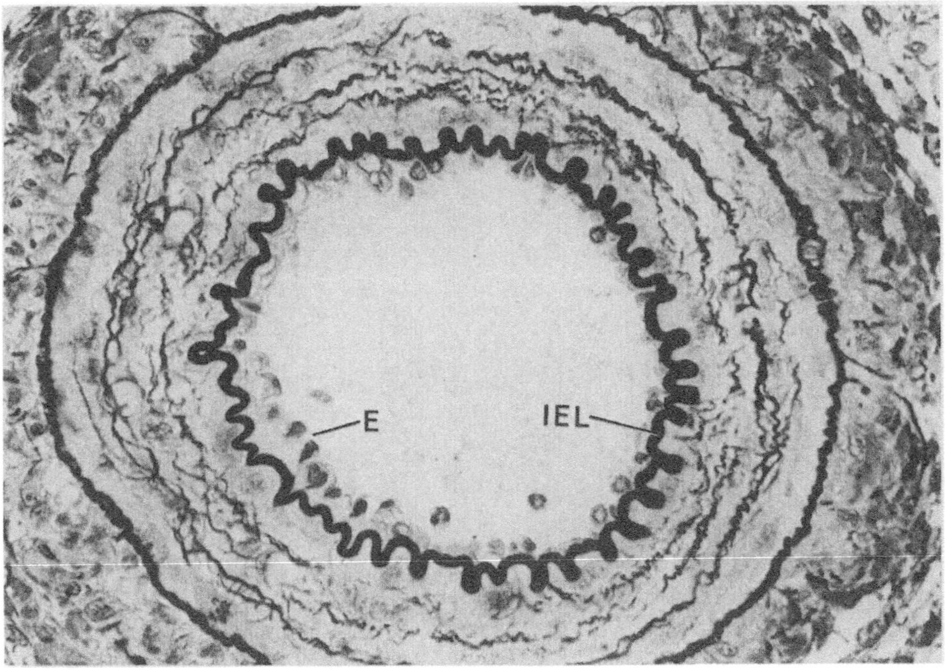

Fig. 5. Biopsy of a mesenteric artery from a Dahl S-rat at the stage of malignant hypertension (BP, 255 mm Hg). The endothelial cell layer *(E)* is partially damaged and uplifted by the underlying fibrin accumulation from the irregularly folded and somewhat distended internal elastic lamina *(IEL)*. EvG; × 290 [18]. (With kind permission of Editio Cantor)

blood pressure, vascular fibrinoid exacerbations were prevented and existing intramural fibrin insudates were completely or partially removed. Lamellar fibroelastosis of the intima occurred as a characteristic of repair.

Such therapeutic effects in malignant hypertensive Dahl S-rats could not be achieved by a chronic pharmacological vasodilation. Treatment of hypertensive Dahl rats with the strong vasodilator minoxidil resulted only in a transitory blood pressure decrease, without any sustained therapeutic effect [17].

Therefore, it could not be decided whether the salutary effect of nifedipine and its antihypertensive derivatives was entirely due to their intrinsic calcium antagonistic effect on the vascular tissue or whether it is secondary to the effective blood pressure control provided by these drugs. For clarifying this question, additional experiments with another model of malignant hypertension using two calcium antagonists with different effects on blood pressure were performed.

Vascular Damage in Stroke-Prone Spontaneously Hypertensive Rats

Stroke-prone rats (SHR SP) originally derived from the Okamoto strain of spontaneously hypertensive rats develop cerebral infarction at advanced age [19]. Addition of

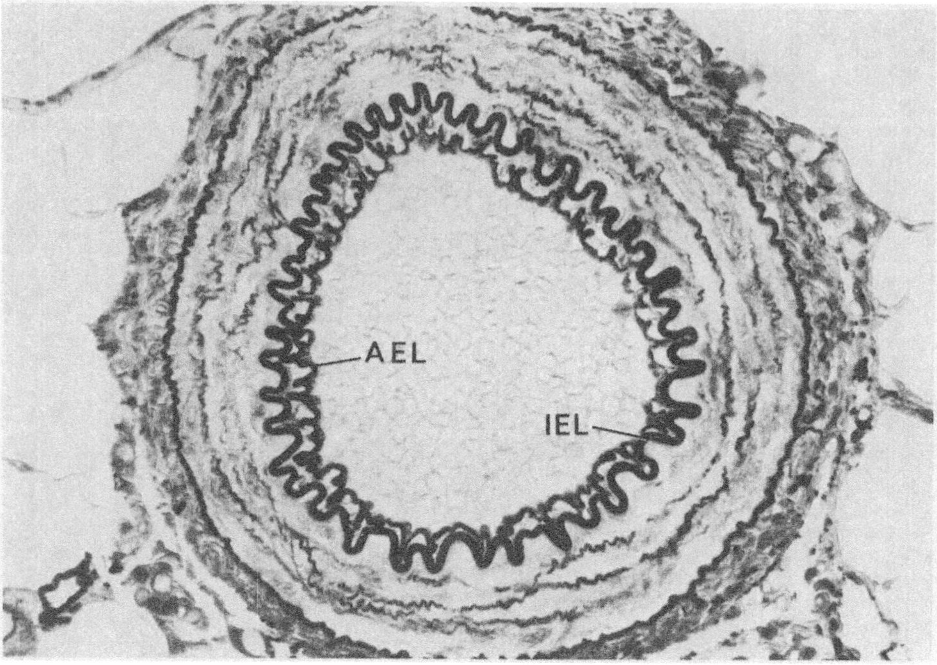

Fig. 6. Mesenteric artery of the same hypertensive Dahl rat as investigated in Fig. 5 after 6-week course of therapy with nifedipine (BP, 160 mm Hg). Intimal fibrin resorption has taken place, supporting reorganization of the endothelium. An additional elastic lamina *(AEL)* in the intima has formed on the luminal side of the original internal elastic lamina *(IEL)*. EvG; × 290 [18]. (With kind permission of Editio Cantor)

1% NaCl to drinking water has been shown to exaggerate hypertension as well as cerebral and renal vascular lesions in young SHR SP [19].

In our experiments, the dietary salt loading of the *adult* SHR SP with already established hypertension drastically accelerated their mortality and produced severe cerebrovascular lesions without causing any marked additional blood pressure increase. After 9 weeks on a diet containing 8% NaCl, 11 of 16 control animals had died and all dead and killed rats had severe renal damage similar to that described in Dahl rats. In addition, most of them had cerebral lesions as arterioral fibrinoid necrosis, cortical aneurysms, hemorrhage, etc.

Effects of Nitrendipine and Nimodipine: Different Influences on High Blood Pressure

In male SHR SP (about 5 months old) treatment with nitrendipine in addition to the high salt diet decreased the high blood pressure only slightly, but completely prevented mortality (Fig. 7) and reduced the incidence and severity of brain and renal lesions [16].

After 9 weeks of observation of the five surviving controls and all the nitrendipine-treated animals, blood samples were taken and the animals were killed. Plasma renin

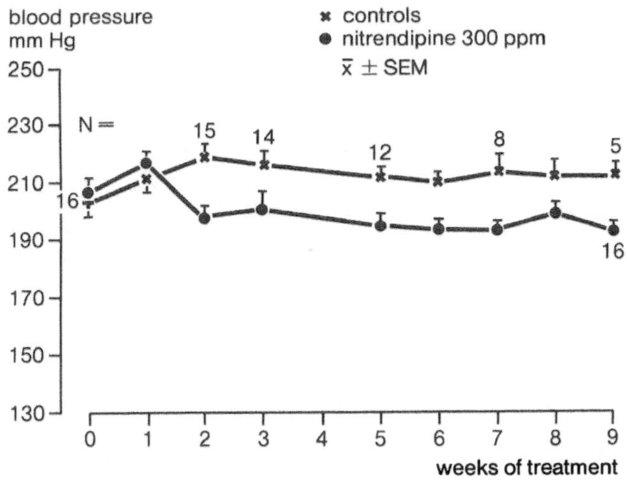

Fig. 7. Systolic blood pressure and mortality (numbers of surviving animals over the curves) in male stroke-prone SHR on high salt (8% NaCl) diet with and without nitrendipine treatment

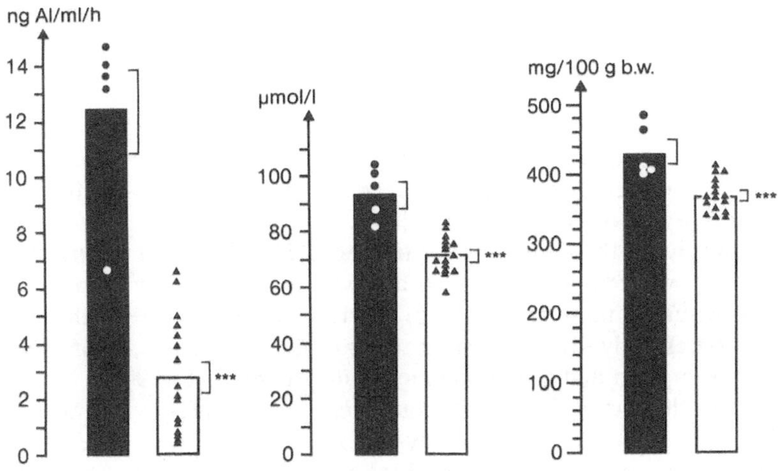

Fig. 8. Plasma renin activity, plasma creatinine concentration, and relative heart weight of SHR SP after 9 weeks on high salt (8% NaCl) diet with and without nitrendipine treatment ($\bar{x} \pm$ SEM; $n = 5$ or 16); *** $P<0.001$; ■ control, □ nitrendipine

activity in the five surviving controls was very high despite permanent salt load. The average serum creatinine concentration was higher in the controls, although those animals that had already died were probably the most damaged but could not be assessed in these investigations. The nitrendipine-treated animals, being under the same salt load, had normal creatinine levels. Moreover, plasma renin activity was extremely low in the nitrendipine-treated animals (Fig. 8). Obviously, high renin levels in the untreated controls were due to the severe renal ischemia, stimulating renin release. Nitrendipine treatment primarily prevented ischemic renal damage and the renin release remained supressed by the high sodium intake.

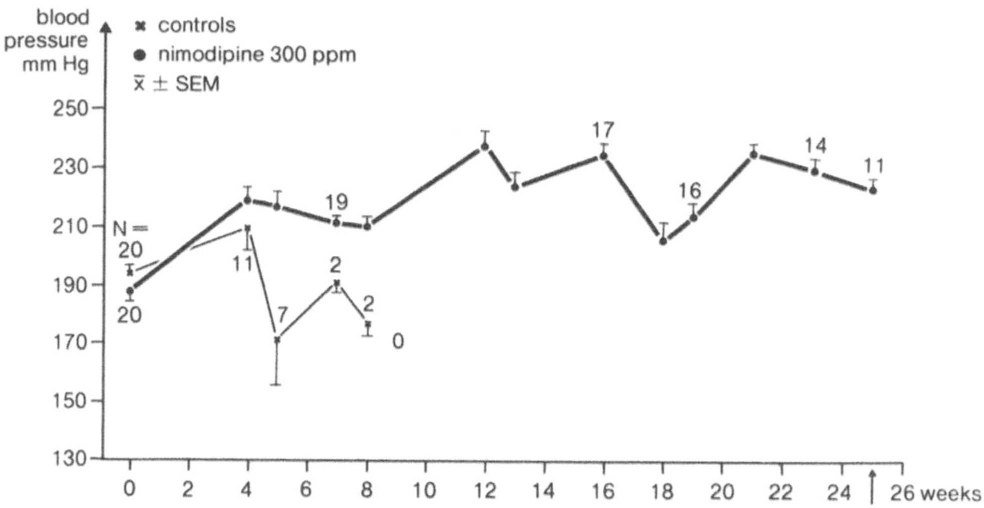

Fig. 9. Development of systolic blood pressure and mortality in SHR SP on high salt diet (8% NaCl): controls and nimodipine-treated rats (numbers over the curves indicate the number of surviving animals)

Similar life-saving and tissue-protective effects have been achieved in stroke-prone SHR using another dihydropyridine derivative nimodipine. Nimodipine is a calcium antagonist with preferential effect on cerebral vessels and has little effect on peripheral blood vessels and on blood pressure [20].

In this experiment, more than a half of the treated SHR SP animals survived 25 weeks on high salt diet, whereas all control rats died within 8 weeks. Nimodipine did not reduce blood pressure in these rats at all. In contrast, blood pressure of the seriously ill controls progressively dropped ante finem so that, on average, their blood pressure was even lower than that of nimodipine-treated animals (Fig. 9).

Based on results of these experiments, it seems clear that the life-saving effect of the dihydropyridine derivatives in malignant hypertensive stroke-prone SHR rats is not primarily due to their effect on the high blood pressure. It has been shown by Fleckenstein et al. [21] that in hypertensive rats – at least in SHR – the calcium content of the arterial wall is very much increased. The excess calcium is mainly concentrated in the arterial media, preferentially in vascular smooth muscle as shown by electron microscope investigation [21]. The calcium overload seems to play a decisive role in the molecular pathway of cell damage and death [21].

For further exploration, another kind of experiment was performed.

Effect of Surgical Parathyroidectomy

Parathyroid hormone is known to regulate calcium influx and transport into the cell not only in bones, but also in contractile tissues [22]. Moreover, it has been claimed that parathyroidectomy (PTX) ameliorates vascular lesions induced by deoxycorticosterone in rats [23].

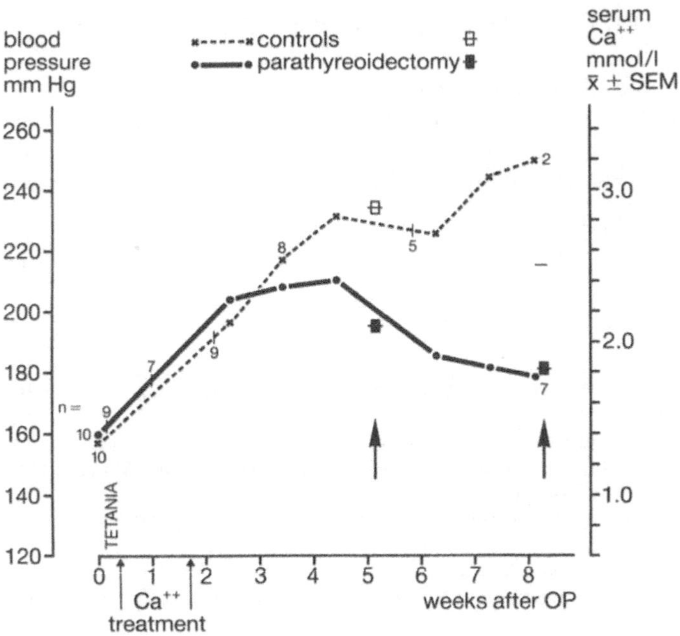

Fig. 10. Effect of bilateral parathyroidectomy on blood pressure, survival rate (numbers over the curves), and total serum calcium concentration in young, male stroke-prone SHR on 8% NaCl diet. All animals subjected to surgery developed tetany and three out of ten died within the first week after parathyroidectomy

It was therefore decided to investigate the effect of salt load in SHR SP with and without PTX. In the preliminary experiments we performed surgical PTX in young male SHR SP and investigated the effect of high salt diet in them and in the intact controls.

All PTX animals developed tetania immediately after the surgery, and three out of ten of them died. In both groups, which were in the developmental stage of hypertension, sodium load accelerated the increase in blood pressure.

At a later stage in the control animals blood pressure continued to increase, and they died successively. The blood pressure of the PTX animals remained in the range of 200–180 mm Hg and all of them survived the 8 weeks of observation (Fig. 10). Signs of a malignant hypertension were completely absent in the PTX rats. Histological examination revealed severe renal and cerebral damage in all control rats, whereas all the PTX animals were completely intact.

In this sense, PTX mimics the effects of calcium antagonistic dihydropyridines in malignant hypertension. Therefore, a similar mechanism of both interventions may be postulated.

Conclusions

Two fundamental conclusions can be drawn from the presented experiments.

1. High intravascular pressure alone is not the detrimental factor in malignant hypertension. High blood pressure is doubtless the prerequisite for hypertensive

tissue injury, but obviously some additional factors are decisive for malignancy of hypertension.

2. The tissue-protective and life-saving effect of the calcium antagonistic dihydropyridines in malignant hypertension is not primarily due to their vasodilating and blood pressure lowering effects. Presumably, these drugs prevent early tissue ischemia and damage by specific inhibition of the deleterious calcium overload in renal and cerebral vessels.

References

1. Fleckenstein A, Fleckenstein-Grün G (1980) Cardiovascular protection by Ca^{2+}-antagonists. Eur Heart J [Suppl B] 1:15–21
2. Nayler WG, Ferrari F, Slade A (1980) Cardioprotective actions of calcium-antagonists in myocardial anoxia and ischaemia. In: Fleckenstein A, Roskamm H (eds) Calcium-Antagonismus. Springer, Berlin Heidelberg New York, pp 119–137
3. Dahl LK (1961) Effect of chronic salt feeding. Induction of selfsustaining hypertension in rats. J Exp Med 114:231–235
4. Dahl LK, Heine M, Tassinari L (1962) Effect of chronic salt ingestion. Evidence that genetic factors play an important role in susceptibility to experimental hypertension. J Exp Med 115: 1173–1190
5. Dahl LK, Heine M, Thompson K (1972) Genetic influence of renal homografts on blood pressure of rats from different strains. Proc Soc Exp Biol Med 140:852–854
6. Tobian L, Lange J, Azar S, Iwai J, Koop D, Coffee K, Johnson MA (1978) Reduction of natriuretic capacity and renin-release in isolated, blood perfused kidneys of Dahl hypertension-prone rats. Circ Res [Suppl 1] 43:I–92–I–98
7. Tobian L, Lange J, Iwai J, Hiller K, Johnson MA, Goossens P (1979) Prevention with thiazide of NaCl-induced hypertension in Dahl "S" rats. Evidence for a Na-retaining agent in "S" rats. Hypertension 1:316–323
8. Jaffé S, Sutherland LE, Barker DM, Dahl LK (1970) Effect of chronic salt ingestion. Morphologic findings in kidneys of rats with differing genetic susceptibilities to hypertension. Arch Pathol 90:1–16
9. Luckhaus G, Garthoff B, Kazda S (1982) Prevention of hypertensive vasculopathy by nifedipine in salt-loaded Dahl rats. Arzneimittelforsch 32:1421–1425
10. Kazda S, Garthoff B, Luckhaus G, Nash G (1982) Influence of nifedipine on hypertensive morphological changes in rats. In: Kaltenbach M, Neufeld HN (eds) 5th International Adalat Symposium. New therapy of ischaemic heart disease and hypertension. Excerpta Medica, Amsterdam, pp 133–143
11. Kazda S, Garthoff B, Dycka J, Iwai I (1982) Prevention of malignant hypertension in salt-loaded "S" Dahl rats with the calcium antagonist nifedipine. Clin Exp Hypertens [A] 4(7):1231–1241
12. Garthoff B, Kazda S (1982) Prevention and reversal of salt-induced hypertension in DS-Dahl rats by nisoldipine. Fed Proc 41:1664
13. Kazda S, Garthoff B, Knorr A (1983) Nitrendipine and other calcium entry blockers (calcium antagonists) in hypertension. Fed Proc 42:196–200
14. Rapp JR (1982) Dahl salt susceptible and salt resistant rats: a review. Hypertension 4:753–763
15. Kazda S, Garthoff B (1982) Management of salt-induced hypertension in Dahl-rats by use of the calcium antagonist nifedipine. In: Iwai J (ed) Salt and hypertension. Igaku-Shoin, Tokyo, pp 51–53
16. Kazda S, Garthoff B, Luckhaus G, Nash G (1983) The calcium antagonist nifedipine and its analogues preserve tissue integrity and increase life span in experimental malignant hypertension. In: Hashimoto K, Kawai C (eds) Asian Pacific Adalat Symposium. New Therapy of Ischemic Heart Disease and Hypertension. Medical Tribune, Tokyo, pp 50–62
17. Kazda S, Garthoff B, Luckhaus G (1983) Calcium antagonists in hypertensive disease: experimental evidence for a new therapeutic concept. Postgrad Med J [Suppl 2] 59:78–83

18. Luckhaus G, Nash G, Garthoff B, Kazda S, Feller W (1985) Healing of malignant hypertensive arteriopathy in Dahl rats by nifedipine. Arzneimittelforsch 35: 115–121
19. Okamoto K, Yamori Y, Nagaoka A (1974) Establishment of the stroke-prone spontaneously hypertensive rat (SHR) Circ Res [Suppl 1] 34/35: 143–153
20. Kazda S, Hoffmeister F, Garthoff B, Towart R (1979) Prevention of the postischaemic impaired reperfusion on the brain by nimodipine (BAY E 9736). Acuta Neurol Scand [Suppl 72] 60: 302–303
21. Fleckenstein A, Frey M, von Witzleben H (1983) Vascular calcium overload – a pathogenic factor in arteriosclerosis and its neutralization by calcium antagonists. In: Kaltenbach M, Neufeld HN (eds) 5th International Adalat Symposium. New therapy of ischaemic heart disease and hypertension. Excerpta Medica, Amsterdam, pp 36–54
22. Borle AB (1973) Calcium metabolism at the cellular level. Fed Proc 32: 1944–1950
23. Nickerson PA, Conran RM (1981) Parathyroidectomy ameliorates vascular lesions induced by deoxycorticosterone in the rat. Am J Pathol 105: 185–190

Trends in Arteriosclerosis in Treated and Untreated Hypertensive Patients

S. Heyden[1], J. G. Fodor[2], and K. A. Schneider[1]

Introduction

The development of arteriosclerosis among hypertensive patients largely occurs in two major vascular beds, the cerebral and coronary arteries. Several pathways for the development of arteriosclerotic complications in the cerebral arteries have been discussed [5]. Hypertension will lead to an increase of the predisposition of major intracranial arteries to arteriosclerosis; hypertension may also be involved with smaller intracerebral vessels. Miliary aneurysms of the small penetrating cerebral arteries have been described as being a direct consequence of hypertension. In addition, small arteries (in the basal ganglia, thalamus, and pons) may show macrophages and fibrin in the intima.

The remarkable decline in cerebrovascular mortality in western industrialized societies began in the 1950s (Fig. 1). Most interpreters see this phenomenon as a combination of environmental changes and the emergence of effective antihypertensive therapy. The massive reduction of age-standardized stroke mortality in the USA by 60% between 1968 and 1977, and in Australia by 46% for persons 40–69 years old was accompanied by a decline in deaths due to coronary heart disease in both countries. This decline in coronary death rates amounted to 35% in the USA between 1962 and 1981 and 25% in Australia for the same period. Thus, the downward trend in coronary mortality was not as strong as that observed for cerebrovascular mortality: The decrease in coronary mortality is roughly one-half of the decrease in cerebrovascular mortality. We now have evidence that these population trends are paralleled by treated and well-controlled hypertensive patients in some [3, 8–13, 17, 26] of the recently completed randomized hypertension intervention trials.

Japan, in contrast to other industrialized nations, is still known to harbor an unusually high prevalence of hypertension in combination with well-known population-wide low cholesterol concentrations. In the absence of hypercholesterolemia, the Japanese mortality statistics are still recording a low coronary mortality (Fig. 2) in the 1980s in spite of the high prevalence of hypertension [6]; however, the stroke mortality exceeds that of western industrialized countries. Likewise, blacks in South Africa and in the USA still have a higher incidence of cerebrovascular disease and lower coronary mortality than whites, with a significantly higher prevalence of hypertension, but more favorable lipid concentrations than found among whites.

[1] Duke University Medical Centre, Durham, NC 27710, USA.
[2] Memorial University of Newfoundland, St. John's, Nfld., Canada, A1B 3V6.

Primary Hypertension
Ed. by W. Kaufmann et al.

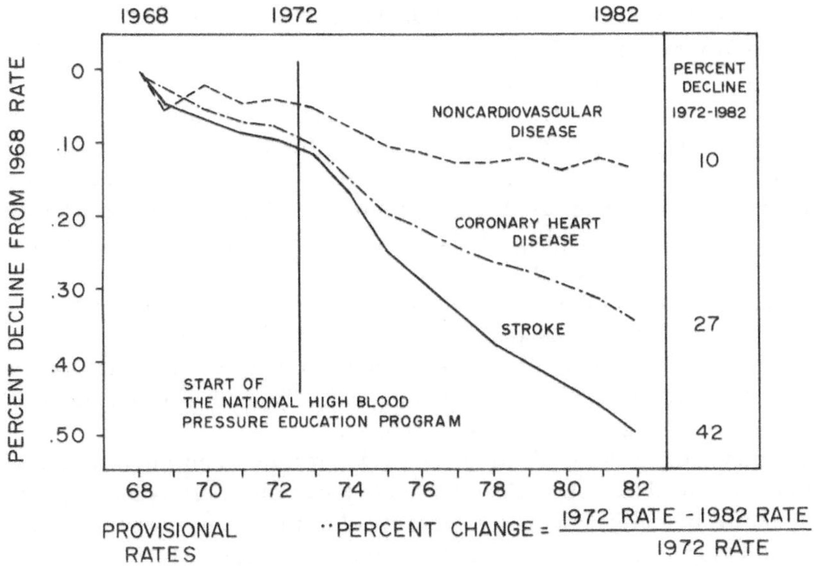

Fig. 1. Differences in the decline between coronary and cerebrovascular mortality in the USA (National Center for Health Statistics and the National Heart, Lung and Blood Institute)

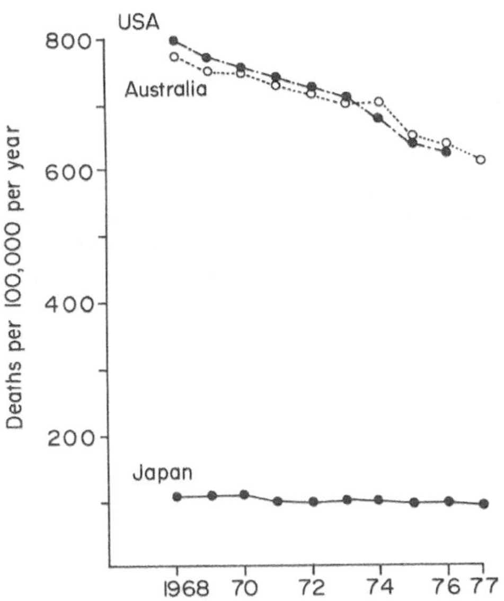

Fig. 2. Differences in the coronary mortality between Japan, Australia, and the United States of America [abbreviated from G. Rose, Br Med J 282:1847 (1981), Fig. 1]

Thus, the population differences in coronary death rates depend in large part on the sine qua non of atherogenesis, hyperlipidemia. In conjunction with hypertension, the clinical manifestations of coronary arteriosclerosis are apparently increasing, while cerebrovascular complications appear to have been declining in the Western hemisphere over the past two decades.

Manifestations of Arteriosclerosis Among Hypertensive Patients in Randomized Intervention Trials

The hardest end point of any study, total mortality, has been reported by all long-term experimental trials involving patients under drug therapy and patients in control groups. An overview of the mortality in four recent hypertension intervention trials is presented in Table 1. The very low total number of deaths in three studies [7, 17, 21] contrasts with the much higher number of deaths in the Hypertension Detection and Follow-up Program (HDFP). To make hypertensive patients from the HDFP trial [4] more comparable to the all-white patients of the other three trials, it would be necessary to exclude black patients from HDFP. Even after removing the black hypertensive men and women from the stepped care group, the death rate at the end of the trial is seven times greater among white hypertensive patients than among the patients of the other three trials (Table 2).

This discrepancy among the trials in all-cause death rates is an important basis from which to review the different results reported in these four trials. A major reason for the discrepancy is that HDFP had no exclusion policy for prospective participants except life-threatening diseases, whereas the other intervention studies had very strict exclusion criteria admitting only otherwise healthy hypertensives into the trials. The HDFP [9] was conducted from 1973 to 1979 and involved 14 communities across the USA. All hypertensives in these communities were eligible, including those with:

Antihypertensive treatment (26%); history of myocardial infarction (5%); history of stroke (2.5%) and/or TIA; left ventricular hypertrophy on ECG (5%); diabetes (7%); heart disease (cardiovascular, congestive, valvular) and/or intermittent claudication; cardiomegaly; retinopathy; renal and hepatic disease; gout; asthma; rheumatoid arthritis; endocrine disorders; obvious alcohol abuse.

Table 1. Death from all causes in four hypertension intervention trials

Randomized intervention trials	Active therapy, stepped care n (%)	Placebo or referred care n (%)
Oslo [7], Australia [17], U.S. Public Health Service [21]	2320	2281
Total deaths	21 (0.9)	32 (1.4)
HDFP (USA) [9]	5485	5455
Total deaths	349 (6.4)	419 (7.7)

Table 2. Comparison of HDFP and three other trials

White hypertensives	HDFP stepped care [9]	Three trials on active therapy [7, 17, 21]
Duration of treatment	5 years	3.8–7 years
Randomized patients (*n*)	2772	2320
Mortality at end of trial (*n*)	168	21
Mortality at end of trial (%)	6.1	0.9

Hypertension Detection and Follow-up Program

The HDFP followed almost 11000 patients between 30 and 69 years of age for 5 years [9]. The HDFP control group after randomization was not placebo treated, but patients were referred back to their usual sources of care. In every category of arteriosclerotic complications, a marked and often significant reduction occurred in stepped care (SC) in comparison with referred care (RC) (Table 3). Among SC patients, fatal complications in the cerebral arteries were reduced more effectively than were coronary complications.

In the HDFP [10], SC participants experienced a reduction in mortality and morbidity from stroke in all patients of every race-sex and age group. The reduction also favored white women in SC with a 30% lower incidence than among white women in RC, and younger patients (ages 30–49 years at entry) with a 27% reduction. A 45% reduction in the incidence of stroke morbidity and mortality was found among SC participants who entered the study at ages 60–69 years. This latter finding presents the answer to the much debated question of whether stroke can be prevented by an aggressive treatment program in an elderly population (which was 65–74 years of age by the time the study ended).

Table 4 shows the normalization of diastolic blood pressure (DBP) levels in white SC patients. They became comparable in their DBP levels to those of the general US population in a similar age range. The annual cerebrovascular disease mortality in HDFP SC was then compared with the white male population of the USA during the same time period between 1974 and 1978 (Table 5). A remarkable similarity was demonstrated. For white women, the numbers of strokes in the SC group were too small to lend themselves to comparison with the general female population.

When the patients with mild hypertension, i.e., baseline DBP level 90–104 mmHg, were analyzed, it became evident that cerebrovascular mortality was as much reduced among SC patients as was death from myocardial infarction – in both instances almost 50% compared with RC (Table 6).

The total cerebrovascular fatal and nonfatal events in SC and RC are contrasted with total fatal coronary heart disease and nonfatal myocardial infarcts in Table 7. A major shift of the hypertensive arteriosclerotic complications from the cerebral vasculature to the coronary vascular bed is discernable [11]. In the HDFP white popula-

Table 3. Deaths from all cardiovascular and noncardiovascular diseases for all HDFP patients at 5 years [9]

Cause of death	Stepped care ($n = 5485$)		Referred care ($n = 5455$)	
	(n)	(%)	(n)	(%)
All cardiovascular diseases	195	(3.6)	240	(4.4)
Cerebrovascular disease	29	(0.5)	52	(1.0)
Myocardial infarction and other CHD	131	(2.4)	148	(2.7)
Other cardiovascular diseases	35	(0.7)	40	(0.7)
All non-cardiovascular diseases	154	(2.8)	179	(3.3)
Total (all causes of death)	349	(6.4)	419	(7.7)

Table 4. Achieved diastolic blood pressure (DBP) for hypertensives under treatment and DBP found in the general US white population

	DBP range (mm Hg)	
	HDFP, stepped care [10] 5 years (30–69 years)	HANES survey [25] 1973–1974 (40–74 years)
White men	86.3–84.0	86.2
White women	85.3–82.2	83.8

Table 5. Annual cerebrovascular disease mortality in US population (1974–1978) and HDFP (1974–1979), stepped care (SC), white men per 1000 [10]

Age group (years)	55–64	65–74	35–74
US population	0.87	3.17	0.84
HDFP (SC)	0.89	3.08	0.95

Table 6. Cardiovascular mortality among patients with "mild" hypertension at entry (HDFP at 5 years; DBP, 90–104 mm Hg) [9]

Fatal events	Stepped care (3903)	Referred care (3922)
Cerebrovascular disease	17	31
Myocardial infarction	30	56
Other ischemic heart disease	56	51
Hypertensive heart disease	5	5
Other cardiovascular disease	12	19
Other hypertensive disease	2	3
All cardiovascular diseases	122 (3.1%)	165 (4.2%)

tion aged 30–69 years at entry, fatal and nonfatal coronary events are four to five times more frequent than cerebrovascular events.

Table 8 demonstrates particularly rewarding results of SC therapy for hypertensive patients in comparison with RC [11]. Patients free of target organ damage at baseline (no history or ECG evidence of myocardial infarction, no stroke or peripheral vascular disease, normal ECG and creatinine level) had a 5-year incidence of fatal and nonfatal coronary heart disease which was one-fourth lower in SC than in RC. In contrast, hypertensive patients who demonstrated signs and symptoms of target organ damage in either the heart, brain, or kidney at entry into the trial, showed no difference in coronary heart disease incidence between SC and RC after 5 years. The only exception was the group of hypertensives with myocardial infarction at the beginning of the trial, randomized into SC and RC. By protocol, the SC patients were treated much more vigorously than RC. A reduction of 23% in SC in total mortality was achieved in comparison with RC. Not totally unexpected, the

Table 7. Total fatal and nonfatal strokes [10]; total fatal coronary heart disease and nonfatal myocardial infarcts in 5 years [11] among white hypertensives free of cerebrovascular disease and coronary heart disease at baseline

	Stepped care		Referred care	
	Sample	Events	Sample	Events
Strokes	3077	46	3017	73
Coronary disease	2772	240	2729	285

Table 8. Results achieved in HDFP: 5-year observations on coronary heart disease (for both blacks and whites) [11]

Coronary events	Stepped care (sample/events)	Referred care (sample/events)	Reduction in favor of SC
Fatal coronary heart disease and nonfatal myocardial infarction, no end-organ damage or antihypertensive therapy at baseline	3439 / 237	3501 / 320	25%
A. pectoris among patients free of A. pectoris at baseline	5071 / 325	5062 / 449	28%
Death from all causes in patients with myocardial infarction at baseline	512 / 63	506 / 81	23%

Table 9. The age factor in the prevention of coronary heart disease in both blacks and whites (HDFP at 5 years) [11]

Fatal coronary heart disease and nonfatal myocardial infarction by age (years)	Stepped care (sample/events)	Referred care (sample/events)	Reduction in favor of stepped care
30–49	2263/154	2203/203	26%
50–69	1665/161	1712/185	10%
60–69	1045/116	1034/125	7%

younger SC hypertensives had a much greater reduction of fatal coronary heart disease and nonfatal myocardial infarction than older hypertensive patients (approximately four times better than the older age group 60–69 years old; Table 9). Interestingly, cholesterol levels in the HDFP population decreased from an initial value of 235 to 220 mg/dl, and thus paralleled the decline of cholesterol levels among the American population during the same 5 years.

The US Public Health Service Hospitals Study

Male and female hypertensives, 21–55 years old (averaging 44 years) were followed for a little over 7 years in an SC and placebo-treated group [21]. The results definitely favor the treatment group (Table 10). Coronary events were not significantly re-

Table 10. Nonfatal complications: noncoronary events (US Public Health Service at 7 years) [21]

Events	Active therapy ($n = 193$)	Placebo ($n = 196$)
Stroke	1	6
Congestive heart failure	0	2
Left ventricular hypertrophy (ECG)	13	25
Left ventricular strain	14	37
Cardiomegaly (X-ray)	16	23
Retinopathy	1	9
Renal insufficiency	1	2
All noncoronary events	46 (24%)	104 (53%)
Total events	87 (45%)	159 (84%)

Table 11. Fatal and nonfatal complications: coronary events (US Public Health Service at 7 years) [21]

Events	Active therapy ($n = 193$)	Placebo ($n = 196$)
Nonfatal myocardial infarction	13	14
Sudden death and fatal myocardial infarction	2	4
Other coronary heart disease	26	37
All coronary events	41 (21%)	55 (28%)

duced under active therapy, but the total number of events was significantly decreased by the SC regimen (Table 11). Three caveats are indicated regarding the nonsignificant reduction of coronary events in the active treatment group:

1. This study, like the previous Veterans Administration (VA) Study, because of its small numbers (264 and 259 men in the VA treatment and placebo groups, respectively) was not considered adequate to reach valid conclusions – even had both studies continued for a much longer observation period. "The sample size needed for assessing the coronary question was actually more than 10 times the size used in that study" [23].

2. In coronary artery disease, we are trying to reverse a long-standing process that has evolved over several decades. The situation is not the same as in heart failure, where a prompt effect occurs as soon as the load is taken off the ventricle. Similarly, the fast effectiveness of lowering blood pressure on the cerebrovascular system requires only short-term experiments for demonstration of the prevention of strokes by antihypertensive therapy.

3. The exclusion criteria provided for the admission of essentially "healthy" hypertensive patients into the trial, and prevented patients from entering with a positive history for cardiovascular symptoms, a positive resting and exercise ECG as well as hypercholesterolemia. Because of this selection process, hypertensive patients in

this trial are unlikely to be representative of the hypertensives seen in the communities with all possible additional risk factors and comorbidity. The exclusion criteria in this study [21] were clinical history of or findings of:

Previous arterial thrombosis or vascular insufficiency (coronary, cerebral, peripheral); congestive heart failure; angina pectoris; valvular heart disease; abnormal ECG; radiographically evident cardiomegaly; retinopathy; diabetes; renal insufficiency; hypercholesterolemia ≥350 mg/dl.

The Oslo Study

In the Oslo study, only male hypertensives, aged 40–49 years and asymptomatic at entry were followed for 5 years [7]. During the trial 65 of 379 men forming the "untreated" control group experienced blood pressure increases ≥180 mmHg systolic and/or ≥110 mmHg diastolic, i.e, 17% of the control group. The "untreated" control group had a number of fatal and nonfatal vascular complications outside the coronary artery system which were absent in the treated group of 406 patients (Table 12). However, unexpectedly, coronary heart disease was found more frequently in the actively treated group (Table 13). Helgeland [7] states: "The controls in this trial actually are not quite untreated (they all received a regular long-term health control and the 17% who experienced increase in blood pressure were started on drug treatment)." Therefore, it is entirely speculative whether and if so, what kind of cardiac-

Table 12. Fatal and nonfatal noncoronary complications in relatively young hypertensive men (Oslo Study at 5 years) [7]

Events	Active therapy ($n = 406$)	Control group ($n = 379$)
Fatal subarachnoid hemorrhage	0	2
Major stroke	0	3
Transient ischemic attacks	0	2
Fatal aortic dissection	0	2
Congestive heart failure	0	1
Subclavian aneurysm	0	1
Left bundel brunch block (ECG)	0	1
Marked left ventricular hypertrophy (ECG)	0	7
Noncoronary events	0	19

Table 13. Fatal and nonfatal coronary complications (Oslo Study at 5 years) [7]

Events	Active therapy	Control group
Sudden death	6	2
Definite myocardial infarction	8	8
"Coronary events without myocardial necrosis"	3	1
A. pectoris with positive exercise ECG	3	2
All coronary events	20	13
Total coronary and noncoronary events	20	32

coronary prevention measures were applied to the control group. The author himself warns not to place too much emphasis on the findings in view of the small sample size. The power of the study to demonstrate a statistically significant 20% reduction in total mortality was only 0.14 (i.e, the beta error is 86%). In the judgement of the Canadian Hypertension Society [14], "Unfortunately, this trial was far too small to have sufficient power to permit any firm conclusions on overall events or on cardiovascular mortality." The investigators measured cholesterol levels at baseline and at completion of the trial. Total cholesterol levels were the highest reported in any of the international hypertension intervention studies, i.e., >270 mg/dl, and no dietary or lipid-lowering drug treatment for hypercholesterolemia was provided. Therefore, no beneficial impact of antihypertensive treatment on coronary disease could be expected. Beyond the strict exclusion criteria at entry and the uncertainty of the treatment received by the control group, it is impressive to see in relatively young men, below 50 years of age, the development of strokes and fatal aortic dissection in seven cases, and sudden death in eight men in both groups. The exclusion criteria applied in this study [7] were:

> Heart disease (coronary, cardiovascular, valvular, congestive); intermittent claudication; ECG abnormalities at rest; some drug treatments (for hypertension, retinopathy, renal disease including proteinuria); diabetes; hepatic disease; rheumatoid arthritis; endocrine disorders; psychosis; severe neurosis; obvious alcohol abuse.

The Australian Study

Again, as in the two previously described trials, exclusion criteria in the Australian study were strict (Table 14) and, according to the one-time director of this study, Dr. Abernethy [1] they were "designed to yield a low-risk population with a correspondingly low expectation of benefit from treatment. The number recruited into the trial – 3427 – gave a sufficient power to test for global treatment benefit only, so that the detection of treatment effects in various subgroups categorized by blood pressure, sex, or age was not feasible."

The number of total events was significantly lower in the active treatment regimen [17] in comparison with the placebo group (Table 15). The coronary events were reduced in the treatment group, but not significantly so (Table 16). The same trend was observed in a subgroup of the Australian patients aged 60–69 years (median aged 64 at entry) (Table 17).

Table 14. Stepwise removal of patients with comorbidity prior to randomization (Australian Study, exclusion criteria) [17]

	Exclusion criteria
1st screening	On treatment for hypertension
2nd screening	A. pectoris; history of myocardial infarction in past 3 months; history of stroke; treatment with estrogen and progesterone; asthma; diabetes; gout
Clinic	TIA; plasma creatinine >2 mg/dl; ECG evidence of myocardial ischemia; complications of hypertension

Table 15. Unexpectedly low rate of complications among hypertensives (Australian Study at 3.8 years) [17]

Noncoronary events	Active therapy ($n = 1721$)	Placebo ($n = 1706$)
Fatal stroke	2	4
Nonfatal stroke	7	13
Transient ischemic attacks	3	8
Aortic aneurysm	0	1
Congestive heart failure	2	1
Retinopathy	1	4
Renal failure	1	2
All noncoronary events	16	33
Total events	86 (5%)	121 (7%)

Table 16. Opposite results in reducing manifestations of coronary heart disease in comparison with the Oslo Study (Australian Study at 3.8 years; see Table 13) [17]

Events	Active therapy ($n = 1721$)	Placebo ($n = 1706$)
Ischemic heart disease:		
Fatal	2	8
Nonfatal myocardial infarction	18	17
Nonfatal other coronary heart disease	50	63
All coronary events	70 (4%)	88 (5%)

Table 17. Effect of normalization of blood pressure in elderly hypertensives in Australia (aged 60–69 years; mean DBP at entry, 100 mm Hg) [16]

Mean DBP on trial	Active therapy ($n = 279$) 87 mm Hg	Placebo ($n = 275$) 94 mm Hg
Fatal and nonfatal ischemic heart disease	19	26
Nonfatal cerebrovascular disease (no fatal cerebrovascular disease)	7	11
All events (including noncardiovascular)	27	42

Abernethy [1] takes issue with the "numerous reviews of the management of mild hypertension which have attempted to support deferral of treatment for mild hypertensive individuals" on the basis of the Australian trial. It is implied that a substantial proportion of supposed mild hypertensive individuals become normotensive in the long term and therefore are not in need of treatment. Abernethy points out that the

Table 18. Placebo patients in the Australian study (from [24])

Third-year status	*n*	%
BP <95 mm Hg	462	35.5
DBP 95–109 mm Hg	326	25.1
DBP ≥110 mm Hg	78	6.0
Trial end point	79	6.1
Premature withdrawal	356	27.4
Total	1301	100.0

so-called evidence of a falling trend in blood pressure is based on readings at a single visit – which are known to be highly variable. "To put the proportion of single-visit blood pressure readings below 95 mm Hg in perspective, these points should be noted: As early as the initial clinic visit after screening, 38% of the placebo group were below 95 mm Hg on that day. By protocol, these subjects, like their counterparts in the active treatment group, were deemed ineligible for treatment, that is, they received placebo tablets until such time as their blood pressure reached the 95 mm Hg threshold again. In fact, most of the 38% recrossed the threshold."

The unfavorable experience of the group with "mild" hypertension in Australia prompted Stamler and Stamler [24] to compile a tabulation of the placebo patients' status at their third annual examination (Table 18). "Six % of those who originally had DBP of 90–104 mm Hg had experienced an average increase in diastolic pressure to 110 or higher. Another 6.1% had already experienced a trial end point, i.e. a major cardiovascular event, fatal or nonfatal. In addition, an unspecified proportion of the 27.4% withdrawn from the study by 3 years had been placed on medication, presumably because of a pressure rise. *Even these data may underestimate the risk of a marked rise in pressure since the study originally excluded persons with any cardiovascular complication.*"

Abernethy [1] concluded: "The data cannot be used to justify the position that a *substantial* proportion of mild hypertensive subjects later become normotensive. Rather, the data suggest, that patients with mild hypertension (DBP 90–104 mm Hg) may demonstrate fluctuations in blood pressure."

Finally, Abernethy opposes the opinion, expressed by reviewers of the Australian trial, that no significant treatment benefit was elicited in subjects with entry DBP of 95–99 mm Hg at the low end of the entry pressure range. A favorable trend *was* demonstrated: 15.6 fatal and nonfatal end points per 1000 patient-years in the active group vs 22.3 in the placebo group, a 30% reduction.

The Problem with White Female Hypertensives

Only limited experience on the fate of white women has been accumulated from recent prospective randomized hypertension intervention studies. Among white women in the HDFP, only the group with "mild" hypertension at entry (90–104 mm Hg) showed a significant benefit in all-cause death rates among SC patients [12, 22]. But in the two higher BP strata beyond DBP 105 mm Hg, more SC patients died than women in the RC group (Table 19). Several reasons have been evoked to

Table 19. Death from all causes. White females at 5 years HDFP (per cent) [12]

DBP mm Hg	Stepped care		Referred care	
	Sample	Deaths	Sample	Deaths
90–104	908	34 (3.8)	917	47 (5.1)
105–114	203	15 (7.4)[a]	183	6 (3.3)[b]
≥115	69	10 (14.5)[a]	50	2 (4.0)[b]

[a] 25 deaths in 272 women with severe hypertension.
[b] 8 deaths in 233 women with severe hypertension.

Table 20. Differences between white females in SC and RC in DBP stratum ≥105 mm Hg [12]

	Stepped care	Referred care
Sample = 3% of total HDFP population	203	183
On treatment at baseline (%)	31	36
Mean age (years)	53.3	51.6
On treatment during 5 years (%)	92	85
	None on beta blockers	Most on beta blockers

explain this apparent anomaly, among others the fact that some very sick women were randomized into the SC group and died shortly after initiation of the trial. Other explanations include the *exceptionally low death rate among RC women, in fact the lowest of any subgroup in all race-sex groups;* and furthermore, chance imbalance in randomization at baseline due to the small numbers in these subgroups. These three facts might suffice to account for some of the discrepant findings in the two upper blood pressure strata. The vigor of treatment in the RC groups is another consideration: In contrast to the RC group of white and black men and black women, the highest percentage treated *and* at blood pressure goal at year 5 was found in the RC group of white women [12]. At year 5, SC patients averaged DBP levels as follows: Black males 86.5 mm Hg, black females 83.9 mm Hg, white males 84.0 mm Hg, white females 82.4 mm Hg. RC patients averaged DBP levels of 91.9, 90.4, 88.5, and 85.4 respectively [9]. Aside from the 3-mm Hg difference in achieved DBP reduction between the two groups, women in RC were mostly treated with beta-blockers which were nearly unavailable to SC patients [22] (Table 20).

In addition to these possible explanations, multiple logistic analysis of baseline characteristics showed that SC white women were at slightly higher risk at baseline than RC women (Table 21). There was "no evidence that excess lowering of blood pressure was causal of the reverse death rates; *survivors had blood pressure lowered to a greater extent than those who died in both SC and RC.* Analysis of both underlying and contributing causes of death and analysis of side effects do not explain these mortality findings" [22]. Smoller [22] concluded on behalf of the HDFP Cooperative Group: "The reverse mortality trend is likely to be a chance finding."

Three observations are relevant in this context:

1. Overall mortality of white women has been the lowest in all four race-sex groups [9]. The comparative figures for stepped care vs referred care are: black

Table 21. Unexpected differences in baseline characteristics and treatment between white females in SC and RC in DBP stratum ≥115 mmHg [22]

	Stepped care	Referred care
Sample = 1% of total HDFP population	69	50
Cigarette smokers (%)	33	24
Stroke at baseline (%)	9	(0)
Receiving treatment for 5 years (%)	98	88
	None on beta blockers	Most on beta blockers

men,112 vs 140; black women,70 vs 98; white men, 109 vs 126; and white women, 58 vs 55. How much reduction in mortality may one achieve if the all-cause death rate is already significantly lower than in all other race-sex groups?

2. The stroke incidence of white women in SC was 30% lower than in RC [10]. Since there are few other risk factors besides hypertension known to be predisposing to stroke, it is mandatory to eliminate this risk in order to prevent strokes.

3. The leading cause of death in Western societies, for both white men and women, is coronary heart disease. Although in general, women develop atherosclerotic disease of the heart about 10 years later than men do, the same factors contribute to premature ischemic heart disease, i.e., smoking, hypercholesterolemia, diabetes and, of course, hypertension.

The three intervention trials discussed [7, 17, 21] offer no help in determining whether treatment of hypertensive white females is of great, little, or no value. The Australian trial randomized 636 women into active treatment and 621 women into placebo groups. Fatal and nonfatal end points after 3.8 years amounted to 24 in the treatment patients and to 36 in placebo patients, a nonsignificant difference. In contrast, the difference among men in the two groups was significant ($P<0.05$), since 67 trial end points occurred among actively treated men and 91 among placebo treated men. The Oslo study only followed male patients and the U. S. Public Health Service Hospitals study had but 45 women under active drug regimen and 33 under placebo treatment. A separate analysis was not felt to be appropriate.

The prevalence of hypertension is broadly the same for both men and women. Without further research into this important public health problem, it would be very unfortunate, indeed, if general practitioners continued to apply different treatment policies to the two sexes. No predictor or set of multiple predictors is presently available from which it becomes possible to determine the low or excess risk of a given white female hypertensive patient to develop cardiovascular complications. The exceptions to this statement are, of course, the diabetic female patient and the smoker, who develop elevated blood pressure. Both the hypertensive diabetic and the smoking women require vigorous treatment.

If the risk of a hypertensive black woman had been much different from the risk of a black hypertensive man, i.e., much lower for stroke and myocardial infarction, one might have found an argument for discussing the hormonal protection of women even in the presence of hypertension. However, for black women, the efficiency of treatment of hypertension is clearly established – in the HDFP, with the highest percent reduction of death in SC compared with RC, a 28% lower total mortality in SC black women was recorded [9].

The recent recommendation in an editorial [20] "to treat women with DBP >105 mm Hg as vigorously as men but not to give active treatment in mild to moderate hypertension," is not borne out by the HDFP data among white female patients with DBP below 105 mm Hg, as Table 19 indicates. We have identified a research area of major clinical and public health importance. Data from the MRC [4, 19] and IPPPSH [13] studies do not shed any new light on the question of treating white women. Only the European Working Party (EWP) investigation in elderly hypertensive patients [2, 3] indicates a definite benefit of treatment for white women.

Three New Hypertension Intervention Trials

International Prospective Primary Prevention Study in Hypertension

The IPPPSH [13] demonstrated that both beta-blockers and diuretics were able to reduce coronary mortality in men and women, but smokers did not benefit from beta-blocker therapy. The baseline cholesterol levels in the subjects of this study averaged 234 mg/dl, and after a treatment period of 3–5 years mean cholesterol levels of 242 mg/dl were recorded. No attempts were made to lower serum cholesterol concentrations among the 6357 hypertensive men and women. It may be recalled that one conclusion of the Lipid Research Clinics Coronary Primary Prevention Trial was that lowering cholesterol levels in hypercholesterolemic normotensive individuals by 1% reduced the risk of coronary heart disease by 2%. The IPPPSH study yielded an interesting finding in hypertensives, with increasing cholesterol levels; that is to say, "an increase of cholesterol levels by 40 mg/dl among hypertensives increases the risk of myocardial infarction by 20%."

Medical Research Council Trial [19]

The MRC study [19] followed 17354 hypertensive men and women in three treatment groups (placebo, beta-blockers, diuretics) over a 5½-year period. No difference was seen in the incidence of coronary events, with 222 cases in the active treatment group and 232 cases in the placebo group. Almost twice as many coronary events occurred in smokers as in non-smokers. In view of what the investigators refer to as "perhaps the most interesting aspect of these analyses, the difference between results for smokers and smokers," it is regrettable that no attempt was made to relate the coronary events to differences in cholesterol levels. From the original publication [19, miniprint Table Im], it is evident that mean cholesterol levels were high, especially in women (260 mg/dl) but also in men (245 mg/dl). No dietary intervention or drug treatment for hypercholesterolemic patients was carried out.

Analysis of the results obtained by "intention-to-treat" is accepted as a reliable, objective statistical method. However, some concern may be raised when "substantial percentages of patients were in fact withdrawn from their allocated regimen during follow-up" [19]. For various reasons, including unacceptably high blood pressure levels in the placebo group, dropouts and premature deaths, and emergence of other trial endpoints there were losses of 47% of men and 40% of women assigned to the placebo group. As pointed out in an accompanying editorial to the MRC report [4], if 44% of men and 37% of women from all three treatment groups stopped the treatment to which they were initially randomized, then "these high figures must be kept in mind when we are considering recommendations with respect to individual drugs." The negative outcome of the MRC trial as far as reducing coronary events by drug treatment is concerned must be viewed in light of both high baseline cholesterol levels which remained untreated, and questions on the way the analysis was handled.

European Working Party on High Blood Pressure

In contrast to the results in the British MRC trial, this hypertension intervention study in elderly patients (70% of them women) [2, 3] revealed a significant reduction in cardiovascular mortality rate. Among the 416 men and women randomized to active treatment, 29 died from cardiac causes; in the placebo group with 424 patients, 47 died from cardiac causes. According to the intention-to-treat analysis, these actual numbers amounted to rates of 15‰ and 24‰ respectively, a percentage change for active treatment by −38 percent. In a separate analysis of terminal fatal events by randomized treatment fatal myocardial infarction was found to occur in 7 patients in the active treatment and 16 patients in the placebo group [3].

No information on cholesterol levels is provided in this final report. However, 3 years earlier [2], the same group published a detailed report on the influence of antihypertensive therapy on serum cholesterol in these elderly patients. The authors explained the "marked fall in cholesterol observed in the more severely hypertensive and actively treated patients was due to the effect of treatment, the large reduction of systolic blood pressure being associated with ... a fall in serum cholesterol."

Comments

It is generally accepted that elevated blood pressure levels augment atherosclerosis directly by way of increased pressure, but some investigators have suggested that renin (or a related vasoactive hormone) may be an independent atherogenic factor. The somewhat lower effectiveness of antihypertensive therapy to reduce the incidence of ischemic heart disease in comparison with reduction of cerebrovascular disease "has encouraged the idea that some component of hypertensive pathophysiology other than blood pressure may be atherogenic" [18]. In experiments with baboons, McGill [18] showed the interaction of a moderate elevation of blood pressure (about 30 mmHg) and modest diet-induced hypercholesterolemia (200 mg/dl) in its effect on experimental atherosclerosis. This mild degree of hypertension "increased the extent of atherosclerosis in the carotid arteries threefold and in other arteries twofold, but did not affect atherosclerosis in the thoracic aorta. Multiple regression analyses demonstrated that, in the carotid arteries, lipoprotein cholesterol level combined with blood pressure predicted about 60% of the variance in lesions. These results revive the idea that one or more of the vasoactive hormones in hypertension may influence atherogenesis directly. However, the most remarkable aspect of our experiment was that within 14 months a modest elevation in BP dramatically augmented atherogenesis at selected sites in the presence of plasma cholesterol levels equal to those of the average American" [18].

In determining which vascular bed will be primarily affected by elevated blood pressure, it appears that the combined effect of hypercholesterolemia and hypertension causes premature coronary arteriosclerosis.

By removing from randomized trials those hypertensive patients who exhibit abnormalities in the ECG, and with past history of myocardial infarction and/or stroke, kidney disease, diabetes, and treatment of hypertension, the incidence of all cardiovascular events is markedly reduced in both treated and untreated hypertensives. As three recent, randomized trials with highly selected "healthy" hypertensive individuals have demonstrated, fatal manifestations of arteriosclerosis for actively as well as placebo treated patients become rare, and contradictory findings have emerged from those three experiments as far as coronary heart disease is concerned. The HDFP is the only long-term study which represents the total spectrum of hypertension from the mildest to the most severe degrees, from the undetected to the previously treated, and from patients with to those without end-organ damage in American communities. This trial has focused attention on the changes of the *incidence* of arteriosclerotic complications from the cerebral to the coronary arteries. In an optimal stepped care program, and particularly in the so-called mild DBP stratum (90–104 mm Hg), the manifestations of cerebral *and* coronary arteriosclerosis were significantly reduced in comparison with a less than optimal treatment regimen in the control group – as was commonly practiced in the USA between 1973 and 1979.

The concept of arteriosclerosis as a progressive disease in most individuals with the essential stimuli – hypercholesterolemia and hypertension – is a fact of life in the twentieth century of western civilization. Regression of arteriosclerosis has been demonstrated in several species of animals after withdrawal of atherogenic stimuli in the diet.

"Regression – diagnosed angiographically – has been reported to have occurred in over 100 patients... It is probable that two mechanisms are involved in angiographic regression. The first may occur when hyperlipidemia is partly or totally corrected. The second may be associated with reabsorption of lipids from the arterial wall. The second type seems independent of changes in plasma lipid levels and may involve resolution of thrombi or other undefined arterial wall factors" [15].

No angiographic study with progression or regression of arteriosclerosis in humans or animals with hypertension has been reported. Therefore, it is presently impossible to state whether the removal of the stimulus hypertension will lead to regression of arteriosclerosis in the cerebral and coronary arteries or to the arrest of the arteriosclerotic process, preventing the clinical event from manifesting itself. However, the most promising type of therapy for hypertensive patients in the Western societies, in an attempt to prevent coronary heart disease, appears to be a combination of vigorous cholesterol lowering and antihypertensive treatment. Indirect evidence for this hypothesis is provided from the Japanese experience (see Fig. 2).

References

1. Abernethy JD (1984) The Australian therapeutic trial in mild hypertension (letter to the editor). Hypertension 6:774–776
2. Amery A, Birkenhager W, Bulpitt C, Clement D, Deruyttere M, DeSchaepdryver A, Dollery C, Fagard R, Forette F, Forte J, Hamdy R, Leonetti G, Lund-Johansen P, MacFarlane JPR,

Mutsers A, O'Malley K, Tuomilehto J (1982) Influence of antihypertensive therapy on serum cholesterol in elderly hypertensive patients. Acta Cardiol 37:235–244
3. Amery A, Birkenhager W, Brixco P, Bulpitt C, Clement D, Deruyttere M, De Schaepdryver A, Dollery C, Fagard R, Forette F, Forte J, Hamdy R, Henry JF, Joossens JV, Leonetti G, Lund-Johansen P, O'Malley K, Petrie J, Strasser T, Tuomilehto J, Williams B (1985) Mortality and morbidity results from the European Working Party on High Blood Pressure in the Elderly Trial. Lancet 1:1349–1354
4. Breckenridge A (1985) Treating mild hypertension (Editorial). Br Med J 291:89–90
5. Chobanian AV (1983) The influence of hypertension and other hemodynamic factors in atherogenesis. Prog Cardiovasc Dis 26:177–196
6. Comstock GW, Suzuki T, Stone RW, Crumrine JL, Johnson DH, Sakai Y, Matsuya T, Sasaki S (1985) Cardiovascular risk factors in American and Japanese executives. J R Soc Med 78:536–545
7. Helgeland A (1980) Treatment of mild hypertension. A five-year controlled drug trial. The Oslo Study. Am J Med 69:725–732
8. Heyden S, Schneider K, Fodor JG (1985) Comprehensive health care and noncardiovascular mortality: an unlikely explanation of the findings from the Hypertension Detection and Follow-Up Program. Circulation 72:692–696
9. Hypertension Detection and Follow-up Program Cooperative Group (1979) Five-year findings of the Hypertension Detection and Follow-up Program: I. Reduction in mortality of persons with high blood pressure, including mild hypertension; II. Mortality by race-sex, and age. JAMA 242:2562–2571; 2572–2577
10. Hypertension Detection and Follow-up Program Cooperative Group (1982) Five-year findings of the Hypertension Detection and Follow-up Program: III. Reduction in stroke incidence among persons with high blood pressure. JAMA 247:633–638
11. Hypertension Detection and Follow-up Program Cooperative Group (1984) Effect of stepped care treatment on the incidence of myocardial infarction and angina pectoris. Hypertension [Suppl 1] 6:I-198–I-206
12. Hypertension Detection and Follow-up Program Cooperative Group (1984) Five-year findings of the Hypertension Detection and Follow-up Program: Mortality by race-sex, and blood pressure. A further analysis. J Community Health 9:314–327
13. IPPPSH Collaborative Group (1985) Cardiovascular risk and risk factors in a randomized trial of treatment based on the beta-blocker Oxprenolol: The International Prospective Primary Prevention Study in Hypertension. J Hypertension 3:379–392
14. Logan AG (ed) (1984) Report of the Consensus Development Conference on the Management of Mild Hypertension in Canada. Canadian Hypertension Society, Toronto
15. Malinow MR (1984) Atherosclerosis: Progression, regression and resolution. Am Heart J 108: 1523–1534
16. Management Committee (1981) Report: Treatment of mild hypertension in the elderly. Med J Aust 2:398–401
17. Management Committee (1980) The Australian therapeutic trial in mild hypertension. Lancet 1:1262–1267
18. McGill HC Jr (1984) Persistent problems in the pathogenesis of atherosclerosis. Arteriosclerosis 4:443–451
19. Medical Research Council Working Party (1985) MRC trial on treatment of mild hypertension: principal results. Br Med J 291:97–104
20. Silman AJ (1984) Hypertension in women: a separate case for treatment? Br Med J 289:1021–1022
21. Smith W McFate (1977) Treatment of mild hypertension. Results of a ten-year intervention trial. US Public Health Service Hospitals Cooperative Study Group. Circ Res [Suppl 1] 40:I-98–I-105
22. Smoller SW (1984) Analysis of mortality results from HDFP in white women with moderate or severe hypertension (Abstr). Circulation 70:II-163
23. Stamler J (1978) Mild hypertension: to treat or not to treat. Discussion. Ann NY Acad Sci 304:140
24. Stamler J, Stamler R (1983) "Mild" hypertension: Risks and strategy for control: I. Primary Cardiol 9:150–166
25. US Department of Health, Education and Welfare (1977) Health and nutrition examination survey. US DHEW, Washington (Vital and health statistics, ser 11, no 203)
26. US Department of Health and Human Services, Public Health Service (1982) Implications of the Hypertension Detection and Follow-Up Program. US DHHS, Washington (NIH publication no 83–2116)

Changes in Brain Blood Flow and Organ Function Following Treatment of Primary Hypertension

W.-D. Heiss[1]

Hypertension as a Risk Factor for Cerebrovascular Disease

The importance of antihypertensive treatment is evident from epidemiologic data on hypertension as a risk factor for stroke. According to the Framingham Study [1, 2] the systolic blood pressure is the most important risk factor, followed by diabetes, cardiac insufficiency, nicotine abuse, and hyperlipidemia. A hypertensive person's risk of suffering a stroke within 16 years is seven times that of a normotonic. Incidence of stroke is increased 5 to 30 times depending on severity of hypertension, age, and sex. The risk does not increase proportionally with hypertension (as is the case for myocardial infarction), but rises more than linearly for higher values (>180 mm Hg systolic pressure). Hypertension is especially risky for younger men and older women. Ischemic as well as hemorrhagic strokes are more frequent in hypertensive patients, and the risk may be directly read from the systolic value, where a fast increase within a short period of observation indicates an exceptionally high risk for cerebrovascular disease [3]. The combination of hypertension with other risk factors further increases the incidence of stroke: hypertension with diabetes increases the risk six times, hypertension with cardiac insufficiency, five times, and hypertension with hyperlipidemia in younger patients raises the incidence of stroke to 10 times that in normal controls.

Relationship Between Blood Pressure and Cerebral Blood Flow

The extent of cerebral blood flow is not strictly dependent on the law of Hagen and Poiseuille (flow in pipes is proportional to the fourth power of the radius and inversely related to the length of a pipe and the viscosity of the fluid), but due to autoregulation it is kept constant within a wide range of systemic blood pressure. Autoregulation of cerebral blood flow is achieved by an alteration of the diameter of the resistance vessels (mainly arterioles) according to the local pressure. Within the range of autoregulation – mean arterial blood pressure of 70 mm Hg to 150 mm Hg [4] – the perfusion in the undamaged brain tissue is kept constant by a compensatory vasodilation. The decrease of blood pressure below the lower limit of autoregulation cannot be compensated by a further increase in diameter of maximally dilated vessels, and as a consequence the blood flow is linearly diminished by further pressure decreases. A raise in blood pressure is followed by vasoconstriction until the value

[1] Max-Planck-Institut für neurologische Forschung und Neurologische Klinik des Städtischen Krankenhauses Köln-Merheim, Ostmerheimer Str. 200, D-5000 Köln 91 (Merheim).

Primary Hypertension
Ed. by W. Kaufmann et al.

at which the vessel's wall cannot continue to resist the intravascular pressure: then passive vasodilation is forced up on the vessels and occurs first in small segments, leading to the appearance of constricted and dilated segments following each other ("sausage-string" phenomenon) [5]. Finally, the passive vasodilation is spread out over all resistance vessels and cerebral blood flow increases more than linearly with further raises in pressure. This point is called the breakthrough of autoregulation [6]. In various brain regions, the curve of autoregulation is different, making some areas more resistant (cerebellum) to pressure changes than others (cerebrum, spinal cord) [7]. The forced vasodilation additionally causes the displacement of endothelial cells and the disruption of tight junctions and leads to an impairment of the blood-brain barrier with increased permeability for proteins [8].

Clinical Symptoms of Acute Increases in Blood Pressure

The brain edema resulting from the disruption of the blood-brain barrier, the leakage of blood cells through the endothelial gaps, and in severe cases the small hemorrhages around vessels cause the general and focal neurologic deficits of an acute hypertensive encephalopathy [9, 10]: The increased intracranial blood volume – due to dilated vessels and raised pressure – induces severe headache, while the local brain edema impairs metabolic supply and causes focal neurologic symptoms, disturbance of consiousness, and epileptic seizures. In patients with acute hypertensive encephalopathy regional cerebral blood flow is increased, and these increases are especially marked in areas with disturbed neurologic function. Areas with increased water content and small hemorrhages can be detected using computed tomography. Immediate treatment with fast acting antihypertensive drugs improves clinical deficits and normalizes regionally disturbed perfusion.

Effects of Chronic Hypertension

Chronic hypertension leads to hypertrophy of the muscular vessel wall and to fibrosis of other vascular compartments [11]. Thereby the vessel is better suited to resist the intravascular pressure, and the breakthrough point of autoregulation is moved to higher values [12]. However, the relative increase of the wall in relation to the total diameter and the consequent decrease of vascular opening also shifts the lower threshold of autoregulation to a higher value and thereby the flow decreases already when pressure drops below 100–120 mm Hg. The brain of a hypertensive patient is therefore endangered in both respects: acute pressure peaks are able to overcome autoregulation, they cause hypertensive crisis, and may lead to rupture of previously damaged vessels (microaneurysms) with consecutive small or massive intracerebral hemorrhages; dropping of pressure during circulatory stress decreases cerebral blood flow below the lower threshold of autoregulation and below the threshold for the functional and morphological integrity of the nervous tissue [13], and often leads to ischemic brain damage. The threshold for functional damage is increased proportionally to the blood pressure. Areas whose supplying arteries are stenotic are extremely vulnerable for transient decreases in blood pressure: in these vascular territories perfusion pressure easily drops below the ischemic threshold and neurologic symptoms can develop. Ischemic and hemorrhagic lesions in small regions without localized neurologic function cause chronic hypertensive encephalopathy characterized by progressive dementia.

Effects of Antihypertensive Treatment

Reduction of Blood Pressure and Cerebral Blood Flow

The reduction of raised blood pressure in patients with cerebral ischemia may be harmful, because regional cerebral blood flow is pressure dependent in ischemically damaged tissue and with hypotension flow may fall critically in these regions. Therefore, in some patients neurologic deficits are accentuated or even first appear when hypertensive values are normalized. As a consequence blood pressure should be slowly decreased to systolic values of 150–170 mmHg in the acute stage of an ischemic stroke.

In chronic hypertensives, however, a strict regulation of blood pressure leads to an improvement of the autoregulatory capacity: the lower limit of autoregulation and thereby the threshold for ischemic brain damage could be brought towards the values in normotensive controls [14]. This treatment decreases the risk of these patients suffering an ischemic infarction.

Regulation of hypertension does not necessarily decrease cerebral blood flow: in 10 hypertensive patients without cerebrovascular disease treated by Gottstein [15], mean arterial blood pressure decreased from 138 to 117 mmHg within 3 weeks; during this period mean cerebral blood flow changed insignificantly from 46.6 to 40.6 ml/100 g/min. Meyer et al. [16] treated 13 hypertensive stroke victims with 500 to 750 mg alpha-methyldopa for 14 days; in these patients cerebrovascular resistance decreased significantly and cerebral blood flow was improved (mean BP 125.6 $\pm$ 16.6 to 105.9 $\pm$ 14.6 mmHg; cerebral blood flow 44.5 $\pm$ 11.0 to 48.9 $\pm$ 10.6 ml/100 g/min). However, it must be kept in mind that improvements of neurologic function are also followed by increases in crebral blood flow [17].

The effect of antihypertensive treatment with alpha-methyldopa was also studied by Goldberg et al. [18]: In 13 patients mean arterial pressure decreased significantly while cerebral blood flow did not change; this result was evidence for a marked change of cerebrovascular resistence. A further analysis of the data indicated a diverging response of cerebral blood flow related to age and necessary dosage for an antihypertensive effect: only in young patients in need of low dosage the capability remained to improve autoregulation and as a consequence to normalize blood flow. In older patients and those in whom high dosages were necessary this potential of recovery of regulatory mechanisms was lost, and blood flow further deteriorated with decreases of blood pressure.

Antihypertensive Therapy for Prevention of Stroke

Several investigations studied prospectively the incidence of stroke in treated and untreated hypertension (Table 1): Hamilton [19] observed seven strokes in the placebo group, while no stroke occurred in the treated group within 5 years.

Table 1. Incidence of stroke in treated and nontreated hypertensives

	n	MAP (mm Hg)	Time period (years)	Strokes (fatal)	
				Placebo group	Treated group
Hamilton [19]	61	110–130	5	7	0
Veterans Administration Cooperative Study [20]	143	115–129	1.5	5	1
Veterans Administration Cooperative Study [21]	380	90–114	3.3	7 (7)	1 (1)
Australian Therapeutic Trial [23]	3427	>95	4	31 (6)	17 (3)
Hypertensive Detection and Follow-Up Program[a] [22]	7825	90–104	5	(31)	(17)
	3120	>105	5	(21)	(12)

[a] Comparison of death rates with specific and usual antihypertensive treatment

In the Veterans Administration Cooperative Study [20] five strokes within 1.5 years were seen in the placebo group and one stroke in the treated group of severe hypertension (diastolic pressure 115–129 mm Hg). Untreated mild hypertension (diastolic value 90–114 mm Hg) was followed by four fatal ischemic infarcts and three fatal hemorrhages within 3.3 years; in the treated group only one fatal stroke occurred [21].

The American intervention study of the Hypertension Detection and Follow-up Program Cooperative Group [22] compared hypertensive patients randomly assigned to a special and consequent antihypertensive treatment with those receiving usual treatment of hypertension. Within the observation period of 5 years the stroke mortality rate in the specially treated group was 50% of that in the control group in which normalization of blood pressure was not specifically achieved and controlled. This result was especially striking in the large group of patients with mild hypertension (diastolic value 90:104 mm Hg).

The Australian Therapeutical Trial [23] of controlled intervention in mild hypertension yielded comparable results. In 1721 treated patients, 17 cerebrovascular attacks (three fatal strokes, 10 strokes with permanent neurologic deficits, four transient ischemic attacks) occurred within four years; while in the untreated 1706 hypertensives, 31 attacks (six fatal, 16 completed strokes, nine TIAs) were observed. The differences in the total number of attacks ($P<0.025$) and in the non-fatal strokes ($P<0.005$) are statistically significant. Similar results were reported by the Swiss Intervention Study Group [24].

Effect of Antihypertensive Treatment on Epidemiology of Acute Cerebrovascular Disease

Epidemiologic studies have already demonstrated the influence of antihypertensive treatment on the incidence and mortality rates of acute cerebrovascular disease. In the study from Busselton, West Australia [25] the mortality rate from acute cerebrovascular diseases for normotensives (RR < 160/100 mmHg) was 0.9/1000, for hypertensives (RR > 160/100 mm Hg) 18/1000; sufficient regulation of hypertension decreased mortality to 3.2/1000, while with insufficient treatment of HT mortality was further increased (37/1000). The decrease in total mortality from cerebrovascular accidents observed for the male population of this community (28 men 1967–1972 compared with 20 in 1973–1977) occurred in relation to the improvement of antihypertensive treatment (sufficiently treated in 1966, 12%, and in 1975, 67% of hypertensive men).

In Rochester, USA, a decrease of the annual incidence rate on cerebrovascular disease from 190/100000 during 1945-1949 to 104/100000 during the period 1970–1974 was observed [26]. This change of morbidity occurred in relation to the improvement of antihypertensive treatment, but also changes in smoking habits and alterations of food constituents (decrease of fat) may be important. The decrease in mortality due to cerebrovascular disease between 1960 and 1975, especially after 1968, is also evident in the total USA annual death rates [27]. All these data strikingly prove the importance of systematic antihypertensive treatment in the prevention of cerebrovascular disease.

Summary

Hypertension is the most important risk factor for stroke. By autoregulation cerebral vessels are able to maintain cerebral blood flow in spite of changes in blood pressure over a wide range. Decreases of blood pressure below the lower threshold of autoregulation are followed by pressure-dependent diminution of blood flow. If blood pressure is raised above the upper limit of autoregulation (breakthrough), cerebral blood flow raises more than linearly due to passive vasodilation. The following changes in blood volume and the alteration of the blood-brain barrier cause the symptoms of acute hypertensive encephalopathy (crisis). In chronic hypertension the vessel wall becomes thicker, and thereby hypertensives are partly protected against hypertensive crisis, but more vulnerable to drops in blood pressure.

Treatment of hypertension can restore normal autoregulation of cerebral blood flow, in some instances blood flow may even be normalized by changes in cerebrovascular resistance. Treatment of hypertension is also necessary for the prevention of stroke: In all controlled trials the incidence of stroke was significantly decreased in the treated group. Improvements in annual incidence and mortality from acute cerebrovascular disease are probably due to the improvements achieved in antihypertensive therapy.

References

1. Kannel WB, Dawber TR, Sorlie P, Wolf PA (1976) Components of blood pressure and risk of atherothrombotic brain infarction: The Framingham Study. Stroke 7:327
2. Kannel WB, Wolf PA, McGee DL, Dawber TR, McNamara P, Castelli WP (1981) Systolic blood pressure, arterial rigidity, and risk of stroke: The Framingham Study. JAMA 245:1225

3. Rabkin SW, Mathewson FAL, Tate RB (1978) Long-term changes in blood pressure and risk of cerebrovascular disease. Stroke 9:319
4. Lassen NA (1959) Cerebral blood flow and oxygen consumption in man. Physiol Rev 39:183
5. Farrar JK, Jones JV, Graham DI, Strandgaard S, MacKenzie ET (1976) Evidence against cerebral vasospasm during acutely induced hypertension. Brain Res 104:176
6. Strandgaard S, MacKenzie ET, Sengupta D, Rowan JO, Lassen NA, Harper M (1974) Upper limit of autoregulation of cerebral blood flow in the baboon. Circ Res 34:435
7. Sato M, Pawlik G, Heiss WD (1984) Comparative studies of regional CNS blood flow autoregulation and responses to CO_2 in the cat. Effects of altering arterial blood pressure and $PaCO_2$ on rCBF of cerebrum, cerebellum, and spinal cord. Stroke 15:91
8. Johansson B, Li LC, Olsson Y, Klatzo I (1970) The effect of acute arterial hypertension on the blood-brain barrier to protein tracers. Acta Neuropathol (Berl) 16:117
9. Byrom FB (1969) The hypertensive vascular crisis. Heinemann, London
10. Skinhoj E, Strandgaard S (1973) Pathogenesis of hypertensive encephalopathy. Lancet 2:461
11. Folkow B (1971) The haemodynamic consequences of adaptive structural changes of the resistance vessels in hypertension. Clin Sci 41:1
12. Strandgaard S, Olesen J, Skinhoj E, Lassen NA (1973) Autoregulation of brain circulation in severe arterial hypertension. Br Med J 159:507
13. Heiss WD (1983) Progress in cerebrovascular disease: Flow thresholds for functional and morphological damage of brain tissue. Stroke 14:329
14. Strandgaard S (1976) Autoregulation of cerebral blood flow in hypertensive patients. The modifying influence of prolonged antihypertensive treatment on the tolerance to acute drug induced hypotension. Circulation 53:720
15. Gottstein U (1976) Behandlung der arteriellen Hypertonie bei Patienten mit Stenosen und Obliterationen im Bereich der hirnversorgenden Arterien. In: Zeitler E (ed) Hypertonie – Risikofaktor in der Angiologie. Witzstrock, Baden-Baden
16. Meyer JS, Sawada T, Kitamura A, Toyoda M (1968) Cerebral blood flow after control of hypertension in stroke. Neurology (Minneap) 18:772
17. Heiss WD, Zeiler K, Turnheim M, Podreka I (1976) Flow and compartmental weight in relation to the course of stroke. Stroke 7:399
18. Goldberg H, Weinberger J, Banka R, Reichgott M, Levine P, Reivich M (1979) Effect of methyldopa on cerebral blood flow in hypertension. Acta Neurol Scand [Suppl 72] 60:144
19. Hamilton M (1966) Selection of patients for antihypertensive therapy. In: Gross F (ed) Antihypertensive Therapie. Springer, Berlin Heidelberg New York, p 196
20. Veterans Administration Cooperative Study Group on Antihypertensive Agents (1967) Effects of treatment on morbidity in hypertension. I. Results in patients with diastolic blood pressures averaging 115 through 129 mm Hg. JAMA 202:116
21. Veterans Administration Cooperative Study Group on Antihypertensive Agents (1970) Effects of treatment on morbidity in hypertension. II. Results in patients with diastolic blood pressures averaging 90 through 114 mm Hg. JAMA 213:1143
22. Hypertensive Detection and Follow-Up Program Cooperative Group (1979) Five-year findings of the hypertension detection and follow-up program. I. Reduction in mortality of persons with high blood pressure, including mild hypertension. JAMA 242:2562
23. Report by the Management Committee (1980) Australian therapeutic trial in mild hypertension. Lancet 1:1261
24. Epstein FH (1980) Ergebnisse der Interventionsstudien der Hypertonie. Symposium Moderne Aspekte der Hochdruckbehandlung. Cologne, 9.11.1980
25. Cullen KJ, McCall MG, Stenhouse NS (1979) Changing mortality due to strokes in men following treatment of Busselton hypertensives 1967–77. Int J Epidemiol 8:213
26. Garraway WM, Whisnant JP, Furlan AJ, Phillips LA II, Kurland LT, O'Fallon WM (1979) The declining incidence of stroke. N Engl J Med 300:449
27. Soltero I, Liu K, Cooper R, Stamler J, Garside D (1978) Trends in mortality from cerebrovascular diseases in the United States 1960 to 1975. Stroke 9:549

Changes in Hypertrophy by Treatment in Hypertension: Results of Experimental Research

E. D. FROHLICH[1]

The discussion that follows is concerned with changes in cardiac mass associated with antihypertensive therapy in experimental forms of hypertension. It is important for the reader to bear in mind that data from experimental (and certainly from clinical) studies are simply not available to support the assigned title that implies antihypertensive therapy will produce a reversal of left ventricular hypertrophy. Indeed, the conclusions that are implied are assumptions that are fair to hypothesize, but we must continually bear in mind that reduction in cardiac size, shape, or contour; reduction in wall thicknesses or mass (by echocardiography); changes in cardiac electrophysiological indices (by electrocardiography); or even reduction in the mass of the heart or left ventricle after therapy by actual weight mean just those findings. Left ventricular hypertrophy and its associated changes with therapy have not been confirmed histopathologically.

Left Ventricular Hypertrophy: Inferential Indices

The concept that is offered above embodies an appeal to the reader, the clinician, and the investigator to bear in mind the experimental findings actually reported. Thus, when hypertension is produced experimentally and a sustained elevation of arterial pressure is produced, there is an invariable increase in left ventricular mass [1–5]. However, this increase in mass of the left ventricle has been inconstantly correlated with the height of arterial pressure. Experimental studies have demonstrated clearly a highly significant correlation between the height of arterial pressure and the measured mass of the left ventricle in two-kidney, one renal artery clip Goldblatt hypertension (2K,1C-GH); but less strong correlations exist for other experimental forms of hypertension including desoxycorticosterone (DOC) salt, cellophane encapsulation of the kidney, figure-of-eight ligature of the kidney, or the spontaneously hypertensive rat (SHR). This is not to say that hypertension does not have a causal role in the development of an increased mass of the heart; it only means that a less close correlation that is not significant statistically is the reality. It may mean that the measured elevated arterial pressure in the 2K,1C-GH more clearly reflects the pressure over a full 24-h period; and it may also mean that other factors exist in the participation of the increased left ventricular mass.

[1] Education and Research Alton Ochsner Medical Foundation, 1516 Jefferson Highway, New Orleans, LA 70121, USA.

Primary Hypertension
Ed. by W. Kaufmann et al.

Increased Cardiac Size

A word is also necessary to underscore the reality that an increased size of the heart means just that. If we can hold strictly to this fact, inappropriately derived inferences will not be made from experimental research – and from the clinical investigative laboratories. Thus, a so-called "big heart" must be defined in terms of cardiac (and, more specifically, left ventricular) mass. This also must be differentiated from the roentgenographic appearance of a heart large in shape or contour, although Ungerleider provided pathological correlations from his derived indices [6, 7]. Other studies have employed a large number of electrocardiographically derived indices to define left ventricular hypertrophy. Some have been used to relate electrophysiographically derived measurements to functional and hemodynamic changes associated with the progression of left ventricular hypertrophy [1, 2, 4, 8–10]. But we must also be aware that while some of these changes may reverse themselves with control of arterial pressure [11], they also have been observed with acute reduction in pressure that clearly is not associated with a reversal of the hypertrophy process [12]. Nevertheless, some of the electrocardiographic indices have been utilized to correlate significantly with the echocardiographic measurements of wall thicknesses and chamber dimensions [13]. But we must also realize that these mensurational indices only imply the existence of left ventricular hypertrophy since these studies do not provide the histological counterpart to the conclusion. Thus, the increased mass by weight, measurement, or inference may reflect left ventricular dilation, increased left ventricular muscle mass, or increased left ventricular collagen content; and it is also conceivable that some of the increased muscle mass could be represented by hyperplasia. These concepts are most important to bear in mind since the investigator could make a quantum leap in conclusions if he ascribes a reduction in cardiac size with antihypertensive therapy to a "reversal of left ventricular hypertrophy."

Reversal, Regression

It follows from the foregoing discussion that we must be precise in our terminology for our observations of the changes that take place in cardiac size or mass with pharmacotherapy of hypertension experimentally or clinically. Some studies have reported a "reversal" or "regression" of left ventricular hypertrophy. Let us be precise in describing our observations correctly. If with antihypertensive therapy we find a reduction of cardiac mass as compared with untreated controls, it is fair to ascribe a *reversal* or *regression* of cardiac mass. But if there is no further increase in cardiac mass while the untreated control hypertensive animals increase cardiac mass, this is more precisely termed a *lack of progression*.

Other Pitfalls

The clinician and laboratory investigator must be precise in comparing data from different studies carried out under different conditions. Just as the mechanisms operating in the development of hypertrophy may be highly variable depending up on the type of hypertension, the underlying mechanisms of the hypertension, the rapidity in the development of hypertension, and the associated pathophysiological conditions, so are the mechanisms and conditions important in the reverse of this process. Most experimental studies concerned with the regression of left ventricular mass have been carried out over a relatively short term of therapy (i.e., 3–4 weeks) in the rat. Since the normal life span in the rat is approximately 3 years, and 2 years in the SHR, the foreshortening of life span closely approximates the natural history of the patient with essential hypertension [14]. Thus, a 4-week treatment period in the SHR is roughly equivalent to half a year of constant pharmacologic therapy in man. Moreover, a number of studies in man have demonstrated a reduction in measurements of wall thicknesses and cardiac dimensions well within that time.

Factors Favoring Increased Cardiac Mass in Hypertension

Preliminary laboratory and clinical studies concerned with the SHR and the essential hypertensive patient prompted us to report that a number of factors might be implicated in the development of cardiac enlargement in hypertension [15]. Subsequently, a number of reports have emanated from our laboratory and others that have supported the contention that in addition to the hemodynamic factors associated with the progressively increasing left ventricular afterload imposed upon the left ventricle, other mechanisms are involved in experimental forms of hypertension and in man with essential and other forms of hypertension. Factors involved in the development, maintenance, and regression of experimental and clinical left ventricular hypertrophy associated with arterial hypertension include the following [1–4]:

1. Hemodynamic factors, such as pressure overload, volume overload, augmented ventricular contractility, faster heart rate, and increased total peripheral resistance
2. Humoral (or pressor) factors, such as catecholamines, angiotensin system, or other hormones (e.g., steroids, thyroid, growth)
3. Race
4. Aging
5. Collagen deposition
6. Coexistent diseases, such as atherosclerosis, obesity, diabetes mellitus, or myocardiopathies
7. Antihypertensive therapy

Studies have indicated that cardiac enlargement and regression with therapy varies with the sex of the experimentally hypertensive animal [16, 17]. The race of a patient with essential hypertension also imparts an important determinant on the relationship between the mass of the left ventricle and the hemodynamic alterations in essential hypertension. Thus, a direct relationship between height of arterial pressure and cardiac mass was demonstrated in the black patient, but not in the white [18]. In addition, if the subject is obese, an added factor of volume overload associated with obesity produces an additional structural adaptation in the left ventricle. Thus, the pressure-overloaded left ventricle in hypertension adapts by a concentric form of hypertrophy [19]; the volume overload associated with obesity promotes an eccentric component to this hypertrophy process [20–22]. This dimorphic response to the hypertrophy of the left ventricle in obesity-hypertension may explain the greater cardiovascular morbidity and mortality in this condition [23]. Other studies have shown a definite relationship between age and the development of left ventricular enlargement, even in normotensive individuals [24]. And even when certain pressor substances are infused in subpressor doses or administered to ventricular myocytes in tissue culture, left ventricular hypertrophy is initiated [25–27]. These similar factors presumably are equally important in the regression of left ventricular hypertrophy in addition to consideration of the nature of the therapeutic intervention (e.g., removal of the possible initiating factors such as a clip on the renal artery or the type of antihypertensive pharmacologic agent).

Reversal of Cardiac Enlargement

A standard experimental approach for determining the systemic and regional hemodynamic effects of antihypertensive drugs was deemed necessary if we are to be able to arrive at meaningful comparisons of these agents. Early reports on the effects of prolonged antihypertensive therapy demonstrated regression of cardiac mass, but multiple drugs were administered [28]. Other studies also demonstrated regression of cardiac mass, but treatment was prolonged and the long-term hemodynamic effects could have masked the more immediate effects of the pharmacologic agent in myocardial protein synthesis [28, 29].

A Model

In order to obtain comparable data from one study to another designed to determine the hemodynamic and cardiac structural effects of various antihypertensive agents, we developed an experimental protocol. Our studies employed normotensive Wistar-Kyoto (WKY) and SHR male rats whose ages were between 16 and 20 weeks. The rats were treated daily with an antihypertensive drug provided either in their drinking (tap) water or administered by gastric tube feedings. The control WKY and SHR rats received no therapy. After 3–4 weeks of continuous therapy, catheters were placed into left ventricle and abdominal aorta and into a femoral vein for injection of radioactively tagged microspheres (15 μm in diameter), withdrawal of blood for determination of cardiac output, and administration of other agents (if necessary), respectively [30–32]. Cardiac output was determined using the reference method by withdrawal of aortic blood over a fixed time. Since the number of microspheres and radioactivity injected were known and the total radioactivity of the withdrawn arterial blood was determined, cardiac output could be calculated [31]. Moreover, by determining the radioactivity of microspheres in each organ removed and weighed at the conclusion of each study, organ hemodynamics could be determined.

In other studies involving normotensive WKY rats receiving a sham operation or a similar procedure, but with the placement of a silver clip around a renal artery, the effects of either the later surgical removal of the clip or antihypertensive therapy could be determined [5]. In addition, it was also possible in these studies to determine the pumping ability of the left ventricle by placing an electromagnetic flow probe around the aorta in order to determine the maximum cardiac output achieved during the rapid infusion of Tyrode's solution over a 1-min interval [33].

Using these or similar methods, there were no effects noted with the short-term or more prolonged administration of diuretics in studies from a number of laboratories. However, the effects of other agents have provided more meaningful data and have stimulated new work concerning the development and regression of left ventricular hypertrophy. This review deals with only those agents studied in experimental hypertension, excluding all clinical studies.

Vasodilators

A wide variety of antihypertensive agents dilate arterioles: the adrenergic inhibitors, angiotensin-converting enzyme (ACE) inhibitors, the calcium entry blocking drugs, and the direct acting vascular smooth muscle relaxants. These categories will be considered separately, and this section concerns the latter group of agents that includes hydralazine and minoxidil.

Studies from several laboratories have failed to demonstrate a regression of cardiac mass in the SHR with hydralazine or minoxidil treatment [34–36]. In fact, in one study the left ventricular mass to body weight ratio actually increased in the normotensive WKY rats; this was associated with an increased myocardial blood flow [36]. In both strains, coronary vascular resistance decreased.

Beta-Adrenergic Receptor Blocking Agents

The data concerning the effects of the beta-blocking drugs on cardiac mass in experimental forms of hypertension have been confusing. Most reports indicate that these agents (e.g., propranolol, timolol, sotalol) do not reduce arterial pressure [16, 37]. But even in these studies, the sex of the animal was an important determinant on the hemodynamic and cardiac mass responses. Thus, when male rats were treated from conception there was no reduction in pressure, but the ratio of left ventricular mass to body weight decreased, while the female rats demonstrated the converse effects [16].

Peripheral Adrenergic Inhibitors

As indicated above, prolonged treatment for up to 1 year produced a decrease in cardiac mass when the SHR was treated with reserpine, hydrochlorothiazide, and hydralazine [28], or when treated with guanethidine [29]. However, when the SHR was treated with the postsynaptic alpha$_1$-receptor inhibitor or with the more complex agent urapidil, there were no changes in cardiac mass [38, 39].

Centrally Active Adrenergic Inhibitors

A large number of experimental studies have demonstrated a decrease in cardiac mass with methyldopa therapy [5, 34–36, 40–43]. The earlier studies demonstrated a reduced cardiac mass that was related to a decreased amount of cardiac muscle protein and an increased proportion of collagen [35, 40, 41], suggesting a true loss of muscle mass with treatment. These studies with methyldopa showed reversal in the SHR [35, 40, 41] as well as in 2K,1C-GH rats [5, 42].

Similar findings were reported from our laboratory in SHR and 2K,1C-GH rats [5, 36, 43]. These studies showed further that treatment with clonidine, an agent with similar pharmacologic actions, produced the same hemodynamic changes as methyldopa. However, only methyldopa reduced cardiac mass. Moreover, the decreased heart weight was also observed in the normotensive WKY which demonstrated no change in arterial pressure [36, 43]. However, when the dose of clonidine was tripled, arterial pressure and total peripheral resistance increased, most likely as a result of the peripheral alpha-receptor agonistic effects; and with this dose, cardiac mass decreased. These findings suggested a dissociation between the pharmacologic and hemodynamic effects of these agents from their effects on reducing cardiac mass. It was of further interest that the D-isomer of methyldopa failed to decrease cardiac mass. Finally, there was no change in myocardial blood flow associated with the regression in cardiac mass with methyldopa.

Thus, despite the more salutary hemodynamic effects of the direct-acting smooth muscle vasodilators (hydralazine and minoxidil) than of the centrally acting agents, cardiac mass failed to change with the former agents, but decreased with the latter agents – even in those rats demonstrating no hemodynamic changes.

Angiotensin-Converting Enzyme Inhibitors

In one study, SHR demonstrated a reduced cardiac mass with captopril treatment [44]. This decrease in cardiac mass was confirmed clinically [45]. However, we failed to demonstrate a decreased cardiac mass with enalapril [46], although this was observed clinically in our patients with essential hypertension [47].

Calcium Entry Blocking Drugs

It is probably inappropriate to consider calcium entry blocking drugs as a homogeneous pharmacologic entity. The hemodynamic effects (systemically and regionally) are quite different among the various agents in this group. We have studied two of these, diltiazem and nitrendipine, in the SHR and have observed highly variable hemodynamic changes as well as disparate effects on cardiac mass. In general, the calcium entry blocking drugs reduce arterial pressure through a decrease in total peripheral resistance; however, their effects on the regional circulations have been quite variable depending upon the hemodynamic agent studied [48, 49]. For example nitrendipine produced renovasodilation, but diltiazem did not. The effects of these compounds also produced disparate effects on cardiac mass: nitrendipine decreased cardiac mass, but diltiazem did not. Both agents were administered for the same duration; both agents produced similar systemic hemodynamic effects – but only nitrendipine decreased cardiac mass. It is of further interest that the reduced cardiac mass occurred in the normotensive WKY as well as the SHR.

Effects of Regression on Cardiac Performance

Pumping Ability of the Heart

As indicated above, in some studies the performance of the heart with and without hypertrophy, as well as after regression of hypertrophy, was assessed by determining the maximum pumping ability of the heart during a rapid 1-min infusion of Tyrode's solution or whole blood. The technique has been employed by several laboratories since we adapted it for the rat with hypertension [33]. Utilizing this method, we showed that the normotensive Wistar rat, made hypertensive by placing a clip on one renal artery (2K,1C-GH) demonstrated decreased pumping ability as compared with sham-operated normotensive controls [5, 50]. However, when this hypertension was treated by surgically unclipping the renal artery or by administering methyldopa, normal pumping ability and cardiac performance were restored [5].

However, in earlier studies involving the SHR, we had demonstrated that normal pumping ability was maintained until the rats were past 80 weeks of age [33]. Thus, differences do exist between the cardiac performance of the 2K,1C-GH and SHR with advanced left ventricular hypertrophy. Moreover, in long-term treatment studies with guanethidine or hydralazine, normal pumping ability was preserved even with regression of the hypertrophy process [29].

Questions

Notwithstanding these findings, several important questions remain concerning the findings of normal cardiac performance in hypertensive rats following regression of hypertrophy. First, pumping ability was assessed following regression of hypertrophy, but while arterial pressure was at normal levels, either because a renal arterial clip had been removed or because the antihypertensive effects of the pharmacologic agents persisted until the time of the performance studies, we do not know how well the heart of a hypertensive animal would perform if arterial pressure were to increase to levels observed prior to the institution of antihypertensive therapy. Second, since the heart with regression of myocardial hypertrophy has an increased percentage (by weight) of collagen, would it demonstrate normal pumping ability at its more "natural" increased resting pressures?

Third, how applicable are these findings in the clinical setting to the patient with essential hypertension with left ventricular hypertrophy? Under these circumstances, the process of ventricular hypertrophy takes place over the prolonged natural history of hypertensive cardiovascular disease. The cardiac adaptation is able to provide a long-term state of stable hyperfunction, as described by Meerson [51]. The increase in arterial pressure and left ventricular afterload is slow but unrelenting; and cardiac failure only supervenes when the ventricle can no longer adapt to the increased work and other stress imposed upon it. However, in the experimental (and even clinical) situations [47, 52], regression of ventricular mass can take place in a matter of a few weeks. Thus, in the situation where a patient whose hypertension was severe prior to initiation of therapy suddenly discontinues antihypertensive medications, and the arterial pressure suddenly and precipitously rises, will the ventricular performance under this situation be normal [53]? Is it possible that performance may remain normal while arterial pressure remains controlled, though not when pressure rises with discontinuance of therapy in the heart with regressed hypertrophy? The "acid test" of the cardiac performance must be assessed at the elevated pressure levels. As of this date, no data are available to answer this critical question.

Several subordinate questions are related to the foregoing major concerns. Will the left ventricle that had been hypertrophied followed by regression hypertrophy again? Will this rehypertrophied heart perform normally? What are the biochemical and physiological characteristics of the myocardium with hypertrophy? Are they similar to those of the normal ventricular myocardium? I am certain that as well as these, still other questions will arise as answers are provided. However, one underlying and nagging question remains to be answered after reviewing the above findings: If altered hemodynamic functions are not the sole explanation for the development of left ventricular hypertrophy (experimentally or clinically) and not the sole explanation for its regression with pharmacotherapy – what are these factors?

Mechanisms of Regression

It is of interest that those agents that reduced cardiac mass appeared to affect only myocardial protein synthesis; the mass of other organs was unchanged [5, 36, 43, 48]. A variety of mechanisms have been offered to explain the reduced cardiac mass, including stimulation of the renin-angiotensin system, the adrenergic nervous system, or perhaps inhibition of calcium entry [48]. Tissue culture studies have shown that angiotensin II initiates protein synthesis [27]; and infusion of norepinephrine and other adrenergic agents in subpressor amounts will also initiate ventricular hypertrophy [25, 26]. It is clear that our understanding of this phenomenon is only beginning. Until we understand the cellular biological mechanisms that underlie protein synthesis and those mechanisms that transduce the physiological signal of pressure overload to the biochemical response of myocardial protein synthesis, our understanding will remain incomplete.

References

1. Frohlich ED (1983) The heart in hypertension. In: Genest J, Kuchel O, Hamet P, Cantin M (eds) Hypertension: Physiopathology and treatment, 2nd edn. McGraw-Hill, New York, pp 791–810
2. Frohlich ED (1983) Hemodynamics and other determinants in development of left ventricular hypertrophy: Conflicting factors in its regression. Fed Proc 42:2709–2715
3. Frohlich ED (1983) Physiological considerations in left ventricular hypertrophy. Am J Med 75(3A):94–99
4. Frohlich ED (1983) Cardiac hypertrophy: Stimuli and mechanisms. In: Sleight P (ed) Scientific foundations of cardiology. Heinemann, London, pp 182–190
5. Kuwajima I, Kardon MB, Pegram BL, Sesoko S, Frohlich ED (1982) Regression of left ventricular hypertrophy in two-kidney, one clip Goldblatt hypertension. Hypertension 4:113–118
6. Ungerleider HE, Clark CP (1939) Study of the transverse diameter of the heart silhouette with prediction table based on the teleroentgenogram. Am Heart J 17:92–102
7. Ungerleider HE (1947) Cardiac enlargement. Radiology 48:129–142

8. Frohlich ED, Tarazi RC, Dustan HP (1971) Clinical-physiological correlations in the development of hypertensive heart disease. Circulation 44:446–455
9. Frohlich ED (1982) Hemodynamic factors in the pathogenesis and maintenance of hypertension. Fed Proc 41:2400–2408
10. Frohlich ED (1977) Haemodynamics of hypertension. In: Genest J, Koiw E, Kuchel O (eds) Hypertension: Physiopathology and treatment. McGraw-Hill, New York, pp 15–49
11. Ibrahim MM, Tarazi RC, Dustan HP, Gifford RW Jr (1977) Electrocardiogram in evaluation of resistance to antihypertensive therapy. Arch Intern Med 137:1125–1129
12. Georgopoulos AJ, Vlastaris PA, Proudfit WJ (1961) R-wave voltage changes in relation to arterial pressure in hypertensive patients. Cleve Clin Q 28:46–51
13. Dunn FG, Chandraratna P, de Carvalho JGR, Basta LL, Frohlich ED (1977) Pathophysiologic assessment of hypertensive heart disease with echocardiography. Am J Cardiol 39:789–795
14. Trippodo NC, Frohlich ED (1981) Controversies in cardiovascular research. Similarities of genetic (spontaneous) hypertension: Man and rat. Circ Res 48:309–319
15. Frohlich ED, Tarazi RC (1979) Is arterial pressure the sole factor responsible for hypertensive cardiac hypertrophy? Am J Cardiol 44:959–963
16. Pfeffer MA, Pfeffer JM, Weiss AK, Frohlich ED (1977) Development of SHR hypertension and cardiac hypertrophy during prolonged beta-blocking therapy. Am J Physiol 232:H639–H643
17. Cambotti LJ, Cole FE, Gerall AA, Frohlich ED, MacPhee AA (1984) Neonatal gonadal hormones and blood pressure in the spontaneously hypertensive rat. Am J Physiol 247:E258–E264
18. Dunn FG, Oigman W, Sundgaard-Riise K, Messerli FH, Ventura HO, Reisin E, Frohlich ED (1983) Racial differences in cardiac adaptation to essential hypertension determined by echocardiographic indexes. J Am Coll Cardiol 1:1348–1351
19. Linzbach AJ (1969) Heart failure from the point of view of quantitative anatomy. Am J Cardiol 5:370–382
20. Messerli FH, Sundgaard-Riise K, Reisin E, Dreslinski GR, Dunn FG, Frohlich ED (1983) Disparate cardiovascular effects of obesity and arterial hypertension. Am J Med 74:808–812
21. Frohlich ED, Messerli FH, Reisin E, Dunn FG (1983) The problem of obesity and hypertension. Hypertension 5:III 71–III 78
22. Reisin E, Frohlich ED, Messerli FH, Dreslinski GR, Dunn FG, Jones MM, Batson HM Jr (1983) Cardiovascular changes after weight reduction in obesity hypertension. Ann Intern Med 98:315–319
23. Kannel W, Braud N, Skinner J, Dawber T, McNamara P (1967) Relation of adiposity to blood pressure and development of hypertension: The Framingham Study. Ann Intern Med 67:48–59
24. Lakatta ED (1979) Alterations in the cardiovascular system that occur in advanced age. Fed Proc 38:163–167
25. Gordon AL, Inchiosa MA Jr, Lehr D (1972) Isoproterenol-induced cardiomegaly: Assessment of myocardial protein content, actomyosin ATPase and heart rate. J Mol Cell Cardiol 4:545–557
26. Szakacs JE, Mehlman B (1960) Pathologic changes induced by l-norepinephrine: Quantitative aspects. Am J Cardiol 5:619–627
27. Khairallah PA, Robertson AL, Davila D (1972) Effects of angiotensin II on DNA, RNA, and protein synthesis. In: Genest J, Koiw E (eds) Hypertension '72. Springer, Berlin Heidelberg New York, pp 212–220
28. Freis ED, Regan D, Pillsbury H III, Mathews M (1972) Alterations of the course of hypertension in the spontaneously hypertensive rat. Circ Res 31:1–7
29. Pfeffer JM, Pfeffer MA, Fletcher P, Fishbein M, Braunwald E (1982) Favorable effects of therapy on cardiac performance in spontaneously hypertensive rats. Am J Physiol 242:H776–H784
30. Nishiyama K, Nishiyama A, Frohlich ED (1976) Regional blood flow in normotensive and spontaneously hypertensive rats. Am J Physiol 230:691–698
31. Tsuchiya M, Walsh GM, Frohlich ED (1977) Systemic hemodynamic effects of microspheres in conscious rats. Am J Physiol 233:H617–H621
32. Ishise S, Pegram BL, Yamamoto J, Kitamura Y, Frohlich ED (1980) Reference sample microsphere method: Cardiac output and blood flows in conscious rats. Am J Physiol 239:H443–H449
33. Pfeffer MA, Pfeffer JM, Frohlich ED (1976) Pumping ability of the hypertrophying left ventricle of the spontaneously hypertensive rat. Circ Res 38:423–429
34. Sen S, Tarazi RC, Khairallah PA, Bumpus FM (1974) Cardiac hypertrophy in spontaneously hypertensive rats. Circ Res 35:775–781

35. Sen S, Tarazi RC, Khairallah PA, Bumpus FM (1976) Cardiac hypertrophy and its reversal by antihypertensive drugs in spontaneously hypertensive rats (SHR). Clin Exp Pharmacol Physiol 3:173–177
36. Pegram BL, Ishise S, Frohlich ED (1982) Effect of methyldopa, clonidine, and hydralazine on cardiac mass and haemodynamics in Wistar-Kyoto and spontaneously hypertensive rats. Cardiovasc Res 16:40–46
37. Pfeffer MA, Frohlich ED, Pfeffer JM, Weiss AK (1974) Pathophysiological implications of the increased cardiac output of young spontaneously hypertensive rats. Circ Res 34(1):235–244
38. Kobrin I, Gallo AJ, Pegram BL, Duckworth D, Frohlich ED (1984) Urapidil in normotensive and spontaneously hypertensive rats: Systemic and regional hemodynamics, cardiac mass, and arterial baroreflex sensitivity. J Hypertens 2:317–320
39. Pegram BL, Kobrin I, Natsume T, Gallo AJ, Frohlich ED (1984) Systemic and regional hemodynamic effects of acute and prolonged treatment with urapidil or prazosin in normotensive and spontaneously hypertensive rats. Am J Med 77(4A):64–73
40. Sen S, Bumpus FM (1979) Collagen synthesis in development and reversal of cardiac hypertrophy in spontaneously hypertensive rats. Am J Cardiol 44:954–958
41. Sen S, Tarazi RC, Bumpus FM (1976) Biochemical changes associated with development and reversal of cardiac hypertrophy in spontaneously hypertensive rats. Cardiovasc Res 10:254–261
42. Sen S, Tarazi RC, Bumpus FM (1981) Reversal of cardiac hypertrophy in renal hypertensive rats: medical vs surgical therapy. Am J Physiol 240:H408–H412
43. Ishise S, Pegram BL, Frohlich ED (1980) Disparate effects of methyldopa and clonidine on cardiac mass and haemodynamics in rats. Clin Sci [Suppl 6] 59:449s–452s
44. Pfeffer JM, Pfeffer MA, Mirsky I, Braunwald E (1982) Regression of left ventricular hypertrophy and prevention of left ventricular dysfunction by captopril in the spontaneously hypertensive rat. Proc Natl Acad Sci USA 79:3310–3314
45. Mujais SK, Tarazi RC, Fouad FM, Bravo EL (1983) Reversal of left ventricular hypertrophy with captopril. Clin Cardiol 6:595–602
46. Pegram BL, Frohlich ED (1982) Immediate systemic and regional hemodynamic effects of MK-421 converting enzyme inhibitor in conscious Wistar-Kyoto and spontaneously hypertensive rats. In: Rascher W, Clough D, Genton D (eds) Hypertensive mechanisms of the spontaneously hypertensive rat as a model for human hypertension. Schattauer, Stuttgart, pp 677–680
47. Dunn FG, Oigman W, Ventura HO, Messerli FH, Kobrin I, Frohlich ED (1984) Enalapril improves systemic and renal hemodynamics and allows regression of left ventricular mass in essential hypertension. Am J Cardiol 53:105–108
48. Kobrin I, Sesoko S, Pegram BL, Frohlich ED (1984) Reduced cardiac mass by nitrendipine is dissociated from systemic or regional haemodynamic changes in rats. Cardiovasc Res 3:158–162
49. Frohlich ED (1985) Hemodynamic effects of calcium entry blocking agents in normal and hypertensive rat and man. Am J Cardiol 56:21H–27H
50. Spech M, Ferrario CM, Tarazi RC (1980) Cardiac pumping ability following reversal of hypertrophy and hypertension in spontaneously hypertensive rats. Hypertension 2:75–82
51. Meerson FZ (1969) The myocardium in hyperfunction, hypertrophy and heart failure. Circ Res 25(2):1–163
52. Ventura HO, Frohlich ED, Messerli FH, Kobrin I, Kardon MB (1984) Immediate regional blood flow distribution following angiotensin converting enzyme inhibition in patients with essential hypertension. Am J Med 76:58–61
53. Frohlich ED (1984) Clinical conference: Hypertensive cardiovascular disease. A pathophysiological assessment. Hypertension 6:934–939

Reversal of Left Ventricular and Coronary Hypertrophy Following Antihypertensive Treatment

B. E. Strauer[1], M. Klepzig[1], and W. Motz[1]

Hypertensive Hypertrophy

The heart in hypertension is seen by the clinician in the following three forms: (a) as regular or concentric, (b) as irregular or asymmetric, and (c) as exhibiting dilatative or eccentric left ventricular hypertrophy [17, 19] (Figs. 1 and 2).

As a result of long-standing arterial pressure, concentric myocardial hypertrophy with thickening of the left ventricular (LV) walls, increase in LV total muscle mass, and increment in mass-volume-ratio develops. Due to the resulting constancy in systolic wall stress, i.e., LV afterload, cardiac index, and LV ejection fractions remain normal. Significant alterations in myocardial oxygen demand do not occur. However, coronary resistance is already increased and coronary reserve is markedly impaired even in young hypertensive patients [17, 19, 22].

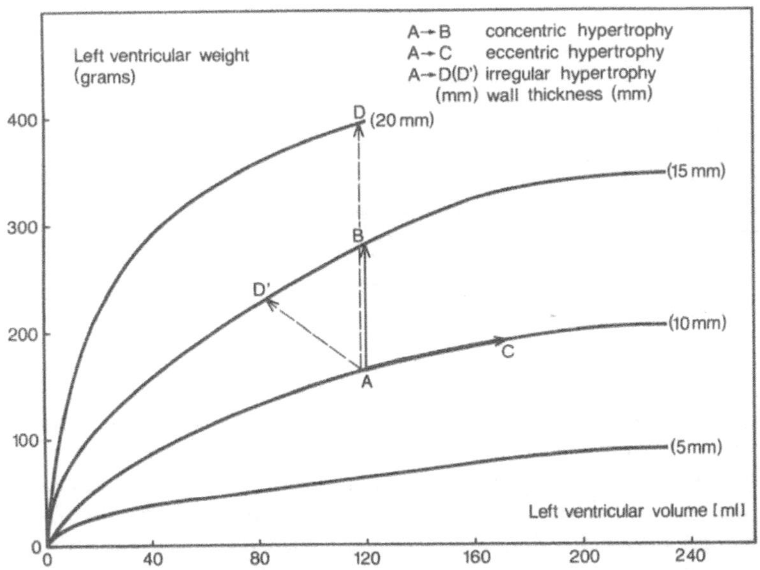

Fig. 1. Classification of left ventricular hypertrophy on the basis of geometric factors: concentric-excentric-irregular left ventricular hypertrophy

[1] Department of Medicine, University of Marburg, Baldingerstrasse, D-3550 Marburg.

Primary Hypertension
Ed. by W. Kaufmann et al.

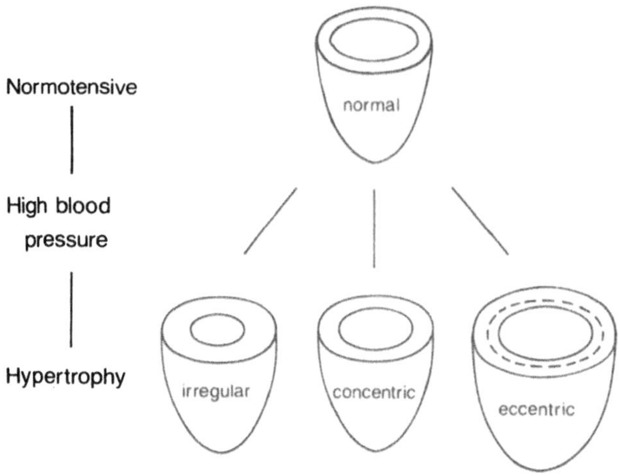

blood pressure	↑	↑	↑
wall thickness	↑↑	↑	→ (↑↓)
ventricular mass ventricular radius	↑ ↓	↑ →	↑ ↑
end-diastolic volume	→↓	→↓	↑
LVMM/EDV	↑↑	↑	→↓
systolic wall stress	↓↓	→	↑
cardiac index ejection fraction	→↓ →↓	→ →	↓ ↓
myocardial oxygen consumption	→↓	→	↑
coronary resistance coronary reserve	↑ ↓	↑ ↓	↑ ↓↓

Fig. 2. Clinical manifestations of the heart in hypertension

In the case of a long-standing pressure load with progressive left ventricular hypertrophy and interstitial myocardial fibrosis, in the presence of coronary artery disease and noncardiac diseases, as well as concomitant myocarditis, myocardial damage with an increase in LV radius, increase in end-diastolic volume, and rise in systolic wall stress may occur. The left ventricle dilates in an eccentric manner. LV pumping indexes, such as cardiac index and ejection fraction, decrease and myocardial oxygen consumption per mass unit rises. As in the case of the other forms of hypertensive hypertrophy, coronary resistance increases due to the rise of its vascular component (hypertensive macro- and microangiopathy). The myocardial factor is also important.

In 14% of cases, patients with arterial hypertension have asymetric ventricular hypertrophy [19]. In the irregularly hypertrophied ventricle, the maximal end-systolic wall thickness is increased by 133% in comparison with normal regions that show only a 58% increase. Cineangiographically, the ventricles look the same as they do in hypertrophic obstructive cardiomyopathy (HOCM). However, an intraventricular obstruction cannot be demonstrated. Since essential hypertension is a widespread disease, essential arterial hypertension represents the most common cause of irregular or asymmetric myocardial hypertrophy [20].

The three forms of left ventricular hypertrophy can develop consecutively (concentric-irregular; concentric-eccentric; irregular-eccentric). All forms may also develop primarily. Consequently, one of these three forms has to be expected when examining a hypertensive patient [17].

Hypertrophy and Heart Failure

The transition from hypertensive hypertrophy to congestive heart failure is caused by numerous, partially still unidentified, mechanisms [3, 20]. Some of these are: excessive left ventricular pressure load with myocardial ischemia and focal necrosis; impairment of O_2 diffusion due to an enlargement of the O_2-diffusion distance between capillary and myocardial cell; reduction of the protein synthesis as well as alterations in the myosin-isoenzyme pattern (V_{1-3}) (until now only experimentally verified); increment in myocardial collagen concentration; decrement in the myosin-ATPase-activity. All these potential mechanisms lead to decrease in myocardial working capacity. Another mechanism, which is important for the pathogenesis of the hypertensive heart failure is the left ventricular dilation due to the chronic pressure load. An increase in left ventricular volume goes along with an increase in left ventricular systolic wall stress, i.e., left ventricular afterload even in the presence of a normotensive systolic blood pressure. An increment in systolic wall stress is almost regularly associated with a decrease in left ventricular function [17, 19]. Accordingly, in the case of hypertensive crisis, a critical or limited O_2 supply may occur.

Hypertrophy and Coronary Circulation

Hypertensive hypertrophy effects not only ventricular myocardium, but also the coronary artery system (Fig. 3). The concentric hypertrophied, "coronary healthy" heart in hypertension presents a significant reduction in coronary reserve (30%–35%) [17, 19, 22] (Fig. 4). With the simultaneous existence of coronary stenosis, impairment of the coronary reserve progressively rises.

Since in the presence of a normal coronary angiography the macroscopically determinable coronary factor is not related to the extent of impairment of the coronary reserve, one can conclude that the increment in the coronary resistance has been caused by a disturbance in the coronary regulation due to involvement, i.e., media-hypertrophy of the small intramurally located coronary resistance vessels [22]. Consequently, in arterial hypertension the left ventricle has to be considered potentially ischemic even with a normal coronary angiogram [22].

The impairment of coronary reserve in these patients reflects the clinical experience; patients with essential hypertension and a normal coronary angiogram may

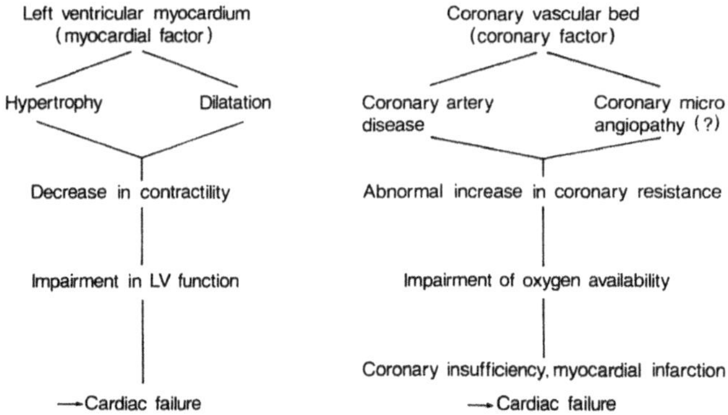

Fig. 3. Cardiac manifestations of arterial hypertension: ventricular myocardium/coronary artery system

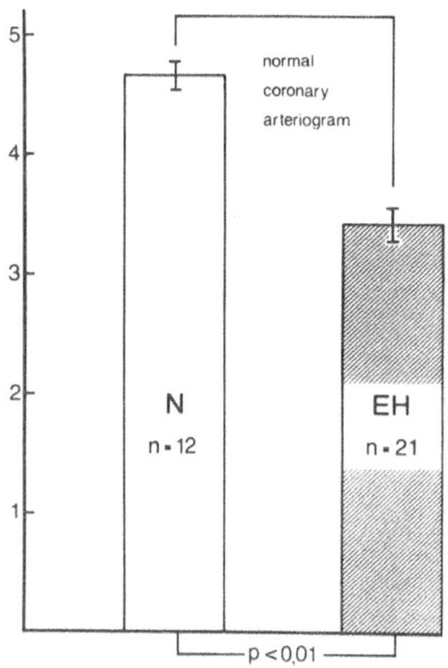

Fig. 4. Coronary reserve (R_{cor}/R_{cor^*}) of normotensive and hypertensive patients with a normal coronary angiogram. *N*, normal; *EH*, essential hypertension

have clinical symptoms which are similar to patients who have a pathological coronary angiogram. Moreover, chronic or sudden blood pressure rises lead to an increase in myocardial oxygen demand, which can be so extensive that myocardial ischemia occurs. Both factors – the impairment of coronary regulation and the increase of the myocardial energy demand – contribute to the pathogenesis of angina in patients with essential hypertension and a normal coronary angiogram.

Based on our experience of 52 patients with essential hypertension, left ventricular hypertrophy and a normal coronary angiogram, about 70% complained of angina

Table 1. Problems and aims of reversal of left ventricular hypertrophy by long-term therapy

1.	Specific mechanism? Unspecific, pressure-independent reduction of LV afterload?
2.	Improvement of LV function? Prevention of hypertensive heart failure?
3.	Normalization of coronary resistance? Improvement of coronary reserve?

pectoris. In the case of severe left ventricular hypertrophy (mass/volume ratio >2.0–2.2), this percentage rose to about 80% [17, 19].

Reversal of Left Ventricular Hypertrophy – Therapeutic Aims

In hypertensive patients left ventricular function may be impaired by at least two factors:

1. Chronic or acute increases in blood pressure result in left ventricular hypertrophy; in later stages left ventricular dilatation, an increase in systolic wall stress, and myocardial oxygen consumption are present. Accordingly, myocardial ischemia may occur.

2. Due to hypertensive small vessel disease, coronary reserve is reduced and myocardial oxygen supply may be impaired.

Both, the myocardial and the coronary factor are closely connected with each other.

From the therapeutic point of view, normalization of left ventricular pressure overload must be achieved. Through blood pressure control both development of left ventricular hypertrophy and heart failure should be prevented. Coronary reserve and coronary vascular resistance should become normal. Treating high blood pressure means treating the etiology of the myocardial and coronary factor in hypertensive heart failure (Table 1).

Regression of Left Ventricular Hypertrophy from the Clinical Point of View

Most important for regression of left ventricular hypertrophy is the control of blood pressure. Regression of left ventricular hypertrophy without lowering blood pressure has not yet been reported. This does not exclude the fact that drug-specific effects play a role: the same reduction in blood pressure can result in different degrees of regression of left ventricular hypertrophy. On the other hand, in normotensive subjects with hypertrophic cardiomyopathies regression in myocardial hypertrophy can be achieved without reduction in blood pressure.

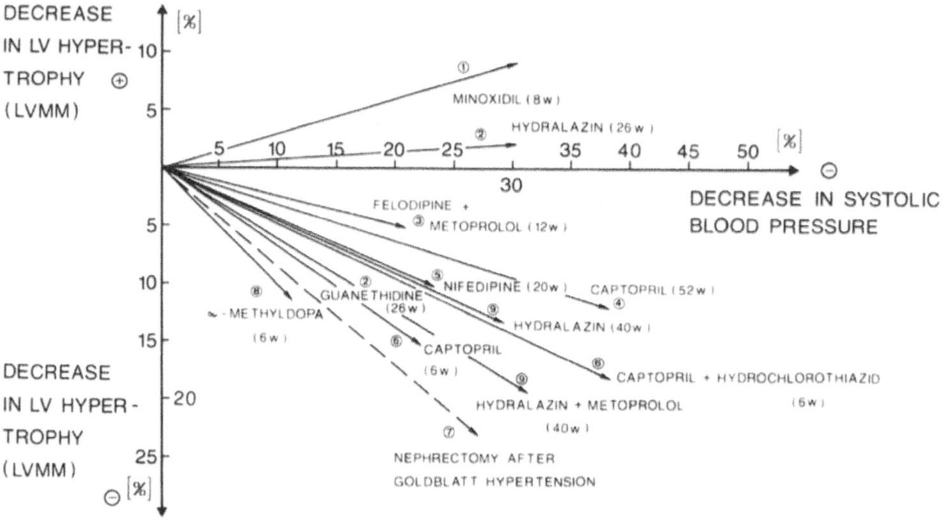

Fig. 5. Relation between blood pressure reduction due to drug therapy and corresponding alterations of cardiac hypertrophy (experimental data): *1,* Sen et al. [13]; *2,* Pfeffer et al. [10]; *3,* Lundin and Hallbäck-Nordlander [6]; *4,* Pfeffer et al. [11]; *5,* Motz et al. [8]; *6,* Sen et al. [14]; *7,* Sen et al. [15]; *8,* Spech et al. [16]; *9,* Motz and Strauer [7]

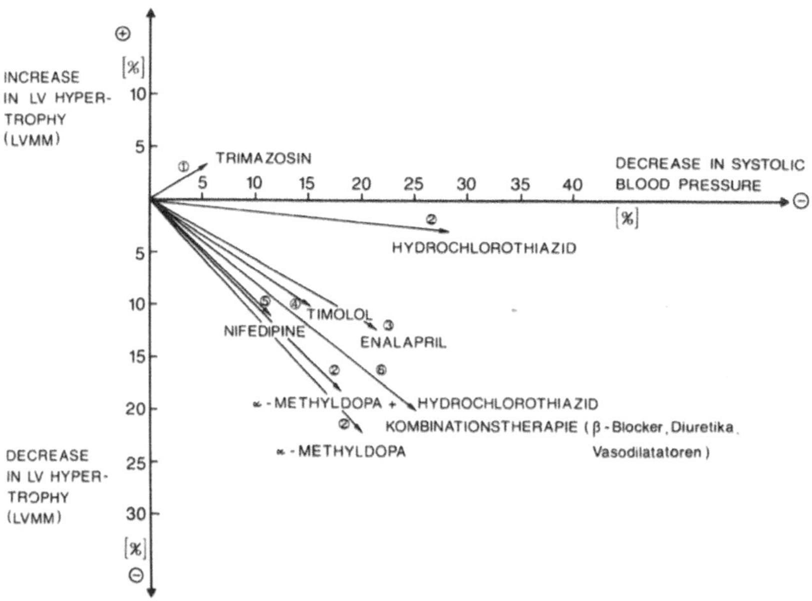

Fig. 6. Relation between blood pressure reduction due to drug therapy and corresponding alterations of cardiac hypertrophy (clinical data): *1,* Drayer et al. [1]; *2,* Wollam et al. [23]; *3,* Nakashima et al. [9]; *4,* Rowlands et al. [12]; *5,* Strauer et al. [21]; *6,* Dunn et al. [2]

Experimental Studies

In the model of the spontaneously hypertensive rat (SHR), many authors showed reduction in blood pressure, although the regression in myocardial hypertrophy varied greatly (Figs. 5 and 6). This variation can be explained by the differences in doses, duration of therapy, way the drugs were given, and differences between SHR species. There are prevention and regression studies. Nevertheless, some statements can be made: monotherapy with diuretics or beta-blockers resulted in good control over blood pressure, but there was only a slight regression in hypertrophy. Beta-blockers in combination with hydralazine can be effective in controlling blood pressure and left ventricular hypertrophy. Concerning left ventricular function, excellent results were obtained with calcium channel blockers (nifedipine, verapamil) (Tables 2, 3) and alpha-methyldopa.

Regression in Coronary Small Vessels Disease

Coronary circulation is impaired in hypertensive heart disease, while coronary reserve is reduced. In the experimental model of SHR, similar changes were found: the minimal coronary vascular resistance, an indicator for the vasodilatating capacity, is already significantly increased at the age of 10 weeks [5].

In a prevention study, SHR were treated from the 5th to the 65th week of age with metoprolol, hydralazine, or both drugs simultaneously. Blood pressure was well

Table 2. Changes in LV function and geometry during high-dose nifedipine therapy ($n=5$)

	Before nifedipine	After nifedipine	P
P_{syst} (mm Hg)	138 ± 33	137 ± 23	NS
HR (min^{-1})	62 ± 28	64 ± 6	NS
CI ($l\ min^{-1}\ m^{-2}$)	2.39 ± 2.18	2.74 ± 1.5	NS
SVI ($ml\ beat\ s^{-1}\ m^{-2}$)	33.1 ± 17.1	42 ± 20.8	<0.1
EDV (ml)	79 ± 39	95 ± 45	NS
ESV (ml)	21 ± 14	22 ± 15	NS
EF (%)	73 ± 9	77 ± 12	NS
MNSER ($vol\ s^{-1}$)	2.37 ± 0.8	2.64 ± 0.78	NS
V_{CF} (s^{-1})	1.29 ± 0.49	1.44 ± 0.57	<0.1
d_{LPW} (mm)	12.2 ± 1.9	11.2 ± 0.8	NS
d_{IVS} (mm)	15.2 ± 3.0	12.8 ± 1.8	<0.05
LVMM (g)	218 ± 50	198 ± 59	<0.05
LVMM/EDV ($g\ ml^{-1}$)	2.76 ± 1.04	2.08 ± 0.41	<0.01
d/r	0.58 ± 0.14	0.40 ± 0.12	<0.01
T_{syst} ($10^3\ dyn\ cm^{-2}$)	241 ± 178	279 ± 171	NS

$\bar{x} \pm SD$

Table 3. LV function and LV hypertrophy of 12 patients with hypertensive LV hypertrophy during high-dose nifedipine therapy

	Before nifedipine	After nifedipine	*P*
P_{syst} (mm Hg)	169 ± 35	151 ± 15	<0.05
HR (min^{-1})	65 ± 21	66 ± 8	NS
CI ($l\ min^{-1}\ m^{-2}$)	1.94 ± 1.53	2.19 ± 1.25	<0.05
SVI ($ml\ beat\ s^{-1}\ m^{-2}$)	27.1 ± 13.4	32.5 ± 16.6	<0.05
EDV (ml)	70 ± 30	75 ± 35	NS
ESV (ml)	22 ± 10	18 ± 10	<0.05
EF (%)	67 ± 9	75 ± 9	<0.01
MNSER ($vol\ s^{-1}$)	2.23 ± 0.6	2.56 ± 0.48	<0.05
V_{CF} (s^{-1})	1.18 ± 0.39	1.4 ± 0.38	<0.05
d_{LPW} (mm)	11.1 ± 1.8	10.7 ± 1.3	NS
d_{IVS} (mm)	13.9 ± 2.1	11.8 ± 1.5	<0.01
LVMM (g)	171 ± 59	153 ± 50	<0.05
LVMM/EDV ($g\ ml^{-1}$)	2.44 ± 1.09	2.07 ± 0.78	<0.05
d/r	0.52 ± 0.1	0.47 ± 0.09	<0.05
T_{syst} ($10^3\ dyn\ cm^{-2}$)	261 ± 119	254 ± 113	NS

$\bar{x} \pm SD$

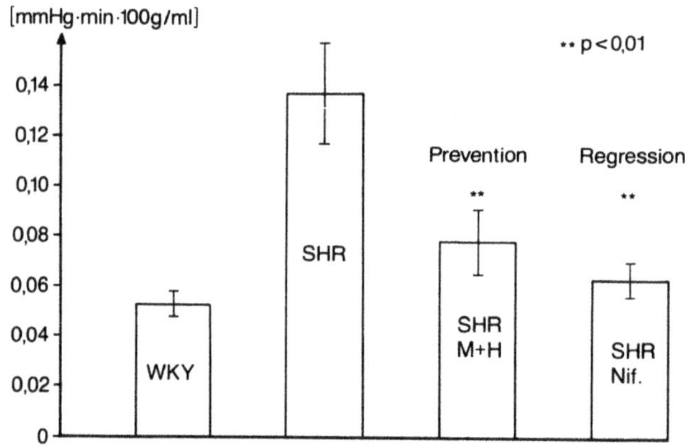

Fig. 7. Minimal coronary artery resistance after a long-term antihypertensive therapy. As in the prevention study, a marked reduction in minimal coronary resistance was achieved after regression of cardiac hypertrophy. [Experiments on the spontaneously hypertensive rat (SHR)]

controlled in all groups. Especially hydralazine treatment prevented the development of myocardial hypertrophy. The minimal coronary vascular resistance was significantly reduced in all groups, although the value of the normotensive control animals was not achieved (Fig. 7).

In the regression study, SHR were treated with nifedipine from the 20th to the 40th week of age. Also in this study, myocardial hypertrophy and minimal coronary resistance were significantly reduced. At least in this model, the control over blood pressure and myocardial hypertrophy resulted in improvement in coronary reserve.

Clinical Results

Also in clinical studies with calcium channel blockers, alpha-methyldopa or angiotensin-converting enzyme (ACE) inhibitors, a reduction in left ventricular muscle mass was achieved. Therapy with diuretics is effective as far as blood pressure is concerned, but there was no regression in left ventricular hypertrophy. Sometimes, differences in clinical results can be explained by the limitations of the methods being applied. Furthermore, during antihypertensive therapy, changes in left ventricular geometry may occur, so that calculations about left ventricular muscle mass may become difficult.

Nevertheless, regression in left ventricular hypertrophy has been shown with nifedipine, captopril, and alpha-methyldopa treatment (Fig. 5). Moreover, long-term therapy with nifedipine, resulted in improvement of left ventricular function. Other calcium channel blockers, like diltiazem and verapamil, may similarly influence the ventricular function.

As the degree of regression of left ventricular hypertrophy varies with different drug therapies, in spite of comparable reductions in wall tension, the question arises whether there are also some pressure-independent factors. The regression of normotensive left ventricular hypertrophy in hypertrophic cardiomyopathies is a strong argument for pressure-independent influences. Especially a long-term therapy with calcium channel blockers, like verapamil [4] and nifedipine [21], resulted in regression of myocardial hypertrophy. Furthermore, there was in the nifedipine-treated patients an improvement in left ventricular function. Possible pressure-independent factors are the prevention of coronary vascular spasms and improvements in microcirculation. Blood viscosity decreases with nifedipine therapy; the formation of thrombocyte aggregates is inhibited. Currently, it cannot be decided to which extent each of these factors contributes to regression of myocardial hypertrophy.

Regression of Left Ventricular Hypertrophy, Clinical Limitations

Left ventricular hypertrophy is a compensating mechanism towards the increased systolic wall tension. Only in the final stages of hypertensive heart disease systolic wall stress increases with ventricular dilatation. Regression in left ventricular hypertrophy results in an improvement of the mass-volume ratio of the left ventricle. Although no regression in left ventricular collagen content in treated hypertensive hypertrophy can be expected, the prognosis of hypertensive heart disease is expected to be improved, when blood pressure is adequately controlled.

On the other hand, one may argue that after a reversal of left ventricular hypertrophy a hypertensive crisis could result in an inappropriate rise in systolic wall stress, so that cardiac decompensation would occur. This therapeutic risk is probably greater in cardiac atrophy like in adriamycine-induced heart failure, because under physiologic and clinical conditions a "steady state" between blood pressure fluctuations and reactive left ventricular hypertrophy will occur.

Conclusions

Reversal of left ventricular hypertrophy, i.e., a causative therapy of the precursor of hypertensive heart failure, can be brought about through differentiated drug treatment. Mainly calcium channel blockers, alpha-methyldopa, ACE inhibitors, as well as combination therapy (beta-receptor, beta-blockers, diuretics, and arterial vasodilators) can be employed. Left ventricular pumping function will be improved and coronary reserve will be significantly enhanced. Consequently, the ischemic risk of the hypertrophied heart muscle is diminished. The pharmacodynamic mechanism is mainly related to an unloading of the pressure loaded left ventricle due to wall stress reduction.

References

1. Drayer DE, Lorenzo B, Werus S, Reidenberg MM (1983) Plasma levels, protein binding, and elimination data of lidocaine and active metabolites in cardiac patients of various ages. Clin Pharmacol Ther 34 (1): 14–22
2. Dunn FG, Bastian B, Lawrie TD, Cozimer AR (1980) Effect of blood pressure control of left ventricular hypertrophy in patients with essential hypertension. Clin Sci 59 [Suppl 6]: 441s–443s
3. Jakob R (ed) (1983) Cardiac adaptation to hemodynamic overload, training and stress. Steinkopff, Darmstadt
4. Kaltenbach M, Epstein S (eds) (1982) Hypertrophic cardiomyopathy. Springer, Berlin Heidelberg New York
5. Klepzig M, Strauer BE (1983) Coronary reserve in spontaneously hypertensive rats: the effect of blood pressure, hypertrophy and long-term vasodilator therapy. In: Jacob R (ed) Cardiac adaptation to hemodynamic overload, training and stress. Steinkopff, Darmstadt, pp 213–219
6. Lundin SA, Hallbäck-Nordlander M (1984) Regression of structural cardiovascular changes by antihypertensive therapy in spontaneously hypertensive rats. J Hypertension 2: 11–18
7. Motz W, Strauer BE (to be published) Prevention of left ventricular hypertrophy by antihypertensive therapy in spontaneously hypertensive rats: effects on systolic wall stress and systolic function. Basis Res Cardiol
8. Motz W, Ploeger M, Ringsgwandl G (1984) Influence of nifedipine on ventricular function and myocardial hypertrophy in spontaneously hypertensive rats. J Cardiovasc Pharmacol 5: 55
9. Nakashima Y, Fouad FM, Tarazi RC (1984) Regression of left ventricular hypertrophy from systemic hypertension by enalapril. Am J Cardiol 53: 1044–1049
10. Pfeffer JM, Pfeffer MA, Fletcher P, Fishbein M, Braunwald E (1982) Favorable effects of therapy on cardiac performance in spontaneously hypertensive rats. Am J Physiol 242: H776–H784
11. Pfeffer JM, Pfeffer MA, Mirsky I, Braunwald E (1982) Regression of left ventricular dysfunction by captopril in the spontaneously hypertensive rat. Proc Natl Acad Sci USA 79 (10): 3310–3314
12. Rowlands DB, Glover DR, Stallard TJ, Littler WA (1982) Control of blood pressure and reduction of echocardiographically assessed left ventricular mass with one-daily timolol. J Clin Pharmacol 14: 89–95
13. Sen S, Tarazi RC, Bumpus FM (1977) Cardiac hypertrophy and antihypertensive therapy. Cardiovasc Res 11: 427–433
14. Sen S, Tarazi RC, Bumpus FM (1980) Effect of converting enzyme inhibitor (SQ 14,225) on myocardial hypertrophy in spontaneously hypertensive rats. Hypertension 2: 169–176
15. Sen S, Tarazi RC, Bumpus FM (1981) Reversal of cardiac hypertrophy in renal hypertensive rats: medical vs. surgical therapy. Am J Physiol 240: H408–H412
16. Spech M, Ferrario CM, Tarazi RC (1980) Cardiac pumping ability following reversal of hypertrophy and hypertension in spontaneously hypertensive rats. Hypertension 2: 75–82
17. Strauer BE (1979a) Myocardial oxygen consumption in chronic heart disease: role of wall stress, hypertrophy and coronary reserve. Am J Cardiol 44: 730–740

18. Strauer BE (1979b) Ventricular function and coronary hemodynamics in hypertensive heart disease. Am J Cardiol 44:999–1006
19. Strauer BE (1983) Das Hochdruckherz, 2nd edn. Springer, Berlin Heidelberg New York
20. Strauer BE (1984) Pathophysiologie und Klinik der Myokardinsuffizienz. Fortschr Med 102: 113–118
21. Strauer BE, Mahmoud MA, Bayer F, Bohn I, Motz U (1984) Reversal of left ventricular hypertrophy and improvement of cardiac function in man by nifedipine. Eur Heart J [Suppl F] 5:53–60
22. Strauer BE, Böhme N, Samtleben W, Schuldig S, Volger E (1984) Clinical approach to disturbances in microcirculation of the heart. Fifth international congress of biorheology, symposium on hemorheological disorders in cardiovascular diseases. Hemorheo 4:45–66
23. Wollam GL, Tarazi RC, Bravo BL, Dustan HP (1982) Diuretic potency of combined hydrochlorothiazide and furosemide therapy in patients with azotemia. Am J Med 72(6) 929–938

The Use of the Dynamic Spatial Reconstructor to Study Renal Function*

M. D. Bentley[1], M. J. Fiksen-Olsen[1], F. G. Knox[1], E. L. Ritman[1], and J. C. Romero[1]

The Historical Need for Dynamic Spatial Reconstruction

It is well known that the discovery of the X-ray represented a major advance in medical science, since it allowed for the first time a non-invasive, direct confirmation of morphological alterations suspected by the physician during physical examination. While the conventional radiograph is a highly valuable method of diagnosis, it is static because fourth-dimensional or dynamic information (i.e., rapid alteration over time) is not provided and third-dimensional information is obscured by the superimposition of anatomic structures. The limitation of the fourth dimension has been solved by following radioopaque tracers through organ systems using rapid-imaging techniques (e.g., cineangiography). However, the problem of superimposition still makes it difficult, and often impossible, to distinguish, unambiguously, one anatomic structure from another, especially when there are only small differences in X-ray density. These kinds of problems are usually overcome by making a number of X-ray pictures from different angles, in which anatomic structures appear in different relationships to one another.

In the last decade or so, advanced imaging techniques have become possible due to the rapid development of sophisticated application of computer technology to medical imaging. In this chapter, we will attempt to explain a method which involves computerized reconstruction of images in three dimensions. By using these techniques along with rapid scanning technology, it is possible to analyze moving elements in the body (dynamic analysis) such as cardiac contraction, organ hemodynamics, and organ function [18]. Since the evaluation of these parameters is of particular interest in hypertensive patients, we will also attempt to illustrate the potential that dynamic spatial reconstruction analysis has in helping the diagnosis, treatment, and follow-up of this disease. Because of the space limitation, we do not intend to be all-inclusive. A more detailed description of different procedures and techniques can be found by interested readers in specialized articles [4, 5, 22].

* These studies were supported with grants from the National Institutes of Health, HL 16496, HL 04664, and RR 02540. Michael Bentley is a Research Fellow supported by the Hypertension Training Program, National Institutes of Health, HL 07296.

[1] Department of Physiology and Biophysics, Mayo Medical School, Mayo Clinic, Rochester, MN 55905, USA.

Primary Hypertension
Ed. by W. Kaufmann et al.

The Summation Method

Two-Dimensional Reconstruction

The history of reconstruction techniques began in 1917 with the publication of a paper by an Austrian mathematician, Radon [16], in which he proved that two- and three-dimensional objects can be reconstructed from an infinite set of projections. In the late 1950s and 1960s, Oldendorf [15], Cormack [3], and Hounsfield [8] utilized such mathematical techniques to make transaxial reconstructions. To appreciate the basic concept of reconstruction, let us reconstruct a transverse section of a cross-shaped object (Fig. 1) by using two orthogonal projections as illustrated in Fig. 2. In the first of these two projections, we orient an energy source at an angle perpendicular to the arms of the cross. Parallel rays of energy emitted by the source are recorded simultaneously on a sensitive film and by a series of photocells aligned along a single transverse plane. It can be seen that the opacity of the projection (ray density) through the cross is proportional to the recorded density. This proportionality is recorded by the photo cells providing an analog display with a relative density of 3, 1, or 0, depending up on the "thickness" of the cross-segment interposed between the photo cells and the energy source. Once this first projection has been recorded,

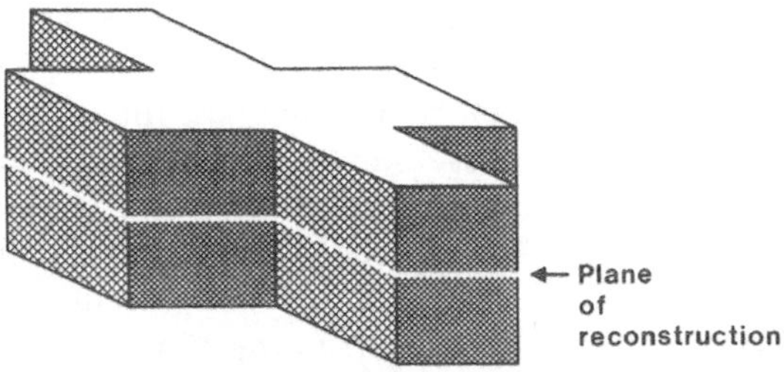

Fig. 1. Original cross-shaped object

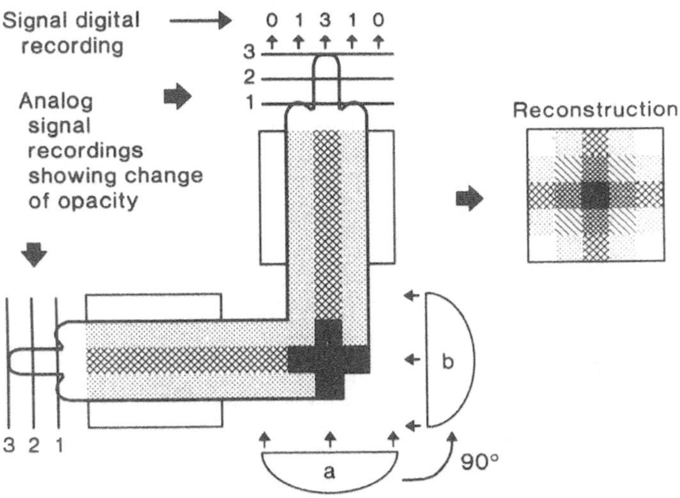

Fig. 2. Reconstruction of transverse section of cross-shaped object from two orthogonal projections

the film and the energy source are rotated 90° to obtain the second projection. As shown in Fig. 2, the ray density of this second projection has the same characteristics as the first projection because of the geometrical homogeneity of the cross. However, when the smeared (i.e., back projected) densities of the second projections are added to those of the first projection, a partially blurred two-dimensional reconstruction of the cross is obtained. In this example (Fig. 2), the accuracy of the reconstruction is low because of the "spread shadows" which are inherent to the limited number of angles of view. We will see later how the quality of the image can be improved by the summation of additional projections taken at many different angles. The "blurring" of the image is further diminished if, prior to summation (back projection), the projections are filtered with a function tailored to the geometry of the scanner system.

Digital Conversion

Figure 3 illustrates the basic principles underlying the conversion of analog recording of density from photocells into a digital display. This can be achieved by arranging a two-dimensional array of numbers, each of which represents the X-ray density of one small square in the picture. Such a square is called a "pixel." As shown in Fig. 3, the density values recorded by photocells during the first projection are uniformly distributed along the series of pixels lying on the same path. In our example, the series of pixels which are lying on a path with a given density value all contain the same number. This yields a one-dimensional array of numbers representing the total X-ray density of the pixels at a given angle of exposure. These numbers are then kept in computer memory while the density values recorded by the photocells in a second angle of projection are recorded in a set of pixels. This second set of values is then added to those obtained during the first projection. This addition is represented in Fig. 3, where the set of numerical values obtained during the first projection is shown

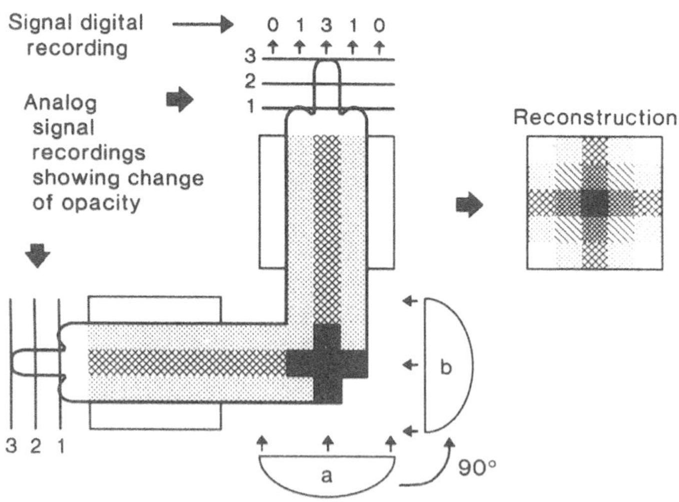

Fig. 3. Conversion of analog density recording of cross-shaped object into a digital array

in the upper side of the square and the set of numerical values obtained during the second projection is represented on the left side of the square. This yields a two-dimensional array of numbers with values corresponding to the summation of density values produced by the two projections. In fact, it can be seen in Fig. 3 that the center pixel of the cross has the highest density in summation (i.e., numerical value of 6) and pixels corresponding to the arms of the cross have less density (i.e., numerical value of 4). Similarly, the two-dimensional array of numbers has spread lesser values (below the numerical value of 4), which correspond to the blurring.

From this example we can see how an algorithm or computer program for a two-dimensional array of numbers can be developed to add-up iteratively all successive density values produced by the photocells during a multitude of projection angles. During this procedure, any given number displayed in the two-dimensional array of pixels will be constantly modified by subsequent projections until the relative density stops changing. This notion is illustrated in Fig. 4 which represents the successive change of density in a two-dimensional array of pixels during eight rotations at 45° angles. As in previous examples, the initial projection indicated in Fig. 4 shows a distribution of numbers that corresponds fairly well to the relative density. It can be seen how these initial numerical values are modified by summation in each of the subsequent rotations. At the end of the eight rotations, the pixels representing the cross in the reconstructed figure all have numerical values of 16; whereas all the values of pixels located outside the cross are equal to or less than 6. An accurate reconstruction can be obtained if the computer is programmed to filter the original data prior to the backprojection summation process. We have used in our example of a two-dimensional reconstruction a cross-shaped object that is a simple geometric structure; however, when analyzing more complex and numerous structures, there

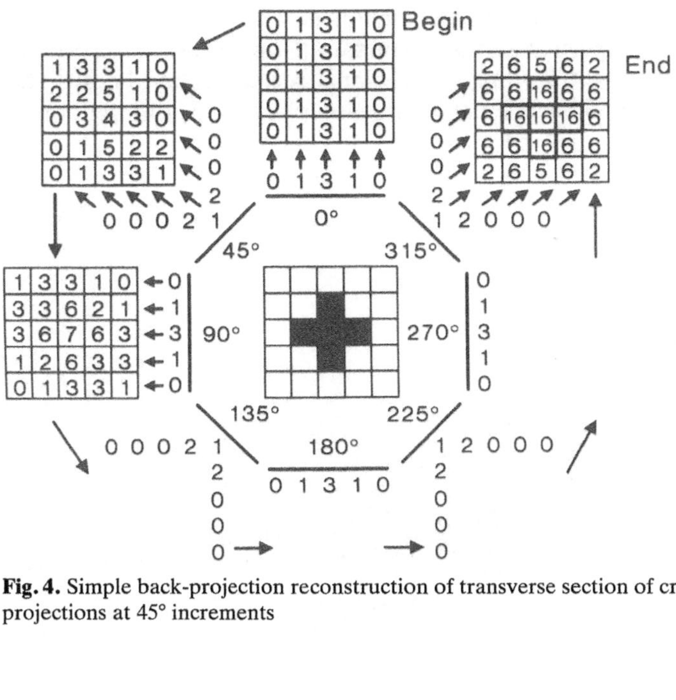

Fig. 4. Simple back-projection reconstruction of transverse section of cross-shaped object from eight projections at 45° increments

are always experimental errors and fluctuations in the number of X-ray photons which show up in the data as "noise" [20]. It is important to mention here that the summation method used in our example is a very simplified version of a so-called filtered back-projection technique. There are however, other methods for reconstructing images that involve algebraic reconstruction and Fourier analysis-based methods [4]. Description of these methods are beyond the scope of this chapter.

Three-Dimensional Reconstruction

Two-dimensional reconstruction of images offers information on the shape of any particular structure and its relationship with others contained in the same plane. Additional information on the three-dimensional shape of the structure and its relationship in planes located above or below will require repeating similar scans to provide data for two-dimensional reconstruction in the desired adjacent planes. A three-dimensional reconstruction of a cross-shaped figure is obtained by "stacking" multiple two-dimensional reconstructions at intervals along the third dimension as indicated in Fig. 5. It can be seen that in agreement with the previous example, the pixels located within each of the four two-dimensional reconstructions exhibit the same numerical ray-density value. The figure also shows that a numerical value of pixels located above or below the planes contained in the cross-shaped structure was zero because no interception of the ray's beams occurred in these planes.

From "stacked" two-dimensional reconstructions, one can obtain a three-dimensional reconstruction of the cross-shaped structure similar to the original. In such a three-dimensional reconstruction, there is a new basic image element consisting of cubes composed of pixels stacked at intervals in the third dimension. These cubes are called "voxels."

A series of two-dimensionally reconstructed planes are usually obtained in computerized axial tomography when searching for tumors or when attempting to define the lower and upper limit of a particular organ structure. However, such a procedure generally does not allow for a true three-dimensional reconstruction because the chosen planes may be separated by unequal or large intervals and by different times.

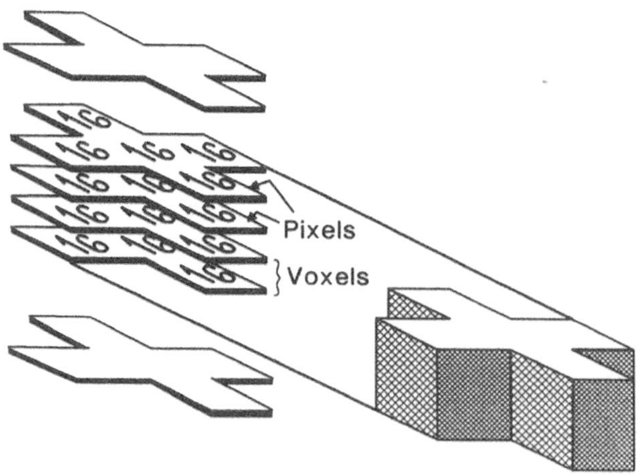

Fig. 5. Three-dimensional reconstruction of cross-shaped object by stacking successive reconstructed planes

In such a case, the accuracy of the three-dimensional reconstruction can be impaired by anatomic movement such as respiration.

An instrument capable of producing three-dimensional reconstructions from simultaneous multiple (synchronous) two-dimensional reconstructions has been developed at the Mayo Clinic. This instrument is called the Dynamic Spatial Reconstructor (DSR). The interval of time needed to complete a scan of complete three-dimensional volume (temporal resolution) is 1/100 s and this can be repeated 60 times per second for up to 20 s, or a large duration of the scans repeated less frequently (e.g., 120 s at 10 times/s).

The Dynamic Spatial Reconstructor

The DSR is a high temporal-resolution, volumetric, roentgenographic, computer-tomographic scanner [18]. Figure 6 shows an artist's representation of the DSR. The scanner consists of a rotating cylindrical gantry on which are mounted 14 rotating anode X-ray tubes which are spaced around a semicircle. The optical images are formed from conical projections of the rays onto a hemi-cylindrical fluorescent screen positioned opposite the X-ray tubes. These images are then recorded by video cameras and stored on video discs [12]. The cylindrical volume scanned by the DSR is 21–39 cm in the transaxial direction and 21 cm in the axial direction. In adult humans, the amount of radiation exposure at the skin in the area of the body that is directly exposed to the X-rays is about 1 R/s DSR time [11]. The rotating gantry with the X-ray tubes, the fluorescent screens, video cameras, and related electronics

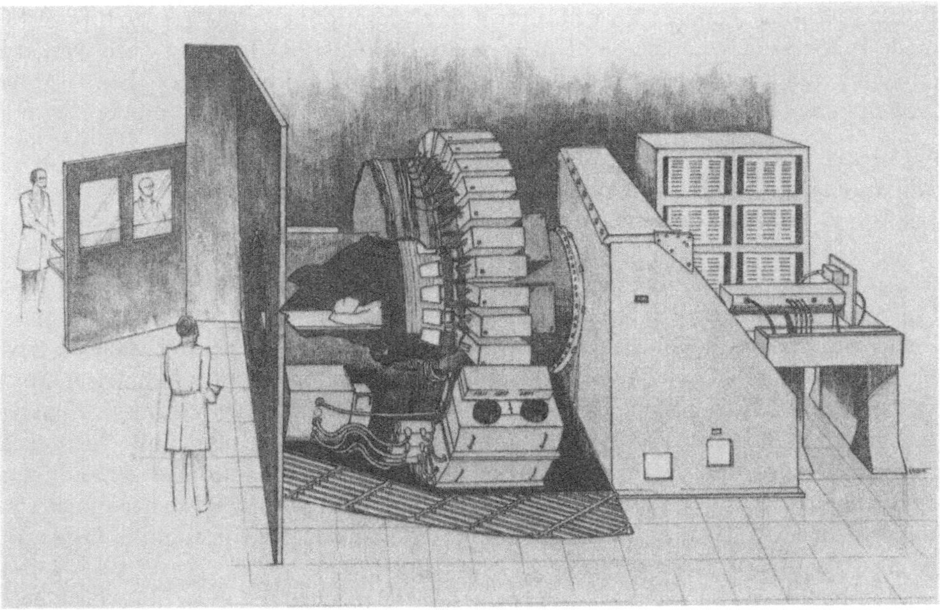

Fig. 6. Artist's representation of a dynamic spatial reconstructor. [19]

weighs 13 tons and turns around on a horizontal axis at 15 revolutions per minute (1 revolution every 4 s).

Each volume image obtained from the 14 video cameras is composed of 120 horizontal scan lines, each line representing the projection of a cross-section spaced 1.8 mm apart in the body. The changes in X-ray density in each of the lines constitute the analog signal stored on video discs which is later digitalized by an analog to digital converter. After subsequent digitization and interpolation (to achieve cubic voxels), each volume image is usually composed of approximately 100 sections each having voxels with minimal dimensions of 0.5–3.0 mm [6]. The actual size depends upon the size of the volume reconstructed.

The DSR is generally programmed to generate raw data at a rate of 50 million picture samples per second [18]. In addition, the arithmetic processes required for converting these data into images are very computation intensive. For scans of 4- to 10-s durations, several thousand cross sections have to be reconstructed. Even for a 2-s scan, many units of computer time are required. With recent advances in microprocessors and special array processors, this long computation time can be substantially shortened.

Estimation of Organ Blood Flow, Organ Tissue Perfusion, and Organ Function Using the DSR

After establishing the technical characteristics of the DSR, we are now in a position to define the experimental circumstances and the rationale underlying the design of computer programs that will allow a dynamic analysis of physiological parameters. The intrinsic characteristics of the DSR allow quantitative estimation of blood flow and perfusion of organ systems, especially for the heart, lung, and kidney [13, 18]. In the following sections, we will offer a brief description of the research progress made in the kidney and some of the potential applications to study cardiovascular dynamics. The interest in these two systems is enhanced because of their obvious participation in hypertension.

Estimations of Renal Blood Flow, Renal Blood Flow Distribution, and Renal Tubular Function Using the DSR

The principles behind the analysis of renal hemodynamics and renal function from synchronous volumetric reconstruction of the kidney during the passage of contrast media can perhaps be understood by considering some of the features that we have already explained about three-dimensional reconstruction of the geometrical cross-shaped figure. Let us assume that we intend to examine blood flow through renal tissue by representing part of the renal arteries and renal parenchyma into the voxels that comprise two perpendicular arms of the cross-shaped figure. The three-dimensional reconstruction of these arms is depicted in Fig. 7, where we have assumed, for the sake of pictorial clarity, a complete three-dimensional reconstruction of planes, a, b, c, d, and e.

The figure also shows that once the complete reconstruction has been achieved we can "play back" the tape and obtain equal complete reconstruction of horizontal

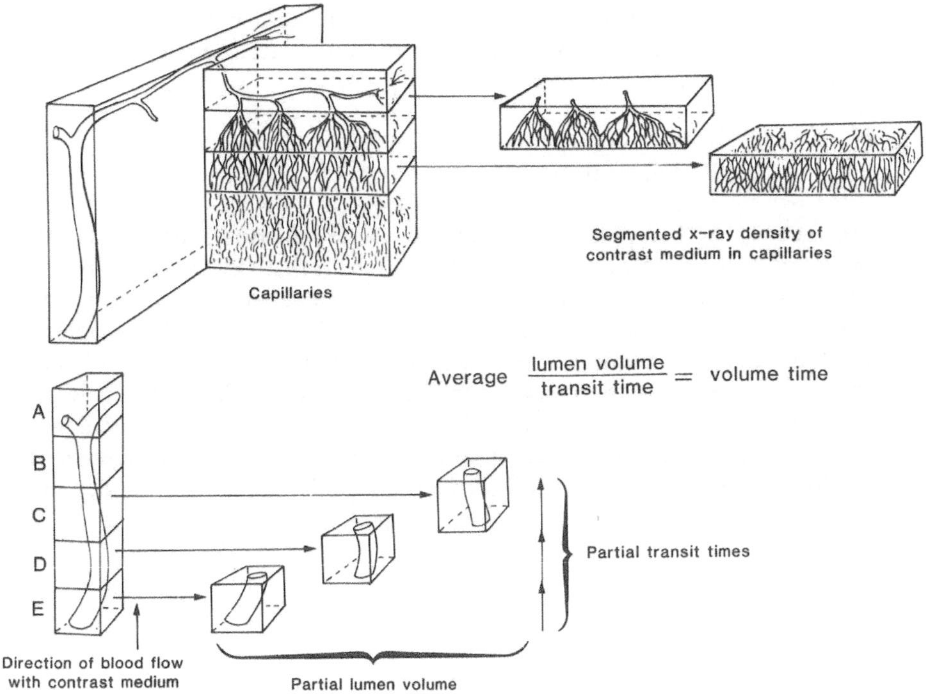

Fig. 7. Schematic drawing of three-dimensional imaging of renal vascular anatomy

or vertical segments of the cross branches by stacking selected voxels in the computer. Let us further assume that, as depicted in Fig. 7, the voxels composing the two branches of these three-dimensional cross structures contain an interlobar renal artery that branches into an arcuate artery; an interlobular artery emerges with its multiple glomerular afferent and efferent arterioles and the peritubular capillaries. According to Fig. 7, the interlobar and arcuate arteries are contained in the same plane, which is positioned perpendicular to the plane containing the interlobular artery with its glomerular afferent and efferent arterioles and the peritubular capillaries. The characterization of all these vascular structures is hypothetical because their X-ray density is not much different from that of the surrounding renal parenchyma. However, these segments of the renal vasculature can be fully characterized when they are filled by an intraarterial injection of an X-ray contrast media such as Renovist [10]. Furthermore, if a contrast media has been administered as an intraarterial bolus injection, then we can examine the partial transit through successive arterial segments. This is possible with the DSR which obtains a complete three-dimensional reconstruction every 1/60 s. Such an analysis can be accomplished, as shown in Fig. 7, by identifying the voxels containing equal segments of the interlobar artery and calculating its lumen volume after such a segment has been filled with contrast media. At the same time, the computation of multiple planes every 1/60 s allows us to estimate the respective times at which the bolus of contrast media passes through each of these arterial segments. A comparable method is to measure the volume of vessel transversed by the bolus during a selected interval (e.g., 1/60 s). In this manner, the relationship between partial lumen volume and partial transit times allows us to calculate the blood flow volume through any arterial segment according to the following equation (Fig. 7):

$$\text{Flow volume} = \frac{\text{Partial lumen volume}}{\text{Partial transit time}}$$

Such an analysis can be applied to any artery whose structure is enclosed in the cylindrical volume scanned by the DSR reconstruction. If the bolus injection of contrast media is given in the root of the aorta, then we can calculate cardiac output and/or blood flow of any of the aortic branches such as subclavian, carotid, mesenteric, renal, etc. A limitation to the use of this technique is imposed by arteries of small diameters whose dimensions are below the spatial resolution of the DSR images, or when the small artery that is to be analyzed is surrounded by large abdominal mass which results in impaired signal detection. Such is the case both for interlobular arteries contained in the renal cortex and for the peritubular capillaries. Under such

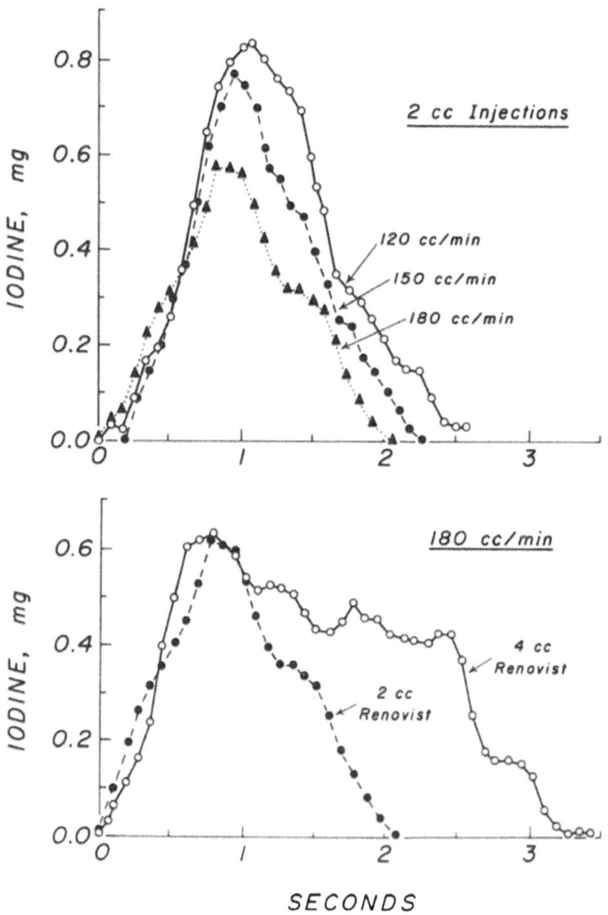

Fig. 8. Effect of altered blood flow velocity *(top)* and amount of injected contrast media on dilution curve characteristics. [21]

circumstances we can observe changes in roentgen density as the contrast media fills the vessel, but cannot resolve the vessel. Hence, the maximal density of contrast media is directly proportional to blood perfusion per unit tissue volume (Fig. 7).

Experiments have been performed to ascertain the manner in which dilution curves of contrast media obtained from arterial reconstruction are affected by changes in blood flow velocity or by changes in the amount of contrast medium (Fig. 8). For this purpose the external carotid blood flow was controlled by a perfusion pump which drew blood from a femoral artery. A 2 ml-bolus injection of an X-ray contrast medium (Renovist) was given at constant velocity at carotid flow rates of 120, 150, and 180 ml/min (Fig. 8). Alternatively varying amounts of Renovist contrast media of 2 and 4 ml were given when carotid blood flow was set at a rate of 180 ml/min (Fig. 8). The results represented in Fig. 8 show that the area under the dilution curves varies appreciably as required for application of the Hamilton Stewart indicator dilution method. These characteristics have been observed for the renal artery, but the physiologic validity of these preliminary data is questionable because renal blood flow is significantly affected by the velocity at which the contrast medium is injected into the renal artery. These problems are inherent to the variability of manually operated injections, which alter the circulation front of contrast media. During this experiment, however, we were capable of obtaining excellent dilution curves of media in cortical sections of renal parenchyma.

Figure 9 illustrates images of midline transverse, coronal, and sagittal sections of the kidney scanned during the passage of contrast medium through the kidney. From these sections, videodensitometric curves for any particular area of the renal cortex and/or renal medulla can be measured. For the purposes of illustration, a kidney was

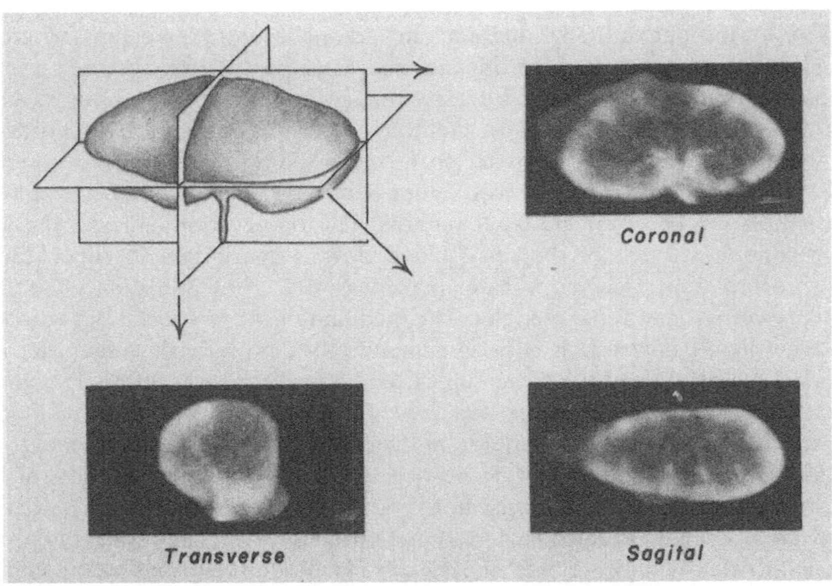

Fig. 9. Transverse-, coronal-, and sagittal-plane reconstructions of dog kidney. Dog 19 kg, 2 cc renovist I/A, pentothal anesthesia (5 mm thick slices, 0.127 s DSR scan aperture). [10]

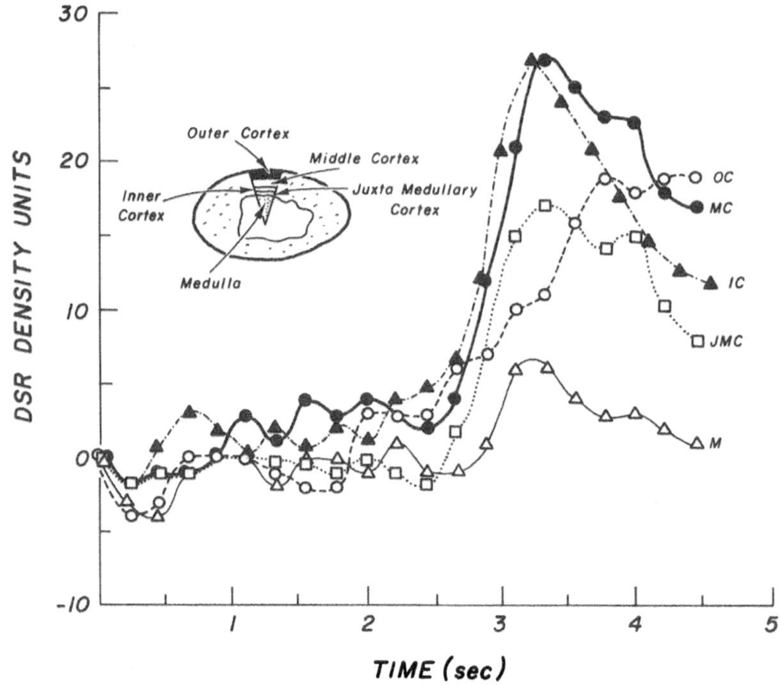

Fig. 10. Dilution curve characteristics of outer cortex *(OC)*, middle cortex *(MC)*, inner cortex *(IC)*, juxta-medullary cortex *(JMC)*, and medulla *(M)* in dog kidney. (Sagittal slice, 4 mm thick, 2 cc renovist injected into renal artery, dog 14 kg.) [10]

exteriorized through a flank incision and scanned during injection of contrast medium into the renal artery. In this instance, images of the renal cortex were sectioned to permit measurement of density (image brightness) in the outer, middle, inner, and juxtamedullary cortex. In addition, density of the medulla was estimated.

It can be seen in Fig. 10 that the peak of the dilution curve in the superficial, middle, and inner cortical areas was higher than the peaks recorded for either the juxtamedullary zone or for the renal medulla. This observation indicates that under resting conditions most of the renal blood flow is distributed to superficial and middle cortical zones leaving a lesser percent of blood for perfusion of the juxtamedullary cortex, and renal medulla. The medullary flow represents 4%–6% of the total renal blood flow which is in agreement with data published by other investigators. The circulation time of the superficial cortical zone was different from other areas of the kidney. This superficial zone filled more slowly with medium and reached its highest density at a later time than did other zones of the kidney.

Many more experiments will be needed to establish definite patterns of blood flow distribution during resting conditions and the manner in which such patterns can be altered by changes in renal perfusion pressure. However, the results of our initial experiments clearly indicate that analysis of renal blood flow distribution within the renal cortex is feasible with the DSR [10]. Furthermore, the DSR offers a great potential for assessing the magnitude and direction of changes during renovascular

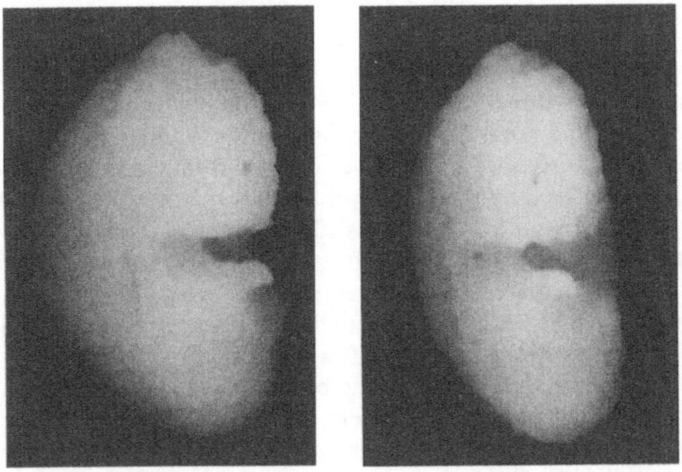

20° RAO, lateral view   Lateral view

Fig. 11. Three-dimensional reconstruction of whole kidney computer generated surface display

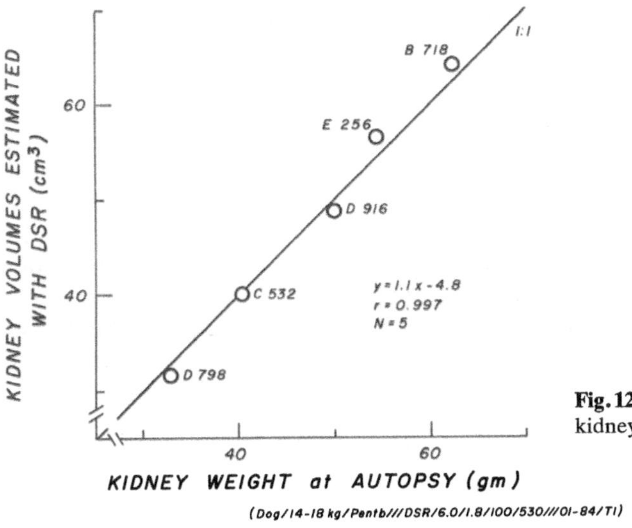

Fig. 12. Correlation of reconstructed kidney volume with kidney weight. [10]

stenosis or during other circumstances where distribution of blood flow may represent an adaptive response from the kidney (e.g., changes in dietary sodium, secondary aldosteronism, etc.).

A computer-generated three-dimensional surface display of a kidney was constructed from the DSR scan data illustrated in Fig. 11. The volume contained by the outer surface of the kidney is readily computed. Figure 12 shows that the volumes of kidneys estimated from DSR reconstructions correlate very well with the recorded weight of the kidneys.

Potentials for Evaluation of Renal Tubular Function

In our previous example we have shown the manner in which videodensitometric changes could be used in dynamic three-dimensional reconstruction to obtain information about renal blood flow and renal blood flow distribution within the kidney. This analysis is based on characteristic dilution curves derived from contrast media which are predominantly not filtered by the glomeruli and not removed from renal circulation by the renal tubules. In our example, the estimated transit-time of a non-filtrable substance through the kidney was estimated to be 2–4 s. However, the use of a contrast media which can be completely removed from the renal circulation by both glomerular filtration and tubular secretion (e.g., iodinated para-amino-hippurate) will offer dilution curve characteristics which are different from those produced by non-filtrable contrast media. These differences are determined by the differences in flow rate between the intravascular renal compartment and the intraluminal tubular compartment. In fact, vascular transit time is much shorter (2–4 s) [10, 14] than the tubular transit time (3–5 min) [24]. From these considerations, it can be assumed that dilution curves of contrast media taken up by the tubules will offer a unique opportunity to determine not only the tubular distribution of media, but also adaptive changes in tubular transit times. It is well known, for example, that the extraction of para-amino-hippurate by the proximal tubules is proportional to the renal flow in the peritubular capillary circulation [1]. From this it follows that the maximal tubular distribution of contrast media (between 10 and 20 s) should agree with the intrarenal distribution of blood flow.

In renographic studies, Britton and Brown [1] used I^{131}-hippuran to study regional blood flow and tubular transit in the kidneys of humans on high and low sodium intakes. Their results suggested that there was an increase in the amount of I^{131}-hippuran transported by juxtamedullary nephrons in response to an increase in salt intake. Similar directional changes in blood flow distribution have been found using microspheres in animals undergoing saline diuresis [23]. These results support the notion that sodium loading increases the appearance of hippuran in deeper nephrons which is facilitated by a corresponding increase in plasma flow to the same nephrons. Because of the limitation inherent to transit renography, these studies could not determine whether the change in transit times represented a shift of transit time within the same nephron population or a shift between different populations with constant transit times.

Such problems can be appropriately resolved by three-dimensional reconstruction with the DSR since it has sufficient resolution to distinguish superficial, cortical, and juxtamedullary transit times [13]. The determination of these patterns goes beyond academic interest since alteration may be a sensitive indicator of changes in intratubular pressure resulting from renovascular constriction or partial ureteral obstruction. Transit times may also be altered in glomerulopathies affecting a significant number of nephrons.

Application of DSR to Determine Cardiac Dynamics

The procedure underlying the three-dimensional dynamic reconstruction in the kidney can be used to study cardiac dynamics [18]. Figure 13 illustrates the steps fol-

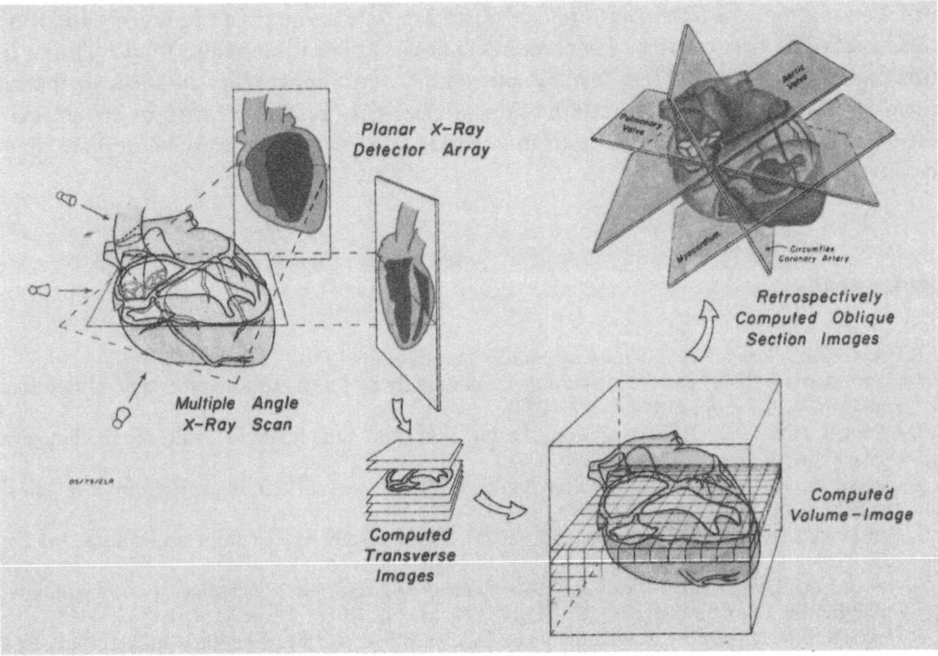

Fig. 13. Schematic flowchart illustrating noninvasive numerical dissection of the heart. [17]

lowed by a three-dimensional reconstruction of the heart which can be sliced in coronal, sagittal, horizontal, or oblique sections. Because of the temporal resolution of DSR reconstructions, it is possible to obtain valuable information concerning changes in the endocardium, epicardium, and myocardium during cardiac motion. As shown in Fig. 13, appropriate sectioning of cardiac chambers filled with contrast media offers a unique opportunity to determine chamber volume [7], myocardial mass [9], and ejection volume. As with the kidney, coronary blood flow can be determined by computing partial transit times and partial filling volumes of coronary arterial segments. Measurements of myocardial mass using DSR imaging techniques can quantitate the cardiac hypertrophy. It would not be overly optimistic to predict from this preliminary work performed at the Mayo Clinic, that the DSR will allow calculation of many important cardiac hemodynamic and contractile parameters using a relatively noninvasive technique.

Summary

In the last decade the use of roentgenographic computer tomographic scanners has produced significant advances in diagnostic methods of cardiovascular disease. The development of modern technology has also enabled synchronous three-dimensional reconstruction which offers very accurate information concerning anatomical relationships. The capability for synchronous volumetric reconstruction with high temporal resolution was first envisioned as a need to determine organ functions and fluid dynamics. The first of these instruments is now in operation at the Mayo Clinic. In this paper we discussed the "modus operandi" and applicability of such an instrument to study cardiac and renal function. Preliminary results of work in progress indicate that the use of such an instrument may open up a new area in medical diagnosis.

References

1. Britton KE, Brown NJG (1971) Clinical renography. Lloyd-Luke, London
2. Cormack AM (1963) Representation of a function by its line integrals, with some radiological applications. I. J Appl Phys 34:2722–2727
3. Cormack AM (1964) Representation of a function by its time integrals, with some radiological applications. II. J Appl Phys 35:2908–2913
4. Gordon R, Herman GT (1974) Three-dimensional reconstruction from projections: a review of algorithms. Int Rev Cytol 38:111–151
5. Gordon R, Herman GT, Johnson SA (1975) Image reconstruction from projections. Sci Am 233:56–68
6. Harris LD, Ritman EL, Robb RA (1983) Computer generated 3-D display of x-ray computed tomographic volume image data. SPIE 312:176–181
7. Hoffman EA, Ritman EL (1985) Shape and dimensions of cardiac computed tomography. Role of image slice thickness and orientation. Radiology 115(3):739–744
8. Hounsfield GN (1973) Computerized transverse axial scanning (tomography). Part I. Description of system. Br J Radiol 46:1016–1022
9. Iwasaki T, Sinak LJ, Hoffman EA, Robb RA, Harris LD, Bahn RC, Ritman EL (1984) Mass of left ventricular myocardium estimated with the dynamic spatial reconstructor. Am J Physiol 246:H138–H142
10. Iwasaki T, Ritman EL, Fiksen-Olsen MJ, Romero JC, Knox FG (1985) Renal cortical perfusion – preliminary experience with the dynamic spatial reconstructor (DSR). Ann Biomed Eng 13: 259–271
11. Kinsey JH, Orvis AL (1981) High repetition rate volumetric x-ray CT scanning. IEEE Trans Nucl Sci 28:1732–1735
12. Kinsey JH, Hansen CR, Roessler RW, Rhyner MH, Ritman EL (1983) Technical characteristics of the x-ray video imaging chain of the DSR system. In: Heintzen PH, Brennicke R (eds) Digital imaging in cardiovascular radiology. Thieme, Stuttgart
13. Knox FG, Ritman EL, Romero JC (1984) Intrarenal distribution of blood flow: evolution of a new approach to measurement. Kidney Int 25:473–479
14. Kramer K, Thurau K, Deetjen P (1960) Hämodynamik des Nierenmarks. I. Capillare Passagezeit, Blutvolumen, Durchblutung, Gewebshämatokrit und O_2-Verbrauch des Nierenmarks in situ. Pflügers Arch 270:251–269
15. Oldendorf WH (1961) Isolated flying spot detection of radiodensity discontinuities – displaying the internal structural pattern of a complex object. IRE Trans Biomed Electron 8:68–72
16. Radon J (1917) Über die Bestimmung von Funktionen durch ihre Integralwerte längs gewisser Mannigfaltigkeiten. Ber Sachs Akad Wiss Math Phys Kl (Leipzig) 69:262–277
17. Ritman EL, Harris LD, Padijar R, Chevalier PA, Robb RA (1979) Noninvasive visualization and quantitation of cardiovascular structure and function. Physiologist 22:39–43
18. Ritman EL, Robb RA, Harris LD (1985) Imaging physiological functions: experience with the DSR. Praeger, Philadelphia
19. Schwartz RS, Ritman EL (1983) Computed tomography in cardiac imaging. Pract Cardiol 9:224–238
20. Shepp LA, Stein JA (1977) Simulated reconstruction artifacts in computerized x-ray tomography. In: Ter-Pogossian MM (ed) Reconstruction tomography in diagnostic radiology and nuclear medicine. University Park Press, Baltimore

21. Sinak LI, Ritman EL (1983) Dynamic Spatial Reconstructor. In: Higgin CD (ed) Computerized transmission tomography of the heart and great vessels – Experimental evaluation and clinical application. Futura Publishing Co, Mt. Kisco, NY
22. Snyder DL, Cox JR (1977) An overview of reconstructive tomography and limitations imposed by a finite number of projections. In: Ter-Pogassian (ed) Reconstruction tomography in diagnostic radiology and nuclear medicine. University Park Press, Baltimore
23. Stein JH, Osgood RW, Ferris TF (1972) Effect of volume expansions on distribution of glomerular filtrate and renal cortical blood flow in the dog. Am J Physiol 223: 984
24. Zum Winkel K, Hallwachs O, Steinhausen M (1968) Kameraszintigraphie und Isotopennephrographie an der Hundeniere und deren Überprüfung durch die Intravitalmikroskopie. Fortschr Geb Rontgenstr 108: 382–393

Critical Review of Antihypertensive Pharmacotherapy

Cardiovascular Intervention Studies: Problems and Perspectives

U. LAASER[1] and P. ALLHOFF[2]

Three decades of medical and epidemiological research lead to the establishment of firm "cardiovascular risk factors" which make an important, if not decisive contribution to the pathogenesis of atherosclerotic disease [1]. The cardiovascular risk-concept, therefore, is not based upon a few large studies only, but relates to a coherent international body of argued and accepted knowledge [2]. However, neither do the main (primary) risk factors explain the total variation of cardiovascular disease (CVD), nor is there one unanimously accepted model of action and interaction of risk factors upon the vessel wall [3]. The final step in the proof of the role risk factors play in the genesis of cardiovascular disease therefore is to show the reversibility of the atherosclerotic process and to demonstrate the therapeutic potential for a reduction of cardiovascular complications. One of the first studies to demonstrate this impressively for a major risk factor was the Veterans Administration Study on diastolic blood pressures between 115–129 and between 90–114 mmHg [4, 5]. Yet the superiority of a certain treatment as shown in a classical controlled clinical trial – double-blind and randomized – does not necessarily hold, if transferred into the general health care system and diluted by faulty indication and incomplete compliance, not to speak of the heterogeneity of real target populations as compared with usually very strongly selected and non-representative study participants. Therefore, even after experimental studies for the development of causal models and clinical trials to show effectiveness under specified conditions, we still need research into the transfer of scientific results into every-day use, which could be described as a process of finding out how to assure the quality of care in special patient groups, epidemiologically speaking, in high-risk groups. Undoubtedly epidemiological observation can contribute to the clarification of causal mechanisms, but we also need intervention studies in total or representative populations in order to investigate the effect of the introduction of certain treatments upon the whole health care system and to analyse the interaction between individuals, either positively supporting or negatively distracting from the real effects of treatment. This is especially true, if we attempt life-style changes in the framework of health education programs, where social interaction is a key element of the interventive strategy. Those intervention studies relate to primary prevention as clinical trials relate to curative approaches. Table 1 is an attempt to assemble the historical steps from (a) experimental studies with high internal validity, but limited generalizability to (b) studies with high external validity, but lesser rigidity of design.

[1] German Institute for High Blood Pressure Research, P.O.B. 101409, D-6900 Heidelberg.
[2] Working Party for Interdisciplinary Health Research, Imbach 27, D-5090 Leverkusen 3.

Primary Hypertension
Ed. by W. Kaufmann et al.

Table 1. Sequence of research steps in the development of cardiovascular prevention

	Subpopulations	Total populations
Research into cause	Experimental studies	Epidemiological observation studies
Research into change	Clinical trials	Intervention studies
Research into transfer	Studies on quality assurance in the care of high-risk groups	Monitoring of programs on general health education

Table 2. Assessment of preventive concepts

High risk approach		Population approach
Specific approach adapted to the individual	⇄	Broad primordial prevention
Relative risk attractive for individual	⇄	Population-wide reduction of attributable risk
Pharmalogical therapeutic approach	⇄	Behavioural approch
High motivation of physician	⇄	Increased array of medical tasks

Rose [6] introduced the well-known concepts of high relative risk and high population attributable risk. The former suggests a truncation of the distribution of risk, while the latter is the sum of a larger number of individuals with small relative risks. This leads to the so-called preventive paradox, which implies that it might be more effective to shift the mean of a distribution than to truncate its upper end. However, one can look upon these two concepts also in terms of implementation in an established health care system, as given in Table 2. According to this viewpoint the high-risk approach has better chances for optimum implementation because (a) as a specific approach it can be adapted to the individual much more readily than overall programs, (b) the relative risk is impressive and motivating information for the individual person, (c) the pharmacologic approach – if available – is relatively easy to handle and does not constitute an ethical problem if weighted against the immediate dangers, and last not least, (d) it might be easier to achieve higher motivation on the part of the physician if clear therapeutic instruments are offered, applicable within the framework of the classical doctor-patient relationship. On the other hand, the population approach while offering an increased array of medical tasks also requires more pronounced physician's involvement in public issues. If we leave out the scenario of pharmacologic mass treatment, then the alternative of "induced behavioral change," is much more demanding for the physician and for other professions specifically trained in this regard (e.g., psychologists), especially if we think of general life-style change. The very important assets of the population approach refer to the really population-wide reduction of disease and the more causal approach in terms of pri-

Table 3. Large trials on the reduction of cardiovascular borderline risks

Study	Design	Sample (n)		Follow-up (years)	End points
$CLOF_{13.2}$	R DB PL	10600	VOL	13	CHD[a]
LRC	R DB PL	3800	VOL	7–10	CHD[a] *
$ANBPS_{INT.}$	R SB PL	3400	VOL	3– 4	CVD[a] *
$HDFP_{90-104}$	R ST	7800	REP	5	TM **
$EWPHE_{INT}$	R DB PL	800	VOL	7	CVD[b] *
MRC_{INT}	R SB PL	17600	VOL	5	CBV[a] **
MRFIT	R ST	12600	VOL	7	CHD[b]
EMFRPT	R ST	49800	REP	6	CHD[b]
COMM.ST.	Quasi ST	40000+	ALL	e.g. 8	CVD[b] ?

CLOF, Clofibrate Study (13.2 years of follow-up); LRC, Lipid Research Clinics Trial; $ANBPS_{INT.}$, Australian National Blood Pressure Study (intention to treat); HDFP, Hypertension Detection and Follow-Up Program (90–104 mm Hg); $EWPHE_{INT}$, European Working Party on Hypertension in the Elderly (intention to treat); MRC_{INT}, Medical Research Council Working Party (intention to treat); MRFIT, Multiple Risk Factor Intervention Trial; EMFRPT, European Multifactorial Risk Prevention Trial; COMM.ST., Community Studies. R, random; DB, double blind; SB, single blind; PL, placebo; ST, standard; VOL, volunteers; REP, representative; TM, total mortality; CHD, coronary heart disease; CVD, cardiovascular disease; CBV, cerebrovascular disease
[a], incidence; [b], mortality; *, $P<0.05$; **, $P<0.01$

mary or better primordial prevention, meaning that the very genesis of risk development is to be inhibited.

Before dealing with intervention studies in total populations, it is of interest to assess the role controlled clinical trials can play in the reduction of border-line risks. There is little doubt about their important contribution to the evaluation of treatments for clinically relevant risks, as typical with manifest hypertension. Table 3 summarizes features of some of the more important clinical trials done in order to show significant reduction of risk factors at borderline levels, i.e., with small relative risks. Admittedly, this is a selection of studies, but it exemplifies the main problems in that only one of the blood pressure studies and the studies on cholesterol reduction, namely the Clofibrate Study [7, 8] and the Lipid Research Clinics Trial [9] are double-blind. Only the Hypertension Detection and Follow-up Program [10] and the European Multifactorial Risk Prevention Trial [11] are representative in the sense that their study population is related to a definable total. Even more important is the fact that only one study (Clofibrate Study) achieved more than 10 years of follow-up and that only one other study (HDFP) put total mortality as a primary study end point, i.e., the sample calculation was based upon the expected reduction of this outcome variable. This clearly limits the potential of such studies to detect compensating effects in the total spectrum of morbidity and mortality, limits their capability of safely excluding long-term toxic side effects (possibly lasting beyond the study's end). Finally, the use of volunteers limits the generalizability of the study results with regard to mass use in the general health care system. The internal validity of many of these studies is impaired by a lack of fulfillment of an essential requirement for ex-

Table 4. Large trials on the reduction of cardiovascular borderline risks (% mortality reduction)

Study	Total mortality	CHD	Non-CVD
$CLOF_{9.6}$	−19**	−9	−27
$CLOF_{13.2}$	−11	−9	−14
LRC	7	24	(−33)
$ANBPS_{INT.}$	29	(55)	4
$HDFP_{90-104}$	20**	20	13
$EWPHE_{INT}$	9	38*	−14
MRC_{INT}	2	−9	0
MRFIT	−2	7	(−10)
EMFRPT	3	7	
UK	−14	−8	
B	17*	21	

Abbreviations are the same as in Table 3. Subscripts indicate years of follow-up; brackets enclose estimated figures; UK, United Kingdom; B, Belgium
* $P<0.05$; ** $P<0.01$

perimental designs: double blinding. Compared with this assessment, quasi-experimental community intervention studies do not do that badly. Of course, this is due to the many difficulties experimental studies of the clinical trial type stipulate in the area of borderline risk, where large study populations are required in order to prove small risk reductions significant at accepted levels.

If we select – in order to compare the results of these studies – reduction of total mortality as the main criterion of success, then it is obvious that the general impression is not at all convincing. As Table 4 makes clear, only one study (Hypertension and Follow-up Program) shows significant reduction of total mortality, whereas the Clofibrate Study at 10 years' follow-up shows significant inverse results, while other study results are insignificantly positive [9, 11, 12, 16, 17] or negative [13]. Due to the insufficient number of events in study populations of limited size, even mortality due to coronary heart disease is significantly reduced only in a single study [17]. On the other hand, non-cardiovascular diseases are inversely increased in the treatment groups in all studies (except for [10, 12]). The absolute increase of non-cardiovascular diseases (about half of the total mortality in the general population) often seems to be even higher than the reduction of coronary heart disease mortality, where achieved. Thus, one essential requirement of research, namely, the repeatibility of positive results, is seriously impaired.

A typical example is the European Multifactorial Risk Prevention Trial, where the reduction of total mortality is in favor of the intervention group. However, total mortality reduction is significant only in Belgium (one of the five participating countries), and is negative (i.e., in favor of the non-treatment group) in the United Kingdom. One of the arguments given in the discussion about these results was that the interventive effort in the United Kingdom has been much less than in Belgium. This

Table 5. The controlled clinical trial in boderline risks

Indication	High attributable risk
Sample	Representativity (volunteers)
	Standardization (multicenter)
	Repetition (generalizability)
	Feasibility (financial means)
Treatment	Effectiveness
	Broad applicability
	Inoffensiveness

does, however, not fully explain the change of sign, significant or not. It has also to be considered in this connection that none of these trials has a high power for confirming the null hypothesis. In most trials only one-sided statistical tests are used (e.g., in the Lipid Research Clinical Trial), thus, not accounting for the possibility that treatments might do harm.

Table 5 summarizes the weaknesses of the concept of controlled clinical trials for the detection of mild-risk reductions. As the required study populations are very large, usually volunteers have to be used who constitute a selection of ready and eager individuals, not necessarily typical of the general population. Usually one clinic or project group has not the capacity to run such a large study, thus the required standardization between participating centers boosts the costs of such trials enormously. High costs make certain studies either unfeasible (e.g., a randomized multifactorial dietary intervention study) and/or prevent repetition, especially if a positive result has been shown in the first study. Beyond this, treatment concepts to be used against mild risks have to show broad mass applicability and long-range inoffensiveness in terms of late toxic effects and (during the reproductive age) genetic damage. These requirements exclude at the present time all non-pharmacologic approaches – in principal better suited to mild risks – and even among the available drugs, only some basic antihypertensive drugs fulfill this criterion.

The milder the risk, the larger, more expensive, and, probably, more inconclusive the research of the clinical trial will be. What is the alternative? If we conceptualize a very simplified pathogenetic chain which leads to cardiovascular disease, then risk factors like hypertension and hypercholesterolemia should be understood as a consequence of unhealthy behaviors in the area of nutrition, physical activity, and smoking. However, such behaviors are not isolated, but form part of a complex pattern which is tied to many aspects of daily life (in that sense, e.g., smoking behavior could be seen as part of a "communication behavior"). In this way, behaviors are a result of personal decisions and influences, mainly from the social environment (psychosocial factors or determinants). The basic structures determining social life are vaguely summarized as "living conditions" (Table 6). A primordial preventive approach should aim at the most basic links of this chain. Therefore, intervention in this sense cannot be restricted to individual persons randomized in a clinical trial, but has to include social ties, social support, neighborhood, and community. We speak

Table 6. Pathogenesis of atherosclerotic cardiovascular disease

Living conditions
▼
Psychosocial determinants
▼
Health behaviors
▼
Risk factors
▼
Morbidity
Mortality

Table 7. Limitations of inference from quasi-experimental intervention studies

No randomization
Open (nonblind)
Lack of independence
Limited comparability
Secular trend
Restricted feasibility
Length of study period

Table 8. Interventional population studies – design elements in support of causal inference

Component	Means
Control	Comparison (pairwise)
Repetition	Stepping (start of programs)
Trend analysis	Distribution of risk factors Development of incidence Change of medical care
Cohorts	Individual change
Dose-response	Variation of program density (maximizing and repetition) Control of program exposition (linkage of component effects)
Pooling	End points

of community-oriented concepts. Thus, a strategy towards mild risks has to involve the general, even the normal population as the understanding of primordial prevention involves the healthy population.

The main difficulty of community intervention studies [14] is that if we use total communities as the basic unit, the individuals at least in the intervention unit are not independent from each other, rather their interdependence forms an essential element of the intervention strategy. Yet total communities cannot be really randomized due to the gigantic effort required in order to provide sufficient numbers of communities for such an endeavor and due to the fact that communities have a collective decision-making process whereby they probably would never accept to remain as controls if intervention seems to become successful. Another difficulty is that given the impossibility of randomization, communities are rarely sufficiently comparable and if so, then their comparability is endangered by external events (e.g., local crises such as unemployment) uncontrollable by a research group. In any case, as important as long-term follow-up is with regard to the detection of subliminal side effects, long study periods may render the final results irrelevant by the time they actually become available (Table 7).

Yet, as we have seen, classical concepts of clinical trials after all do not do so much better with regard to the scientific analysis of the reversibility of borderline risks. On the other hand, even quasi-experimental study designs [18] can compensate for their obvious weaknesses, for example, by using the national frame as a reference, as is the case in the German Cardiovascular Prevention Study [15] and by applying an extensive array of process measurements, as is outlined in Table 8. It is clear that the inherent conceptual and operational weaknesses of research into borderline risks cannot fully be compensated for; however, the degree of plausibility that observed changes are real changes and are due to the applied programs or treatment schemes can be increased to a degree of rendering the likelihood of alternative hypotheses very low indeed.

In summary, it may be said that the classical concept of the controlled clinical trial comes to its conceptual limits if mild and very mild risks are to be approached, and we have to accept that what might turn out to be at best an insufficient fulfillment of essential requirements for causal inference has to be replaced by a sincere analysis of degrees of plausibility. Principally, in qualitative terms this is not so different from a concept of the probability of error – which is the more adequate language to express the establishment of significance.

References

1. Stamler J (1978) Life styles, major risk factors, proof and public policy. Circulation 58(1):3
2. The Pooling Projekt Research Group (1978) Relationship of blood pressure, serum cholesterol, smoking habit, relative weight and ECG abnormalities to incidence of major coronary events: Final Report. J Chronic Dis 31:201
3. McGill MC Jr (1980) Morphologic development of the atherosclerotic plaque. In: Lauer RM, Shekelle RB (eds) Childhood prevention of atherosclerosis and hypertension. Raven, New York
4. Veterans Administration Cooperative Study Group (1967) Effect of treatment on morbidity in hypertension: Results in patients with diastolic blood pressures averaging 115 through 129 mm Hg. JAMA 202:1028
5. Veterans Administration Cooperative Study Group (1970) Effects of treatment on morbidity in hypertension. II. Results in patients with diastolic blood pressures averaging 90 through 114 mm Hg. JAMA 213:1143
6. Rose G (1980) Relative merits of intervening on whole populations versus high-risk individuals only. In: Lauer RM, Shekelle RB (eds) Childhood prevention of atherosclerosis and hypertension. Raven, New York and (1985) Sick individuals and sick populations. Int J Epidem 14/1:32
7. Committee of Principal Investigators (1980) WHO cooperative trial on primary prevention of ischaemic heart disease using clofibrate to lower serum cholesterol: Mortality follow-up. Lancet II:379
8. Committee of Principal Investigators (1984) WHO cooperative trial on primary prevention of ischaemic heart disease with clofibrate to lower serum cholesterol: Final mortality follow-up. Lancet II:600
9. Lipid Research Clinics Program (1984) The lipid research clinics' coronary primary prevention trial results. I. Reduction in incidence of coronary heart disease. JAMA 251(3):351

10. Hypertension Detection and Follow-up Program Cooperative Group (1979) Five-year findings of the hypertension detection and follow-up program. I. Reduction in mortality of persons with high blood pressure, including mild hypertension. JAMA 242(23): 2562
11. World Health Organization European Collaborative Group (1983) Multifactorial trial in the prevention of coronary heart disease. 3. Incidence and mortality results. Eur Heart J 4: 141
12. The Management Committee (1980) The Australian therapeutic trial in mild hypertension. Lancet I: 1263
13. Laaser U (1984) Der Amerikanische Multiple Risk Factor Intervention Trial: Konsequenzen für Praxis und Forschung in der Bundesrepublik. JAMA [D] 1: 53
14. Laaser U (1985) Lay involvement in the primary prevention of cardiovascular disease: The Rhein-Neckar Community Study (GRN). In: Laaser U, Senault R, Viefhues H (eds) Primary health care in the making. Springer, Berlin Heidelberg New York Tokyo
15. Die Projektleiter des Forschungsverbundes DHP (1984) Die Deutsche Herz-Kreislauf-Präventionsstudie (DHP). In: Bundesministerium für Forschung und Technik (Hrsg) Forschung zur Gesundheitsvorsorge, Herz-Kreislauf-Krankheiten. Bundesministerium für Forschung und Technologie, Bonn
16. Medical Research Council Working Party (1985) MRC trial of treatment of mild hypertension: principal results. Brit Med J 291: 97
17. Amery A, Birkenhager W, Brixko P et al (1985) Mortality and morbidity results from the European Working Party on High Blood Pressure in the Elderly trial. Lancet I: 1349
18. Campbell DT, Stanley JC (1963) Experimental and Quasi-Experimental Designs for Research. Rand McNally College Publ Co, Chicago

Indications for Antihypertensive Treatment*

J. Staessen[1], R. Fagard[1], P. Lijnen[1], R. Van hoof[1], and A. Amery[1]

Introduction

The decision of a clinician to treat or not to treat a particular hypertensive patient with hypotensive drugs shall be based on the health status of this patient and on data derived from different sources; the latter can be grouped into two major categories: epidemiological studies and intervention trials.

Epidemiological Studies

The clinician can look at data from epidemiologists, who studied populations without intervening and found that elevated blood pressure is a major and independent risk indicator for mortality, especially cardiovascular mortality and stroke incidence. Epidemiologists have concluded that the higher the pressure, the greater the risk for stroke and this is true not only for diastolic but also, and perhaps to a greater extent, for systolic blood pressure. Based on this evidence, some clinicians concluded that patients with elevated blood pressure should receive hypotensive drugs.

However, there are still open questions:

1. We do not know from the available data whether a reduction of blood pressure by artificial means, such as *hypotensive drugs*, will reduce the cardiovascular morbidity and mortality to the same extent. Indeed, we do not know how long the pressure has to be lowered to obtain this possible beneficial effect, and we should be aware that hypotensive agents may have adverse reactions.

2. If we decide on this basis to start hypotensive drug treatment we should treat not only patients with a systolic blood pressure of 190 mm Hg, but also those with a systolic pressure of 160 mm Hg and even 140 mm Hg, since they, too, are at greater risk than subjects with a systolic pressure of 120 mm Hg. This would mean that the majority of people above age 40 should receive hypertensive drugs. Obviously we should look at other criteria. Could these be derived from intervention trials?

Results of Intervention Trials

The published intervention trials have recently been discussed by Staessen et al. [1]. The overall results are summarized in Tables 1–7.

---

* This and other studies in our laboratory are supported by the National Research Council (NFWO).

[1] Inwendige Geneeskunde – Cardiologie, U.Z. Gasthuisberg, Herestraat 49, B-3000 Leuven.

Primary Hypertension
Ed. by W. Kaufmann et al.

Table 1. Total mortality incidence in different hypertension trials according to treatment regimen[a]

Trial identification	Active	Control	*P* between two groups
Veterans Administration Cooperative Study on Antihypertensive Agents [3–5]			
DBP: 115–129 mm Hg	0/73	4/70	?
DBP: 90–114 mm Hg	10/186	21/194	?
Hypertension-Stroke Cooperative Study [6]	26/233	24/219	>0.1
U.S. Public Health Service Mild Hypertension Trial [7]	2/193	2/196	>0.1
Göteborg Trial [16]	21/635 (3.3%)	24/391 (6.1%)	<0.05
Hypertension Detection and Follow-up Program [11]	349/5485	419/5455	<0.01
Australian Therapeutic Trial in Mild Hypertension [9, 10]	9/1721	19/1706	<0.05
Oslo Study [14]	10/406	9/379	>0.1
Total	427/8932	522/8610	<0.001

[a] In this and the following tables the results were not entered if fewer than 100 patients were admitted in any of the treatment groups

?, a test for significance is not given in this paper; DBP, diastolic blood pressure

Table 2. Incidence of cardiovascular mortality in different trials according to treatment regimen

Trial identification	Active	Control	*P* between two groups
Veterans Administration Cooperative Study on Antihypertensive Agents [3–5]			
DBP: 115–129 mm Hg	0/73	4/70	?
DBP: 90–114 mm Hg	8/186	19/194	?
Hypertension-Stroke Cooperative Study [6]	15/233	19/219	>0.1
U.S. Public Health Service Mild Hypertension Trial [7]	2/193	2/196	>0.1
Göteborg Trial [16]	8/635 (1.3%)	10/391 (2.6%)	N.S.
Hypertension Detection and Follow-up Program [11]	195/5485	240/5455	?
Australian Therapeutic Trial in Mild Hypertension [9, 10]	4/1721	13/1706	<0.025
Oslo Study [14]	7/406	6/379	>0.1
Total	239/8932	313/8610	Not calculated

?, a test for significance is not given in this paper; DBP, diastolic blood pressure; N.S., not significant

Table 3. Deaths from cerebrovascular accidents in different trials according to treatment regimen

Trial identification	Active	Control	*P* between two groups
Veterans Administration Cooperative Study on Antihypertensive Agents [3–5]			
DBP: 115–129 mm Hg	0/73	0/70	?
DBP: 90–114 mm Hg	1/186	7/194	?
Hypertension-Stroke Cooperative Study [6]	6/233	10/219	>0.1
U.S. Public Health Service Mild Hypertension Trial [7]	0/193	0/196	>0.1
Göteborg Trial [16]	2/635 (0.3%)	3/391 (0.8%)	N.S.
Hypertension Detection and Follow-up Program [11]	29/5485	52/5455	?
Australian Therapeutic Trial in Mild Hypertension [9, 10]	2/1721	4/1706	>0.1
Oslo Study [14]	0/406	2/379	?
Total	40/8932	78/8610	Not calculated

?, a test for significance is not given in this paper; DBP, diastolic blood pressure; N.S., not significant

Table 4. Deaths from coronary heart disease (including sudden death) in different trials according to treatment regimen

Trial identification	Active	Control	*P* between two groups
Veterans Administration Cooperative Study on Antihypertensive Agents [3–5]			
DBP: 115–129 mm Hg	0/73	1/70	?
DBP: 90–114 mm Hg	6/186	11/194	?
Hypertension-Stroke Cooperative Study [6]	4/233	7/219	>0.1
U.S. Public Health Service Mild Hypertension Trial [7]	2/193	2/196	>0.1
Göteborg Trial [16]	5/635 (0.8%)	6/391 (2.6%)	N.S.
Hypertension Detection and Follow-up Program [11]	131/5485	148/5455	?
Australian Therapeutic Trial in Mild Hypertension [9, 10]	2/1721	8/1706	0.051
Oslo Study [14]	6/406	2/379	?
Total	156/8932	185/8610	Not calculated

?, a test for significance is not given in this paper; DBP, diastolic blood pressure; N.S., not significant

Table 5. All cerebrovascular events (fatal and nonfatal) in different trials according to treatment regimen

Trial identification	Active	Control	*P* between two groups
Veterans Administration Cooperative Study on Antihypertensive Agents [3–5]			
DBP: 115–129 mm Hg	1/73	4/70	?
DBP: 90–114 mm Hg	5/186	20/194	?
Hypertension-Stroke Cooperative Study [6]	37/233	42/219	>0.1
U.S. Public Health Service Mild Hypertension Trial [7]	0/193	2/196	?
Göteborg Trial [16]	7/635 (1.1%)	7/391 (1.8%)	N.S.
Hypertension Detection and Follow-up Program [11]	?	?	?
Australian Therapeutic Trial in Mild Hypertension [9, 10]	12/1721	25/1706	<0.025
Oslo Study [14]	0/406	7/379	<0.02
Total	62/3447	107/3155	Not calculated

?, a test for significance is not given in this paper; DBP, diastolic blood pressure; N.S., not significant

Table 6. All coronary events (fatal and nonfatal) in different trials according to treatment regimen

Trial identification	Active	Control	*P* between two groups
Veterans Administration Cooperative Study on Antihypertensive Agents [3–5]			
DBP: 115–129 mm Hg	0/73	3/70	?
DBP: 90–114 mm Hg	11/186	13/194	?
Hypertension-Stroke Cooperative Study [6]	7/233	9/219	>0.1
U.S. Public Health Service Mild Hypertension Trial [7]	8/193	7/196	?
Göteborg Trial [16]	23/635 (3.6%)	27/391 (6.9%)	<0.03
Hypertension Detection and Follow-up Program [11]	?	?	?
Australian Therapeutic Trial in Mild Hypertension [9, 10]	0/1721	88/1706	>0.1
Oslo Study [14]	20/406	13/379	>0.1
Total	139/3447	160/3155	Not calculated

?, a test for significance is not given in this paper; DBP, diastolic blood pressure; N.S., not significant

Table 7. Incidence of morbid events in different hypertension trials according to treatment regimen

Trial identification	Specification	Active	Control	*P* between two groups
Veterans Administration Cooperative Study on Antihypertensive Agents [3–5]	Assessable events			
DBP: 115–129 mm Hg		2/73	27/70	0.001
DBP: 90–114 mm Hg		22/186	76/194	$t = 5.0$
Hypertension-Stroke Cooperative Study [6]	End points	112/233	123/219	0.12
U.S. Public Health Service Mild Hypertension Trial [7]	First morbid	56/193	90/196	?
Göteborg Trial [16]	Total mortality + myocardial infarction + stroke	44/635 (6.9%)	49/391 (12.5%)	?
Hypertension Detection and Follow-up Program [11]	Total mortality	349/5485	419/5455	<0.01
Australian Therapeutic Trial in Mild Hypertension [9, 10]	Trial end points	91/1721	127/1706	<0.01
Oslo Study [14]	Cardiovascular events	25/406	34/379	>0.1
Total	Variable	Not calculated	Not calculated	Not calculated

?, a test for significance is not given in this paper; DBP, diastolic blood pressure; N.S., not significant

Since the methodology of these intervention trials is of major importance, they will be grouped accordingly.

Double-Blind Placebo-Controlled Trials

A double-blind placebo-controlled trial uses the most appropriate method to study whether drug treatment is different from placebo treatment. The results of the following double-blind placebo-controlled trials have been published:

1. First double-blind trial [2]
2. Veterans Administration Cooperative Studies [3–5]
3. Hypertension-Stroke Cooperative Study [6]
4. U.S. Public Health Service Trial [7]
5. Japanese trial in the aged [8]

In all five trials there was no significant difference in total mortality or cause-specific mortality between the controls and treated groups. The first two trials [2, 3] showed some advantages in favor of antihypertensive treatment, while the results of trials (3) and (4) [6, 7] did not indicate a clear advantage. The difference in complications in trial (5) [8] was only significant when the blood pressure elevation per se was considered as a complication.

Single-Blind Placebo-Controlled Trials

The Australian Mild Hypertension Trial [9, 10] was a single-blind, placebo-controlled experiment. Because of the number of patients randomized and the methodology, it is the most relevant trial if one wishes to compare the outcome of patients with mild hypertension treated with either placebo or hypotensive drugs.

The trial shows a significant reduction in total mortality, which was the result of the decrease in cardiovascular mortality; the noncardiovascular mortality was unchanged.

Cerebrovascular events were significantly decreased and the same trend was seen for fatal cerebrovascular events, nonfatal hemorrhage of thrombosis, and transient ischemic attacks. On the other hand, over two-thirds of all trial end points were due to ischemic heart disease, but in this category the reduction of all events was only one-fifth.

Open, Randomized Trials Comparing Two Treatment Procedures

The Hypertension Detection and Follow-up Program (HDFP) [11] was an open, randomized program (it was not labeled as a trial) and compared the effects of a systematic antihypertensive treatment program conducted in specialized clinics (stepped care) to the effects of community-based hypertensive treatment (referred care).

In the total number of randomized patients the 5-year mortality from all causes was 17% lower in the stepped than in the referred care. The reduction in mortality was seen not only for cardiovascular mortality (−19%) but also for noncardiovascular mortality (−14%).

In discussing the results of this program, one should take into account its special nature. It was not a placebo-controlled trial; it was also not a comparison between two well-specified drug regimens. It compared two treatment procedures: treatment of hypertensive patients in the regularly available medical practice and treatment in specialized centers where several measures were taken to increase compliance. Also the observers were, at least partially, different: the specialized personnel in the special centers and the regular health workers in the referred care group. The data show very little difference between the decrease in cardiovascular mortality (−19%) and the decrease in non-cardiovascular mortality (−14%), which suggests that factors other than blood pressure reduction, such as general care, may have been important. One wonders, therefore, if the same changes in general care in other parts of the world, such as here in Europe, would produce a similar decrease in mortality.

Open, Randomized Trials Comparing Hypotensive Drug Treatment to a Regimen Without Hypotensive Drug Treatment

Four trials compared the outcome of hypertensive patients randomized to a hypotensive drug treatment group and a group without hypotensive drugs or placebo.

Already 20 years ago, Hamilton et al. [12] reported a reduction in complications in male patients treated with hypotensive drugs, but not in female patients.

Carter [13] showed in his stroke survivors a reduction in mortality in the patients below age 65, but not in the patients above age 65.

In the Oslo study published by Helgeland [14], 785 young men between age 40 and 49 with uncomplicated hypertension were studied. Between both treatment groups no difference was found in total mortality or cardiovascular mortality. The incidence of cardiovascular events was not significantly different, since the decrease in cerebrovascular events on active treatment was partially counterbalanced by the tendency to more coronary events. In interpreting these results, one should keep in mind that the patients were young men with very mild hypertension and that antihypertensive drugs were administered in 17% of the control group.

The trial in elderly patients reported by Sprackling et al. [15] was small, including only 123 patients, and no significant differences in events were obtained.

Open Trials, Without Random Allocation

Several open trials have been reported where the patients were not allocated at random. They will not be discussed in detail here.

The large Göteborg trial [16] was the only trial in hypertension where the incidence of myocardial infarction was significantly reduced on active treatment, whereas stroke was not, even combining fatal and nonfatal stroke.

After review of this impressive number of patients studied, one may hope to find an answer for the vast majority of the patients seen at our clinics. Is this so?

Discussion

Looking at subgroups in trials may be dangerous, especially if no stratification was planned before the start of the trial. "In a flurry of retrospective subgroup analyses, hypotheses and counterhypotheses result from this type of post hoc activity, while the main result may be obscured, for reasons that have little to do with scientific validity" [17].

However, the clinician is faced with specific patients and some of these cases will now be discussed.

The White, Hypertensive Woman

The hypertensive patient seen most often at our outpatient clinics here in Europe is a white woman with uncomplicated essential hypertension. Do the intervention studies prove that by the use of hypotensive drugs we can decrease mortality in general or cardiovascular mortality or even only the incidence of cardiovascular events?

The answer is no, and this can be illustrated by looking at the published intervention studies. Let us start with the double-blind placebo-controlled studies. In the first double-blind trial, published by Wolff and Lindeman [2], mainly blacks were entered, while the Veterans Administration studies coordinated by Freis were restricted to males [3]. Therefore they do not offer an answer to our question. The other three double-blind placebo-controlled trials [6–8] showed no significant benefit in favor of treatment.

In the single-blind placebo-controlled Australian Mild Hypertension Study [9, 10], there was no significant difference in the female group between those actively treated and controls, no significant difference in mortality from all causes, no difference in cardiovascular and cerebrovascular mortality, and even no significant difference in all cardiovascular events combined!

In the U.S. HDFP [11] the largest number of patients was entered, but also here there was no significant difference in mortality in the white female subgroup between the referred care and the stepped care group. This study also does not indicate that we can prolong life expectancy in hypertensive white woman by administering hypotensive drugs.

Let us look at the studies which were not blind, but open, and where the patients were randomly allocated to an active treatment group and to a group without active hypotensive drugs. Hamilton et al. [12] showed a decrease in cerebrovascular events in the treated males, but no significant difference in the female group. The study of Carter [13] does not give a separate analysis by sex and can therefore not be used for our discussion. In the Oslo study by Helgeland [14] only men were entered, and in the "elderly" trial of Sprackling et al. [15] no difference was found between the two groups for the study as a whole.

The many trials where the patients were not allocated at random will not be discussed here in detail, because this lack of randomization makes interpretation more difficult. It should be mentioned that in the Göteborg study [16], which is so often quoted, only men were entered.

Thus, from all the intervention trials, published before the end of 1984, not one indicates that antihypertensive drugs will improve the prognosis of the patient who is in the majority of those seen at the hypertension clinic: the white woman.

The White, Hypertensive Man

Concerning the influence of hypotensive drug therapy on morbidity and mortality, convincing data are lacking in hypertensive men below age 40 or above age 70. In middle-aged men with diastolic blood pressure at repeated examination of 95 mmHg or more, controlled trials have demonstrated that hypotensive drug treatment can improve prognosis. Trials are in progress to study the outcome of isolated systolic hypertension; however, to date no convincing data are available.

Stroke Survivors Above Age 65

Is antihypertensive drug treatment indicated in stroke survivors above age 65? This has been studied more specifically in two trials, namely the trials of Carter [13] and Hoobler [6]. The reoccurrence of stroke could not be significantly decreased by hypotensive drug treatment in these two trials. Of all morbid events, analyzed in the latter study, only the incidence of congestive heart failure was decreased in the study population.

Hypertensive Patients with Other Risk Indicators

In several major epidemiological surveys, besides high blood pressure, other major risk indicators for cardiovascular diseases have been identified in the population at large such as cigarette smoking, hypercholesterolemia, and to a lesser extent obesity, impaired glucose tolerance, and physical inactivity. One is therefore inclined to start hypotensive drug therapy more readily in a given hypertensive patient when other risk indicators are also present.

However, when one risk indicator outweighs the others in a particular individual, do the risk indicators then contribute independently to the overall risk? This was not the case as reported in the paper of Bulpitt et al. [18] who, in studying patients with moderate or severe hypertension, found only age, impaired renal function, systolic blood pressure, and cigarette smoking as independent risk indicators. Furthermore, up to now no trial has shown, or even investigated under controlled conditions, whether in hypertensive patients with risk indicators other than high blood pressure per se hypotensive drugs are more or less effective in decreasing morbidity or mortality rates and therefore improving prognosis. The widespread idea that hypotensive drug treatment should be started more readily in hypertensive patients with additional risk indicators is up to now speculative and therefore needs confirmation from controlled studies.

Concluding Remarks

Based on epidemiological studies, the evidence is overwhelming that both systolic and diastolic blood pressure are major risk indicators for cardiovascular morbidity and mortality. Also an impressive number of patients have been followed over many patient/years in well-controlled intervention trials; therefore, one could hope to find a clearly established rationale for hypotensive drug treatment in our patients.

A detailed analysis of the data, however illustrates, that for the majority of hypertensive patients seen at our European clinics a solid basis is still lacking. It is hoped that the results of ongoing trials, which are likely to be reported in 1985 will broaden the basis on which a clinician can base a decision.

References

1. Staessen J, Cattaert A, Fagard R, Lijnen P, Vanhees L, Amery A (1983) Epidemiology of treated, compared to untreated, hypertension. In: Genest J, et al. (eds) Hypertension, 2nd edn. McGraw-Hill, New York, pp 1069–1093
2. Wolff FW, Lindeman RF (1966) Effects of treatment in hypertension. J Chronic Dis 19:227–240
3. Veterans Administration Cooperative Study Group on Antihypertensive Agents (1967) Effects of treatment on morbidity in hypertension. JAMA 202:1028–1034
4. Veterans Administration Cooperative Study Group on Antihypertensive Agents (1970) Effects of treatment on morbidity in hypertension. JAMA 213:1143–1151
5. Veterans Administration Cooperative Study Group on Antihypertensive Agents (1972) Effects of treatment on morbidity in hypertension. Circulation 45:991–1004
6. Hypertension-Stroke Cooperative Study Group (1974) Effect of antihypertensive treatment on stroke recurrence. JAMA 229:409–418
7. McFate Smith W (1977) Treatment of mild hypertension. Circ Res [Suppl 1] 40:I–98–I–105
8. Kuramoto K, Matsushita S, Kuwajima I, Murakami M (1981) Prospective study on the treatment of mild hypertension in the aged. Jpn Heart J 22:75–85
9. Report by the Management Committee (1980) The Australian therapeutic trial in mild hypertension. Lancet I:1261–1267

10. Report by the Management Committee (1981) Treatment of mild hypertension in the elderly. Med J Aust 2:398–401
11. Hypertension Detection and Follow-up Program Cooperative Group (1979) Five-year findings of the hypertension detection and follow-up program. JAMA 242:2562–2577
12. Hamilton M, Thompson EN, Wisniewski TKM (1964) The role of blood pressure control in preventing complications of hypertension. Lancet I:235–238
13. Carter AB (1970) Hypotensive therapy in stroke survivors. Lancet I:485–489
14. Helgeland A (1980) Treatment of mild hypertension: A five-year controlled drug trial. Am J Med 69:725–732
15. Sprackling ME, Mitchell JRA, Short AH, Watt G (1981) Blood pressure reduction in the elderly: A randomised controlled trial of methyldopa. Br Med J 283:1151–1153
16. Berglund G, Wilhelmsen L, Sannerstedt R, Hansson L, Andersson O, Silvertsson R, Wedel H, Wikstrand J (1978) Coronary heart-disease after treatment of hypertension. Lancet I:1–5
17. Abernethy JD (1984) The Australian therapeutic trial in mild hypertension (letter). Hypertension 6:774–776
18. Bulpitt CJ, Beilin IJ, Clifton P, Coles EC, Dollery CT, Gear JSS, Harper GS, Johnson BF, Munro-Faure AD (1979) Risk factors for death in treated hypertensive patients. Lancet II:134–137

Rationale for Established Antihypertensive Treatment

H. Holzgreve[1] and M. Middeke[1]

Medical science organizations and experts have repeatedly drawn up recommendations for antihypertensive drug therapy. The currently valid stepped-care approach of the American Joint National Committee on Detection, Evaluation and Treatment of High Blood Pressure [15] and the German League against Hypertension [3] agree in recommending diuretics and beta blockers as the treatment of choice in hypertension. The question arises: What are the criteria that should be applied for selecting the initial antihypertensive agents and for the sequence of combining such drugs?

When establishing and implementing such a stepped-care antihypertensive therapy scheme, it must be kept in mind that many highly touted and apparent breakthroughs in therapy later become dubious and short lived. In setting up their stepped-care plan, it was by no means the ambition of the aforementioned organizations to be heralds or pioneers of new therapies, but rather to mediate conclusively established and indisputably confirmed therapeutic modalities.

In view of the broad spectrum of antihypertensive agents, it is difficult to establish compulsory or universally acceptable criteria for the selection of antihypertensives. Several criteria, however, are obvious and mandatory, for example, the feasibility of long-term oral administration. The following criteria are especially significant:

1. Demonstrated efficacy, that is, prevention of the typical long-term complications of hypertension
2. Good tolerance and an acceptable side-effect rate at equally effective doses, as demonstrated in long-term comparative therapeutic studies

Demonstrated Efficacy of Treatment

Several hypertension intervention studies have clearly shown that drug therapy in hypertensive individuals between the ages of about 30 and 65 with diastolic blood pressure values between approximately 95 and 110 mm Hg improves life expectancy and decreases morbidity. These findings stem from four randomized controlled studies, namely, the Veterans Administration study [17], the United States Public Health study [16], the Australian Therapy Study on Mild Hypertension [11], and the Oslo study [4]. Additional studies include the Hypertension Detection and Follow-Up Program Cooperative Group (HDFP) study [6, 7] which, although randomized, involves a control-group population in which 43% to 58% of the persons received

[1] Medizinische Poliklinik, Universität München, Pettenkoferstr. 8a, D-8000 München 2.

Primary Hypertension
Ed. by W. Kaufmann et al.

Table 1. Hypertension intervention trials (May 1985). Change (%) in mortality for all causes (TM), in mortality for cardiovascular disease (CVM), in fatal and nonfatal cerebrovascular accidents (CVA), and in coronary accidents (CHD) in 5 years per 1000 persons by antihypertensive drug treatment

Trial	Change (%)			
	TM	CVM	CVA	CHD
1. VA [17]	−50	−56	−74	−16
2. USPH [16]	−49	−49	−83	−15
3. Berglund [1]	−46	−51	−39	−48
4. HDFP [6, 7]	−17	−19	−36	−12
5. Australien [11]	−29	−56	−46	−11
6. Oslo [4]	+3	−7	−100	+30
Mean	−31	−40	−63	−12
Without 3, 4, 6	−43	−54	−68	−14

VA, Veterans Administration; USPH, United States Public Health; HDFP, Hypertension Detection and Follow-up

antihypertensives, and the study done by Berglund et al. [1], which is not randomized and in which 24% of subjects in the control group were under treatment.

When the results of these studies are expressed in terms of "prevented complications" per 1000 patients over 5 years, the following success rates emerge (Table 1): In these intervention studies the total mortality rate decreased by 17%–50%, and cardiovascular mortality by 7%–56%. The Oslo study was the exception, with a (statistically insignificant) 3% rise in total mortality and only a slight drop of 7% in cardiovascular mortality. The calculated mean reductions were 31% for total mortality and 40% for cardiovascular mortality. Therapy proved particularly favorable in terms of fatal and nonfatal cerebrovascular accidents – a typical complication of high blood pressure – which was reduced by 36%–100%, with a mean decrease of 63%.

For a long time it was not possible, because of the limited number of cases in individual studies, to conclude with equal reliability that the incidence of coronary heart disease and its complications also decreases under the influence of therapy. This uncertainty primarily resulted from the fact that, due to ethical considerations, several studies had to be discontinued at a point in time at which the rate of cerebrovascular complications increased in the untreated control group, while a favorable but statistically not yet significant therapeutic effect on the complications of coronary heart disease was just beginning to emerge. Today, collective evaluation of all studies justifies the statement that antihypertensive treatment prevents fatal and nonfatal myocardial infarction and sudden death to a small, but marked extent. The results of all the cited studies show a mean reduction of 12%, which increases to 20% when the Oslo study [4] – which will be discussed later – is excluded.

It must, however, be borne in mind that in the HDFP [6, 7] and Berglund studies [1] 43%–58% and 24%, respectively, of the control-group subjects were receiving

Table 2. Step 1 and step 2 antihypertensive drugs used in hypertension intervention trials

Trial	Therapy
1. VA [17]	Diuretic – reserpin
2. USPH [16]	Diuretic – reserpin
3. Berglund [1]	Beta blocker (78%) or diuretic
4. HDFP [6, 7]	Diuretic – reserpin or methyldopa
5. Australien [11]	Diuretic – methyldopa or beta blocker (? %)
6. Oslo [4]	Diuretic – methyldopa or beta blocker (25%)

Abbreviations given in Table 1

antihypertensive agents. Naturally, this fact makes it more difficult to demonstrate therapeutic success. When the findings of both of these studies as well as, for reasons which will be explained later, the Oslo study [4] are excluded, the success rates increase from 31% to 43% for total mortality, from 40% to 54% for cardiovascular mortality, from 63% to 68% for cerebrovascular accidents and from 12% to 14% for the complications of coronary heart disease.

Table 2 lists the antihypertensive agents prescribed for mild hypertension in these intervention studies. In the Veterans Administration and United States Public Health studies, a diuretic and reserpine were used, in the HDFP study a diuretic and reserpine or alpha-methyldopa, in the Australian and Oslo studies a diuretic and alpha-methyldopa or beta-blockers, and in the Berglund study diuretics and, for the most part (namely, in 78% of the hypertensive subjects), beta-blockers.

Based on the hypertension intervention studies published to date, proof that fatal and nonfatal hypertensive organ complications can be prevented is most thoroughly documented for diuretics, not quite as thoroughly for beta-blockers, reserpine and alpha-methyldopa, and as yet not at all for several more recent antihypertensives, for example, calcium antagonists and the angiotensin-converting enzyme (ACE) inhibitors.

On the basis of the results of the Multiple Risk Factor Intervention Trial (MRFIT) study [10] and the Oslo study [4] misgivings have repeatedly been expressed concerning the use of diuretics in mild hypertension. The MRFIT study states that in hypertensive individuals with preexisting pathologic ECG changes diuretic treatment is not only ineffective, but also harmful. This conclusion is unacceptable to many statisticians, because the groups were not formed by stratification before the study but rather after the study had been concluded. Besides these statistical considerations, what is much more relevant for the physician is that this claim is in crass contradiction to the findings of other studies (Table 3). In the HDFP study [8], for example, it was possible to prevent 44 deaths (per 1000 subjects over 5 years) in the stepped-care group as compared with the referred-care group employing a diuretic as initial medication, even when at the beginning of the study end-organ damage was present. End-organ damage was defined as left ventricular hypertrophy on ECG, evidence of myocardial infarction from history or the ECG, history of stroke and arterial occlusive disease, or serum creatinine levels of over 1.7 mg/dl. In cases where such complications were absent, only 15 deaths (per 1000 subjects over 5 years) could be prevented.

Table 3. Mortality in the referred-care and stepped-care groups, as well as deaths prevented, per 1000 persons in 5 years of HDFP participation for patients with and without end-organ damage at entry [8]

End-organ damage at entry	Deaths (*n*)		Deaths prevented (*n*, %)
	Referred-care	Stepped-care	
No	58	45	13 (−22.4)
Yes	200	156	44 (−22.0)

End-organ damage: LVH on ECG, evidence of MI (history or ECG), history of stroke or intermittent claudication; creatinine >1.7 mg/dl

Thus, not only was there no harmful effect of diuretics in patients with end-organ damage at entry, but the success in terms of deaths prevented was indeed three times higher than in patients with uncomplicated hypertension.

Furthermore, in the HDFP study, 5173 participants with diastolic blood pressure at 90 to 104 mm Hg met MRFIT eligibility criteria. In patients with and without evidence of resting ECG abnormalities at entry, mortality rates for all causes and for major cardiovascular diseases were consistently lower in the stepped-care group than in the referred-care group [9] – a finding in crass contradiction to the MRFIT results.

Nor does the Oslo study lend support to the claim that antihypertensive treatment with diuretics increases cardiovascular mortality. The author wrote: "Considering the mild degree of hypertension, the small size of the study groups and the short follow-up time, it was not unexpected that both total mortality and morbidity from cardiovascular events were uninfluenced by drug treatment." A study, which the authors themselves considered inconclusive, can hardly be taken as evidence for the assertion that diuretics produce adverse effects.

Breaking numbers down into hypertensives free of end-organ damage at baseline discloses that both the results of HDFP [9] and the Oslo study [5] seem to confirm the MRFIT observations as far as coronary heart disease is concerned. The subgroups of hypertensives with ECG abnormalities according to MRFIT criteria show a higher mortality from coronary heart disease in the stepped-care group [9] and the treated group [5], respectively, than in the referred-care group and the untreated group. However, due to the small numbers in these subgroups, the differences did not reach statistical significance and could be caused by random variation.

Tolerance and Incidence of Side Effects

A second criterion for the selection of antihypertensives is the rate of side effects at equally effective doses. However, it is extremely difficult to determine precisely the rate and significance, the quantity and the quality of side effects. For this reason, evaluation of antihypertensive agents according to this criterion is not independent of subjective factors and personal experience; there is considerable freedom of interpretation and the possibility of misuse.

Since it is difficult to evaluate the tolerance and side effects of drugs from different small-scale studies and since antihypertensive therapy is undeniably a long-term procedure, methodically sound therapeutic studies are mandatory. These must compare the antihypertensive action, tolerance, and side effects of a new preparation with those of standard therapy and must involve sufficiently large patient populations studied over a reasonably long period of time. Furthermore, only in this way can rare but significant side effects be detected and the long-term effects of metabolic and endocrine changes on morbidity and mortality elucidated. A case in point: The fact that diuretics cause impotence in a certain percentage of patients was first recognized in a long-term study, the Medical Research Council (MRC) trial [13].

Besides the long-term intervention studies already described, there are several therapeutic studies, especially those from the Veterans Administration Group [18, 19], which have compared the tolerance and side-effect rates of diuretics, beta-blockers, reserpine, and hydralazine over a period of at least 1 year. Three large-scale multicenter studies comparing the action and side effects of diuretics and beta-blockers are currently in progress or already completed, but not yet published in their final form (May 1985). These include studies by the MRC [12], the Heart Attack Primary Prevention in Hypertension study (HAPPHY) [20], and the International Prospective Primary Prevention Study in Hypertension (IPPPSH) [14]; see Table 4.

Such long-term controlled studies represent the appropriate means for determining the value of a new hypotensive agent in antihypertensive therapy. Unfortunately, studies of this nature testing new antihypertensive substances have not yet been intiated, let alone completed. At any rate, in the future, any new antihypertensive agent or substance group with antihypertensive action claiming a preferential status in antihypertensive treatment will have to be examined in the light of such large-scale therapeutic studies and will have to be compared with diuretics or beta-blockers. Owing to their elaborate nature, this type of study can only be realized

Table 4. Three comparative hypertension intervention trials

Trial		Regime A	Regime B
MRC [12]	Step 1	Propranolol	Bendrofluazide
90–109 mm Hg	Step 2	Methyldopa or guanethidine	Methyldopa or guanethidine
IPPPSH [14]	Step 1	Oxprenolol	Placebo
100–125 mm Hg	Step 2	Hydrochlorothiazide or chlorthalidone	Hydrochlorothiazide or chlorthalidone
	Step 3	Hydralazine or prazosin	Hydralazine or prazosin
HAPPHY [20]	Step 1	Atenolol or metoprolol	Bendrofluazide or hydrochlorothiazide
100–130 mm Hg			
	Step 2	Hydralazine	Hydralazine
	Step 3	Spironolactone	Spironolactone

today with the support of the pharmaceutical industry. But the opportunity to demonstrate the superior long-term efficacy of a promising substance should provide ample stimulus and justify the efforts involved.

Unsuitable Criteria

In agreement with Bock and Anlauf [2], we are of the opinion that various arguments for the classification of antihypertensives are unviable, including, for example, the claim that an antihypertensive drug interferes with the pathogenetic mechanism of hypertension, that blood pressure during exercise is reduced, that left ventricular hypertrophy regresses, that the hemodynamic profile is positively affected, and that the circadian rhythm of blood pressure is physiologically influenced.

Summary

For long-term therapy the most suitable antihypertensives are those that meet the two requirements:

1. Efficacy has been demonstrated, this is, appropriate long-term intervention studies have shown that fatal and nonfatal hypertensive complications are prevented.
2. Tolerance and the rate of side effects have been tested in long-term studies involving sufficiently large patient populations. New agents should be compared with standard therapy.

Today these criteria are best fulfilled by diuretics, as well as beta-blockers – alone or in combination with diuretics – and reserpine in combination with diuretics. Renowned medical organizations, including the American Joint National Committee [15] and the German League Against Hypertension [3], have clearly based their stepped-care approaches for the treatment of hypertension on these criteria: They recommend diuretics and beta-blockers as the treatment of choice.

Addendum: At the time of preparation of the manuscript the MRC-, IPPPSH- and EWPHE-trials were not yet published.

References

1. Berglund G, Wilhelmsen L, Sannerstedt R, Hansson L, Andersson O, Sivertsson R, Wedel H, Wikstrand J (1978) Coronary heart disease after treatment of hypertension. Lancet I: 1–5
2. Bock KD, Anlauf M (1984) Die Qual der Wahl – das Dilemma der Hochdrucktherapie. Munch Med Wochenschr 126: 477–479
3. Deutsche Liga zur Bekämpfung des hohen Blutdruckes (1984) Empfehlungen zur Hochdruckbehandlung in der Praxis und zur Behandlung hypertensiver Notfälle, 6th edn. DLBHB, Heidelberg
4. Helgeland A (1980) Treatment of mild hypertension: a five-year controlled drug trial. The Oslo study. Am J Med 69: 725–732
5. Holme I, Helgeland A, Hjermann I, Leren P, Lund-Larsen PG (1984) Treatment of mild hypertension with diuretics. The importance of ECG abnormalities in the Oslo study and in MRFIT. JAMA 251: 1298–1299

6. Hypertension Detection and Follow-up Program Cooperative Group (1979) Five-year findings of the hypertension detection and follow-up program. I. Reduction in mortality of persons with high blood pressure, including mild hypertension. JAMA 242:2562–2571
7. Hypertension Detection and Follow-up Program Cooperative Group (1979) Five-year findings of the hypertension detection and follow-up program. II. Mortality by race-sex and age. JAMA 242:2572–2577
8. Hypertension Detection and Follow-up Program Cooperative Group (1982) The effect of treatment on mortality in "mild" hypertension. Results of the hypertension detection and follow-up program. N Engl J Med 307:976–980
9. Hypertension Detection and Follow-up Program Cooperative Research Group (1984) The effect of antihypertensive drug treatment on mortality in the presence of resting electrocardiographic abnormalities at baseline: the HDFP experience. Circulation 70:996–1003
10. Multiple Risk Factor Intervention Trial Research Group (1982) Multiple-risk factor intervention trial: Risk factor changes and mortality results. JAMA 248:1465–1477
11. Report by the Management Committee (1980) The Australian therapeutic trial in mild hypertension. Lancet 2:1261–1267
12. Report of Medical Research Council Working Party on Mild to Moderate Hypertension (1977) Randomized controlled trial of treatment for mild hypertension: design and pilot trial. Br Med J I:1437–1440
13. Report of Medical Research Council Working Party on Mild to Moderate Hypertension (1981) Adverse reactions to bendrofluazide and propranolol for the treatment of mild hypertension. Lancet 3:539–543
14. The IPPPSH Collaborative Group (1984) The international prospective primary prevention study in hypertension (IPPPSH): objectives and methods. Eur J Clin Pharmacol 27:379–391
15. The Joint National Committee on Detection, Evaluation, and Treatment of High Blood Pressure (1984) The 1984 report of the Joint National Committee on Detection, Evaluation, and Treatment of High Blood Pressure. Arch Intern Med 144:1045–1057
16. United States Public Health Service Hospitals Cooperative Study Group (1977) Treatment of mild hypertension. Results of a ten-year intervention trial. Circ Res [Suppl I] 40:98–105
17. Veterans Administration Cooperative Study Group on Antihypertensive Agents (1970) Effects of treatment on morbidity in hypertension. II. Results in patients with diastolic blood pressure averaging 90 through 114 mm Hg. JAMA 213:1143–1152
18. Veterans Administration Cooperative Study Group on Antihypertensive Agents (1977) Propranolol in the treatment of essential hypertension. JAMA 237:2303–2310
19. Veterans Administration Cooperative Study Group on Antihypertensive Agents (1982) Comparison of propranolol and hydrochlorothiazide for the initial treatment of hypertension: II. Results of long-term therapy. JAMA 248:2004–2011
20. Wilhelmsen L, Berglund G, Elmfeldt D, Wedel H (1981) β-Blockers versus saluretics in hypertension. Comparison of total mortality, myocardial infarction, and sudden death: study design and early results on blood pressure reduction. Prev Med 10:38–49

Calcium Channel Blockers in the Treatment of Hypertension*

P. WEIDMANN[1], M. P. GNAEDINGER[1], and D. E. UEHLINGER[1]

The central role that calcium (Ca) plays in cardiovascular regulation is well apparent in several clinical situations. Chronic hypercalcemia due to hyperparathyroidism, vitamin C intoxication, or other etiologies is sometimes accompanied by hypertension [1]. Acute hypercalcemia induced by Ca infusion may also increase blood pressure (BP), particularly in patients with impaired renal function [2, 3]. Conversely, acute severe hypocalcemia causes hypotension [4], and a pharmacologic inhibition of transmembranous Ca transport has been noted to lower BP in various forms of hypertension [5–7, 8]. Ca antagonists, as they were termed by their scientific godfather Fleckenstein [9], or calcium channel blockers (CCB), the term in use more recently [10], are agents that inhibit the cellular entry of calcium through a broad group

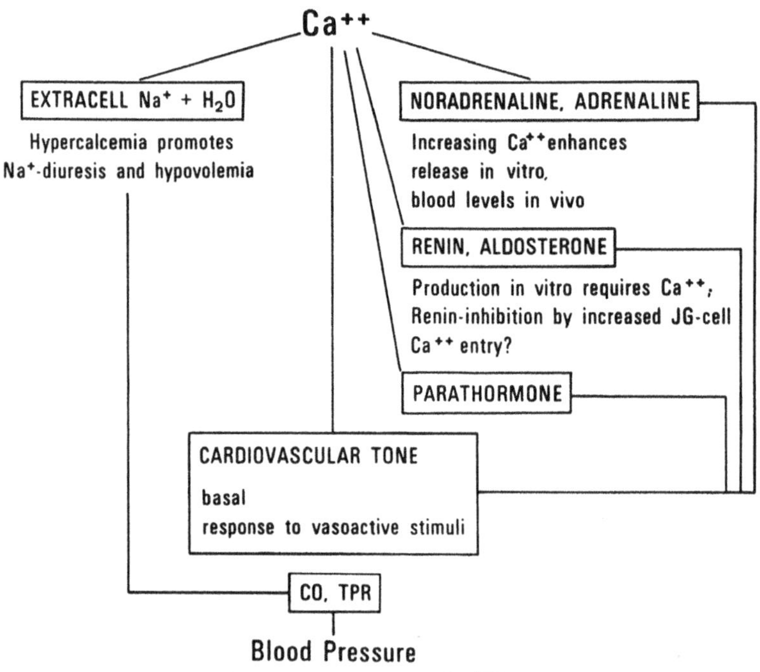

Fig. 1. Possible interactions between calcium (Ca^{2+}) and some blood pressure-regulating factors. *CO*, cardiac output; *TPR*, total peripheral resistance; *JG*, juxtaglomerular

* This work was supported by the Swiss National Science Foundation.

[1] Medizinische Poliklinik, Freiburgstr. 3, CH-3010 Bern.

Primary Hypertension
Ed. by W. Kaufmann et al.

of voltage-dependent and receptor-operated, Ca-selective plasma membrane ion channels [11, 12].

Ca has an intracellular messenger function in excitation-contraction coupling and, thus, determining cardiovascular tone, in regulating cardiac pacemaker activity and atrioventricular conduction, and probably also in modulating the secretion and/or production of additional BP-regulating factors such as the catecholamines, renin, and aldosterone [11, 13] (Fig. 1). On the other hand, the various CCB differ not only in their chemical structure and their exact mechanism of action at the Ca channel and perhaps on other cellular components, but they have also certain end-organ or tissue selectivity [9, 11, 12].

Effects of Calcium Antagonists on Blood Pressure Regulating Factors

Direct Effect on Cardiovascular Function

The dihydropyridine derivative nifedipine (NIF) and the aralkylamine derivatives verapamil (VER) and diltiazem (DIL) are the CCB which so far have been most widely applied. They differ partly in their direct pharmacologic effects on the heart and blood vessels (Table 1) [9, 11]. NIF exerts a more pronounced arteriolar vasodilation and has only a minimal influence on the cardiac pacemakers. VER is a somewhat weaker vasodilator, but it can have a distinct depressant effect on the sinus node automaticity and atrioventricular conduction. DIL resembles VER in its vasodilating potency, while its negative chronotropic and dromotropic effects seem to be somewhere between that of NIF and VER. The potential inhibition of myocardial contractility is perhaps slightly greater with VER than with NIF or DIL. Nevertheless, in vivo these potential negative chronotropic, dromotropic, and inotropic actions of systemically administered CCB may be attenuated by sympathetic cardiovascular reflexes. Although a direct reduction in basal cardiovascular muscle tone appears to be the major and common mechanism by which CCB can influence BP, some additional factors may play a modulating role (Fig. 2).

Effect on Circulating Catecholamines and Renin

The role of Ca in the coupling between the electric signal and the release of norepinephrine from nerve terminals is well known. Moreover, studies in vitro demon-

Table 1. Potential direct effects of therapeutic doses of calcium antagonists on the heart and blood vessels

	NIF	VER	DIL
Coronary arterial vasodilation	++++	+++	+++
Peripheral arterial vasodilation	++++	+++	+++
Inhibition of SA-node automaticity	±	+++	+
Inhibition of AV conduction	±	++++	+++
Inhibition of myocardial contractility	++	+++	++

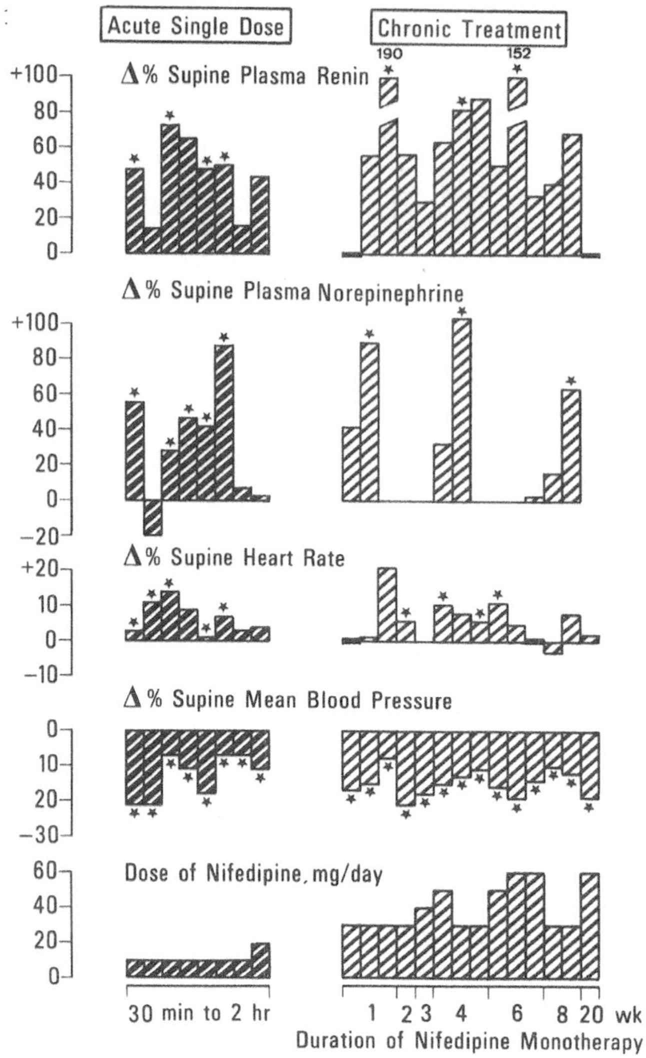

Fig. 2. Percentage responses of supine plasma renin, norepinephrine, heart rate, and mean BP to an acute single dose or chronic monotherapy with NIF in essential hypertension. *Asterisks* indicate changes reported as being statistically significant. In the case of acute single-dose studies, the duration of monotherapy *(bottom)* expresses the interval between drug administration and the illustrated measurements

strated with increasing Ca concentrations in the incubation media a parallel rise in the release of norepinephrine from sympathetic nerves and adrenaline from adrenal medullary tissue (for detailed references, see [13]); while acute hypercalcemia in man was associated with an increase in the blood levels of both catecholamines [2, 14]. Regarding renin and aldosterone, it has been shown that their production in vitro requires Ca (for detailed references, see [13]). On the other hand, an increased entry of Ca into the juxtaglomerular cells of the kidney may inhibit renin release [15].

Most studies of the interaction between CCB and these factors have been conducted with NIF or VER. In order to obtain a reasonably representative profile of the influence of a monotherapy with these agents on plasma catecholamine and renin levels, we performed a comprehensive analysis of published reports. In patients with benign essential hypertension, the administration of NIF either as an acute single dose or chronically for up to 20 weeks duration [7, 8, 16–27] was often associated with distinct increases in plasma renin and norepinephrine (Fig. 2). When VER was given in essential hypertension either as an acute single dose or as a short-term monotherapy of up to 16 weeks duration [17, 21, 22, 24, 28–32] plasma renin values were only slightly and not consistently modified (Fig. 3).

Differences between the humoral effects of NIF and VER are further corroborated by a comparative assessment of the average responses to these agents in the

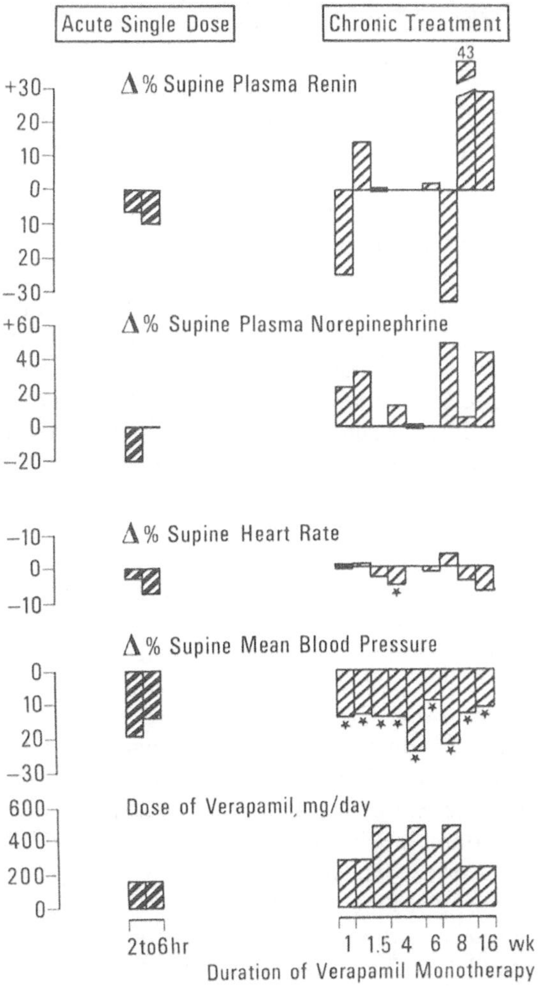

Fig. 3. Percentage responses of supine plasma renin, norepinephrine, heart rate, and mean BP to an acute single dose or chronic monotherapy with VER in essential hypertension. Remaining legend as in Fig. 2

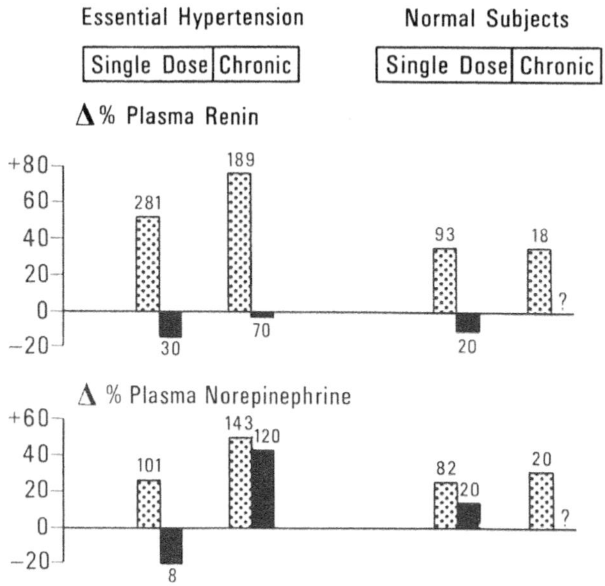

Fig. 4. Comparison of average percentage responses of supine plasma renin and norepinephrine to NIF (□) or VER (■) in essential hypertension or normal subjects. All data shown in Figs. 2 and 3 are incorporated into this analysis. Each *bar* represents the average response of the reported cases; the total numbers of subjects available for analysis are shown above or below the columns

published reports of both patients with essential hypertension (for references, see above) and normal subjects [17, 21, 22, 24, 28–34] (Fig. 4).

NIF, given either acutely or chronically, increased plasma renin by an average of about 60% in patients with essential hypertension and 30% in normal subjects. In contrast, following administration of VER, plasma renin was on average unchanged or even slightly decreased. Plasma norepinephrine also was increased by an average of 25% following an acute single dose of NIF, but largely unchanged after acute administration of VER in both hypertensive and normal subjects. During chronic therapy, plasma norepinephrine tended to be increased slightly on both agents, although perhaps somewhat less on VER. Plasma epinephrine was not modified during treatment with either NIF or VER (for detailed reference, see [35]). Effects of newer dihydropyridines seem to resemble those of NIF.

The mechanisms by which treatment with CCB may influence circulating renin and norepinephrine are not entirely clear. Nevertheless, the increases in plasma norepinephrine following administration of NIF resemble the mild changes induced by direct arteriolar vasodilators, such as the hydralazines, minoxidil, or carprazidil [13]. The degree of sympathetic stimulation by the latter agents appears to be determined largely by the degree of peripheral vasodilation and BP reduction with consecutive activation of the baroreflex-mechanism. Obviously, this does not apply in the case of VER which caused a similar BP reduction as did NIF. Relatively stable plasma norepinephrine levels, despite a distinct fall in BP, following acute administration of VER in essential hypertension raises the possibility that VER per se may acutely inhibit the neural discharge of norepinephrine. Alternative explanations, such as a different effect of NIF and VER on the baroreflex, or the plasma clearance of norepinephrine also deserve further consideration.

The potential of NIF to stimulate plasma renin also appears to be quite comparable to that of the direct arteriolar vasodilators. The increase in sympathetic activity

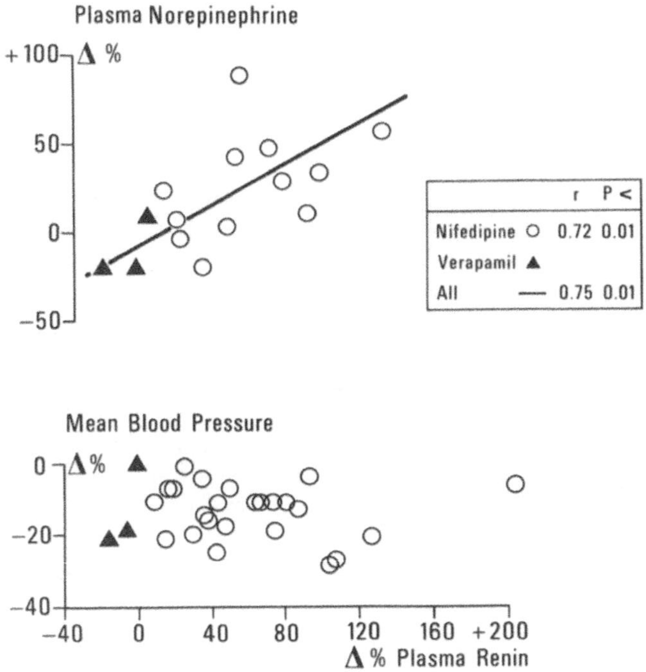

Fig. 5. Relationship between percentage changes in supine plasma renin and plasma norepinephrine levels or mean BP after an acute single dose of NIF or VER in normal or hypertensive subjects. Each data *point* represents the mean value of a reported study (same reports as analyzed in Figs. 2 and 3)

and/or fall in systemic and renal arterial perfusion pressure induced by these vasodilators are known complementary factors which may activate renin secretion through renal beta-receptors, baro-receptors, and perhaps also other mechanisms. Our analysis reveals no consistent relationship between variations in plasma renin and concomitant changes in mean BP induced by the acute administration of NIF or VER in normal or hypertensive subjects (Fig. 5). However, a significant correlation between the induced changes in circulating renin and norepinephrine suggests that renin-variations following acute CCB therapy may closely reflect the individual effects of such drugs on sympathetic activity. Nevertheless, the relative importance of different degrees of renal vasodilation for the contrasting renin effects of NIF and VER cannot be assessed from this analysis, and a direct effect on renin production or release has not been excluded.

The lack of an increase in heart rate on treatment with VER (Fig. 2) is generally attributed to a direct negative dromotropic and chronotropic action [12]. This well-established pharmacologic potential of VER [9] shall not be disputed. However, the finding of a significant correlation between variations in heart rate and concomitant changes in plasma norepinephrine or renin following acute Ca channel blockade in normal or hypertensive subjects (Fig. 6) suggests that the different chronotropic effects of acutely administered NIF or VER may be determined, at least in part, by a different influence of these agents on the sympathetic system.

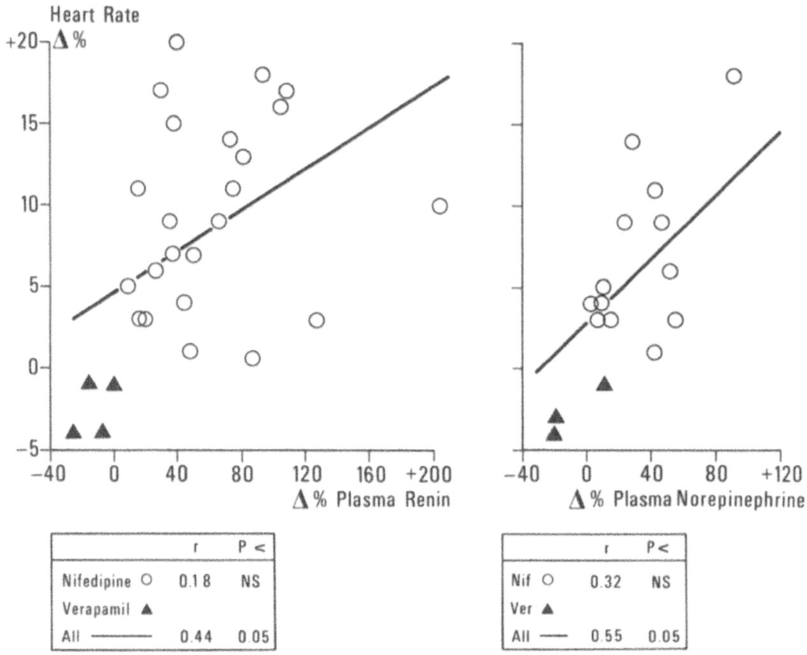

Fig. 6. Relationship between percentage changes in heart rate and plasma renin or norepinephrine levels after an acute single dose of NIF or VER in normal or hypertensive subjects. Remaining legend as in Fig. 5

Effects on Plasma Aldosterone and Electrolytes

Considering NIF, basal plasma aldosterone concentrations tended to be decreased slightly following acute administration [7, 20, 36, 37], but not during chronic administration [7, 21, 22, 27, 38]. An acute inhibition was also noted in patients with primary hyperaldosteronism [39]. Aldosterone responsiveness to infused angiotensin II was decreased acutely in some normal subjects [40], unchanged after 2 weeks of NIF monotherapy in normal or borderline hypertensive subjects [38], and distinctly reduced after 6 to 8 weeks of such treatment in patients with essential hypertension [27]. VER failed to alter basal and angiotensin II-stimulated plasma aldosterone levels in normal subjects acutely, but significantly lowered these values after 5 days of treatment; plasma cortisol levels followed a similar pattern [34].

It is possible that the development of mild hyporesponsiveness of plasma aldosterone on treatment with NIF or VER depend upon duration of treatment, dosage, and the subject's clinical condition. The biological relevance of the adrenal-cortical modifications remains to be determined.

Plasma potassium which may modulate aldosterone release and/or be changed as a consequence of slight variations in plasma aldosterone [41], was not consistently modified following short-term therapy with NIF, VER, or DIL in patients with essential hypertension (for detailed reference, see [13]); plasma sodium levels also were stable.

Effects on Cardiovascular Responsiveness

Certain human conditions are associated with an exaggerated cardiovascular pressor responsiveness to norepinephrine. These include established essential hypertension in which blood levels or norepinephrine and epinephrine are normal or sometimes even slightly increased [42–44]; as well as normotensive offspring of hypertensive families [45] and patients with borderline hypertension [46], nonazotemic diabetes mellitus [47], or mild renal functional impairment [48], in which circulating catecholamines generally are normal. It is possible that the norepinephrine hyperresponsiveness in some normotensive offspring of hypertensive parents represents a familial predisposition for the development of essential hypertension. In early renal failure or diabetes mellitus, the occurrence of cardiovascular hyperresponsiveness could also be a factor contributing to the frequent development of high BP. Therefore, agents that reduce the exaggerated reactivity could possibly provide a rational antihypertensive therapy in these situations.

Ca channels are partly operated by alpha adrenergic receptors [11, 49, 50], and there seems to be a regionally variable dependence of alpha-adrenoceptor-mediated vasoconstriction on transmembranous Ca entry [50]. Therefore, Ca entry blockade may lower not only the basal vascular tone, but also the reactivity of certain blood vessels. Various CCB were found to decrease the norepinephrine-induced contraction of arterial strip preparations and the pressor response to norepinephrine and/or angiotensin II in the experimental animal [35, 49, 50].

Following single-dose NIF administration to normal subjects, a reduction in the BP responses to both norepinephrine and angiotensin II was reported [51]. In per-

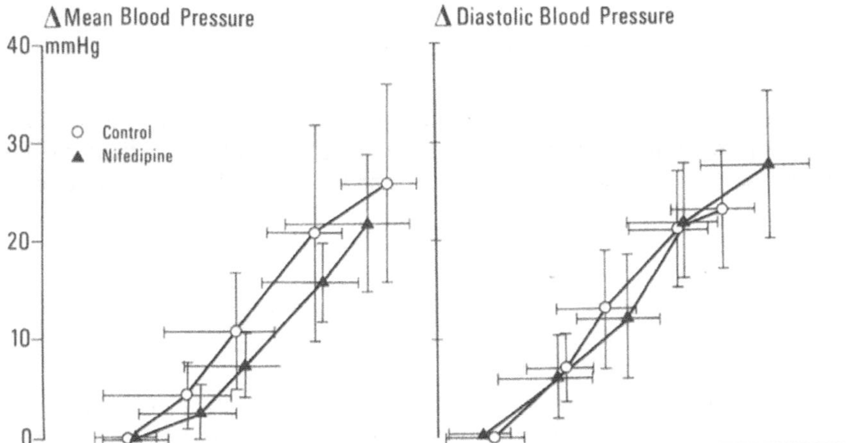

Fig. 7. Relationship between norepinephrine-induced changes in mean BP and plasma norepinephrine concentrations during norepinephrine infusion *(left graph)*, and between angiotensin II-induced changes in diastolic BP and plasma angiotensin II concentrations during angiotensin II-infusion, in 17 normal or borderline hypertensive subjects studied before and after 6–8 weeks of monotherapy with NIF, 30–60 mg per day. *Vertical* and *horizontal lines* indicate SD. From Bianchetti et al. [14]

sons with normal or borderline increased BP, NIF given for 2 weeks in a dose of 30–60 mg per day, reduced BP responsiveness to norepinephrine, as evidenced by a significant shift to the right of the relationship between increases in BP and concomitant increases in plasma norepinephrine induced by a norepinephrine infusion; in contrast, the plasma angiotensin II-pressor response curve during angiotensin II infusion was unchanged (Fig. 7) [14]. A similar constellation has been found in patients with essential hypertension treated for 4 to 5 weeks with NIF [30] or with nitrendipine [52]. The norepinephrine hyperresponsiveness was also improved in hypertensive patients with diabetes mellitus type II treated for 6 weeks with nitrendipine [53]. The data obtained during chronic dihydropyridine treatment in normal man or essential hypertension suggest that noradrenergic BP control mechanisms depend more upon transmembranous Ca transport than do angiotensinergic mechanisms. In fact, the latter may depend more upon sodium influx and activation of the sodium-potassium pump [54]. Nevertheless, VER, 120 mg tid given for 5 days to normal subjects, was reported to reduce the pressor responses to both norepinephrine and angiotensin II infused i.v.; the angiotensin responsiveness also seemed to be blunted following an acute single i.v. dose of VER, but an interpretation is difficult since no measurements of plasma angiotensin concentrations were provided [34].

Effects of CCB on pressor responsiveness may possibly depend not only upon dosage and duration of treatment, but also upon the particular agent. Thus, VER, but not NIF or DIL, has also an affinity for alpha-adrenergic receptors [55]. Moreover, whatever the exact mechanism, an improvement of norepinephrine-hyperreactivity may play a relevant role in the BP-lowering mechanism of certain CCB in essential or diabetes-associated hypertension.

Effects on Cardiac Output and Total Peripheral Resistance

The antihypertensive effect of CCB in essential hypertension is related to a decrease in total peripheral resistance, while cardiac output is unchanged or, particularly during the first few weeks of treatment with NIF or some other dihydropyridine compounds, may be increased [8, 18, 56–62].

Do Calcium Antagonists Correct an Underlying Abnormality in Essential Hypertension?

Whether and to what extent abnormalities in Ca metabolism may play a primary pathogenetic role in hypertensive states not associated with frank hypercalcemia, is presently unclear. Disturbances in blood cell membrane cation metabolism exist both in essential hypertension and in normotensive offspring of hypertensive families [63–65]. Moreover, it has been postulated that spontaneous hypertension in the rat and human essential hypertension are both associated with an increase in free cytosolic Ca in vascular muscle cells, resulting from enhanced transmembranous uptake or diminished cellular extrusion or binding of Ca to the cell membrane or sarcoplasmatic reticulum [56, 65]. Such a mechanism, although still speculative, could produce hypertension [66].

Some observations with CCB have been interpreted in favor of a Ca-dependent dysregulation in essential hypertension. These include (a) a correlation of their BP-lowering effect with the pretreatment BP level and a lack of influence in normotensive subjects [20, 26, 56] (see also below), (b) the possibility that in essential hypertension the abnormally constricted brachial arteries may be dilated more completely by a CCB than by the potent direct vasodilator nitroprusside [67, 68], and (c) the report of a close relationship between BP and blood platelet Ca content before and after treatment with NIF or VER [69]. Nervertheless, BP responses to other antihypertensive drugs, such as diuretics, beta-blockers, and sympatholytics also tend to correlate with pre-treatment BP [70–72], and this as well as an altered platelet Ca content could theoretically represent unspecific phenomena associated with the hypertensive state. Furthermore, the vasodilating, BP-lowering, and platelet Ca-modifying effects of CCB in essential hypertension per se could not give proof for the pathogenic role of a primary disturbance of the calcium metabolism in cardiovascular muscle cells. In fact, Ca is the common intracellular trigger for various pressor substances, and the potential of CCB to lower BP at least acutely in different forms of hypertension (see below) is consistent with this.

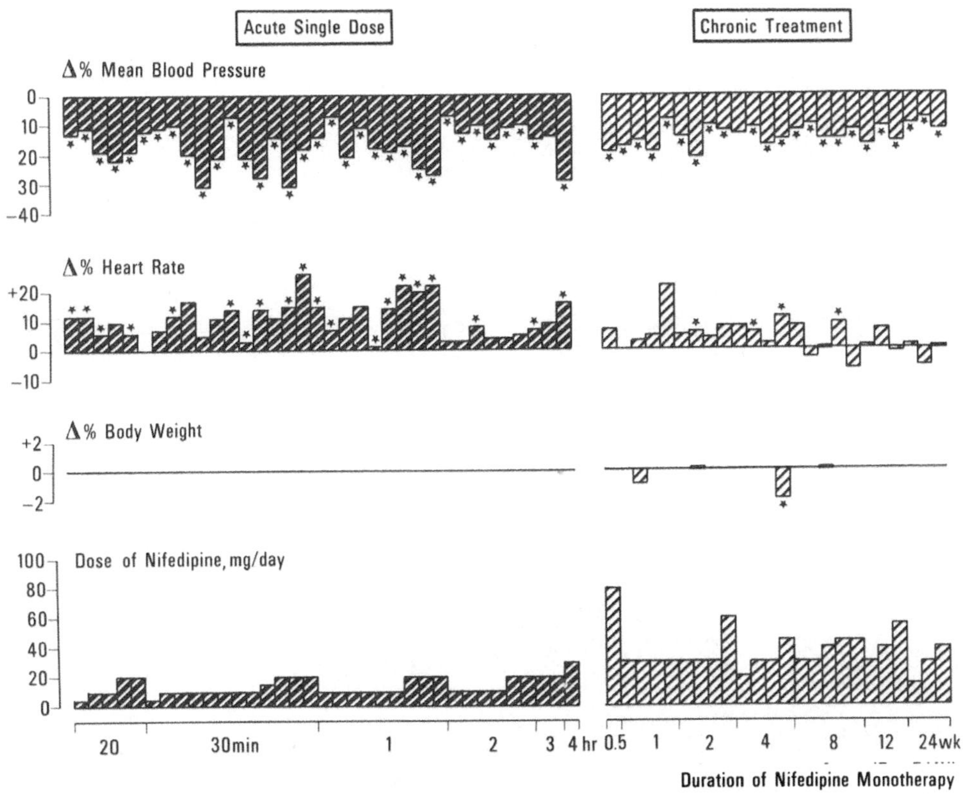

Fig. 8. Percentage responses of mean BP, heart rate, and body weight to an acute single dose or chronic monotherapy with NIF in essential hypertension. Each *column* represents the average percentage change in a report based on a minimal number of six subjects. Remaining legend as in Fig. 2

Antihypertensive Potency

Essential Hypertension

Monotherapy

The potency of a monotherapy with NIF or VER in essential hypertension was assessed by an analysis of published reports with a minimal number of six subjects per study [6–8, 16–30, 32, 36, 37, 56, 59, 73–107].

It is evident that NIF (Fig. 8) lowered supine mean BP on average by about 10% to 30% when given as an acute single dose (5–30 mg sublingually or orally), and by about 10% to 20% during chronic oral treatment of 1–24 weeks duration (15–80 mg/day). Supine heart rate was increased acutely by an verage of about 10%, but this effect tended to dissipate during chronic NIF therapy, despite a persistent BP reduction. The antihypertensive potency and associated chronotropic effects of NIF monotherapy beyond 6 months duration deserve further study.

VER (Fig. 9), given either as an acute single dose (80–160 mg orally) or chronically for up to 2 years (160–480 mg/day), also reduced mean supine BP on average about 10% to 20%; while supine heart rate tended to be slightly decreased.

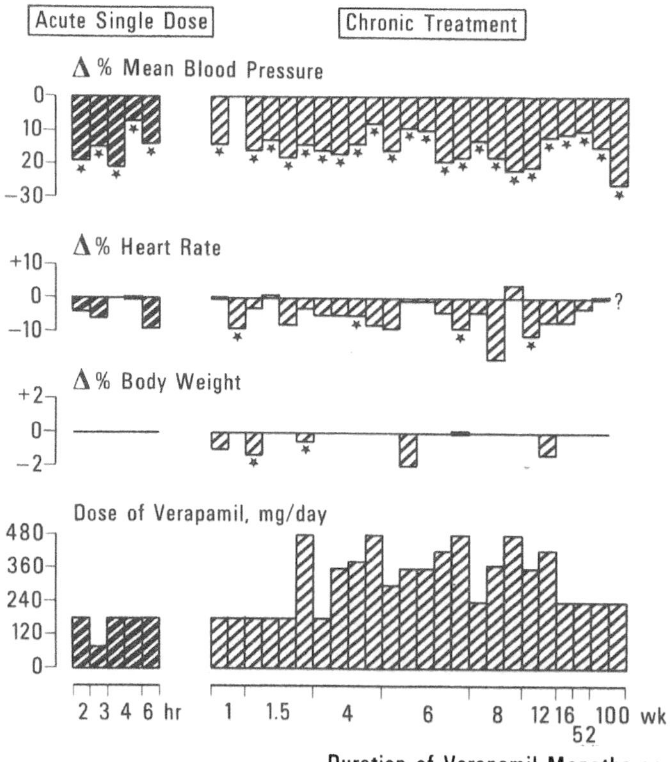

Fig. 9. Percentage responses of mean BP, heart rate, and body weight to an acute single dose or chronic monotherapy with VER in essential hypertension. Remaining legend as in Fig. 2

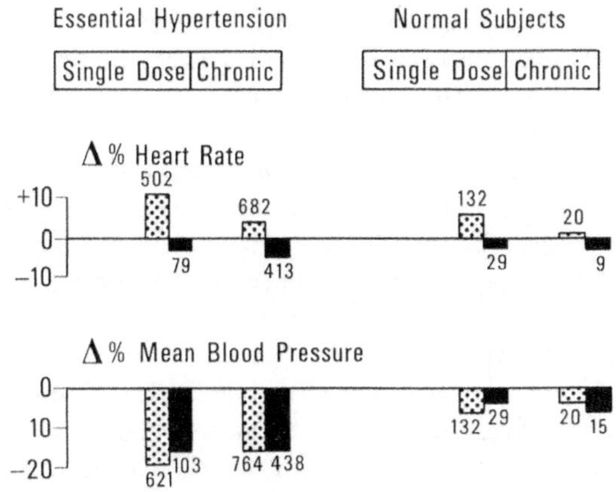

Fig. 10. Comparison of average percentage responses of supine mean BP and heart rate to monotherapy with NIF (□) or VER (■) in essential hypertension or normal subjects. All data shown in Figs. 8 and 9 are incorporated. Each *bar* represents the average response of the reported cases; the total numbers of subjects available for analysis are shown above or below the column

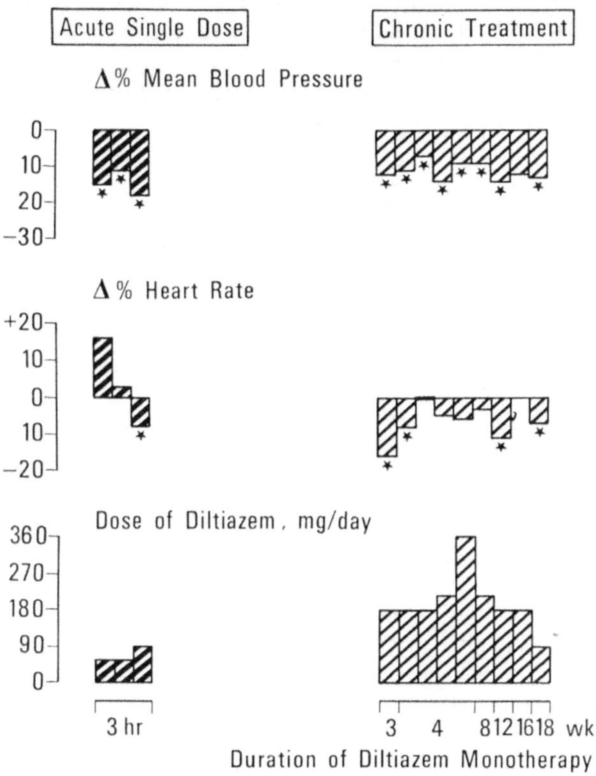

Fig. 11. Percentage responses of mean BP and heart rate to an acute single dose or chronic monotherapy with DIL in essential hypertension. Remaining legend as in Fig. 2

It follows that despite the considerable pharmacologic and pharmacodynamic differences of NIF and VER, these CCB, when given in appropriate dosage, exert a similar BP-lowering effect in essential hypertension; while only minimal BP changes are induced in normal man (Fig. 10) [14–17, 19, 20, 23, 34, 75].

Moreover, various other CCB have also been found to lower BP when given either acutely or more chronically to patients with essential hypertension. These

CCB include the dihydropyridine derivatives (nifedipine group), nicardipine [23, 62] nitrendipine [61, 108], nisoldipine [109, 110], and felodipine [111, 112], the aralkylamine derivatives (the group also including VER), diltiazem (Fig. 11) [56, 57, 91, 113–116], tiapamil [117, 118], and additional agents.

Effects of CCB on upright BP and HR generally resemble their influence on supine values. Nevertheless, orthostatic hypotension and/or dizziness may sometimes occur after emergency application (see below), and we have sporadically encountered it following initiation of CCB therapy in elderly patients. Moreover, during chronic NIF-monotherapy, HR tended to be increased more distinctly in the standing than in the supine position [7, 22, 25].

Although more studies for longer than 6 months to 1 year are needed, the persistence of a stable antihypertensive effect during chronic monotherapy (Figs. 8 and 9) is of practical importance. When body weight was reported, it was on average often unchanged or even decreased slightly during monotherapy with NIF, VER (Figs. 8 and 9) or some other CCB [61, 119, 120]. This may be interpreted as indirect evidence that relevant body sodium-fluid retention, which is a well-known side effect antagonizing at long-term the antihypertensive potency of direct arteriolar vasodilators such as hydralazine, minoxidil, and the like, may not be common with the CCB.

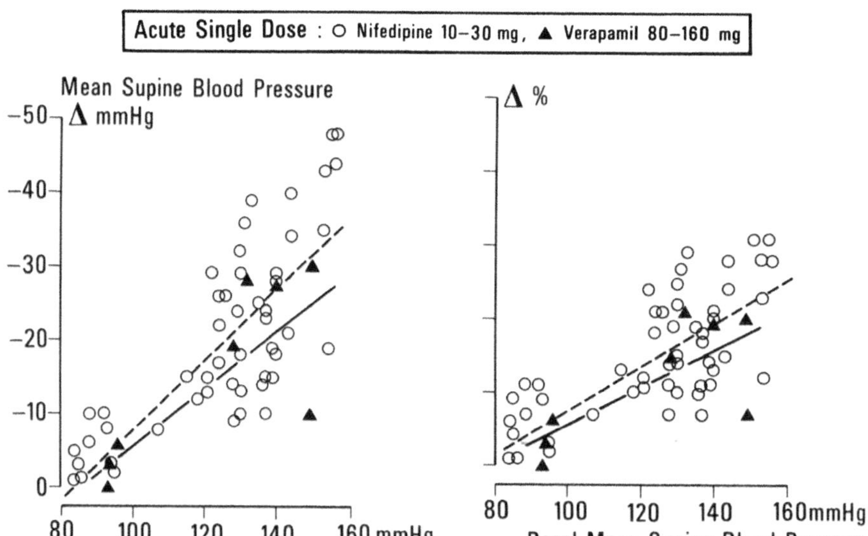

	r	P <
Nifedipine ○	0.78	0.001
Verapamil ▲	0.78	0.05
All	0.77	0.001

	r	P <
Nif ○	0.71	0.001
Ver ▲	0.71	0.05
All	0.75	0.001

Fig. 12. Relationships between supine mean BP before treatment and absolute or percentage BP responses to an acute single dose of NIF or VER in patients with essential hypertension and normal subjects. Each data *point* represents the mean value of a reported study (same studies as in Figs. 8 and 9) and utilizing dosages as specified

In fact, renal sodium excretion may be increased acutely by various CCB [17, 118, 121–124]. Natriuresis probably returns to control values within a few days of chronic calcium channel blockade [123]. Total plasma or blood volume was largely unchanged on chronic therapy with these agents [8, 18, 21, 27, 28]. Nevertheless, a tendency for increased exchangeable body sodium has been noted following 6 to 8 weeks of monotherapy with NIF [27]; interestingly, much of the sodium retained appeared to be distributed to an extracellular compartment [27]. Mild sodium and water retention was reported in some patients on long-term treatment [124]. The observation of a persistent antihypertensive efficacy of a VER monotherapy of up to 2 years' duration [107, 125] (Fig. 9) suggests that sodium-fluid volume retention, if it occurred at all, was not a major antagonistic factor, at least in some patients.

The magnitude of BP responses to CCB monotherapy may depend upon several factors. Comparing the various reported studies of patients with essential hypertension or normal subjects who received NIF or VER acutely or chronically (Fig. 8, 9,

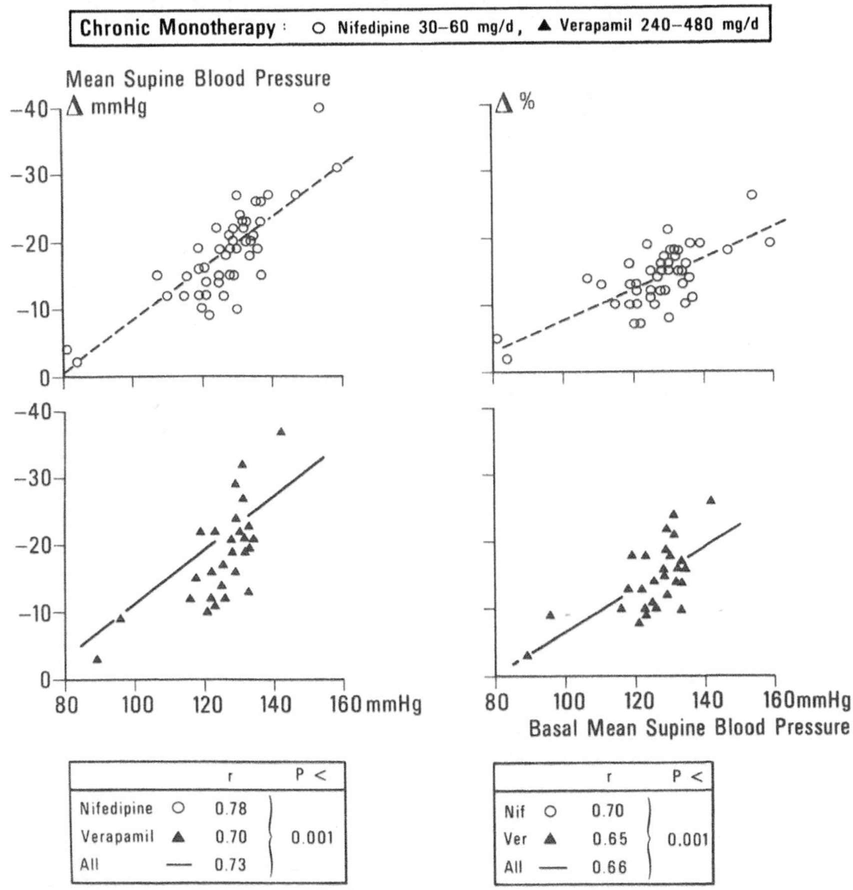

Fig. 13. Relationships between supine mean BP before treatment and absolute or percentage BP responses to chronic monotherapy with NIF or VER in patients with essential hypertension and normal subjects. Each data *point* represents the mean value of a reported study (same studies as in Figs. 8 and 9), utilizing dosages specified

Table 2. Effect of combined treatment with calcium-antagonists and thiazide-type diuretics and/or beta-blockers and other sympatholytics on supine blood pressure and heart rate in patients with essential hypertension

Author	Year	Reference	Patients (n)	Preceding treatment		Combined treatment			
				Initial drug(s)	Duration (weeks)	Drug added	Duration (weeks)	Blood pressure $\Delta\%$ [a]	Heart rate $\Delta\%$ [a]
Ca-antagonist and thiazide type diuretic									
Anavekar et al.	1981	[32]	17	D	2	VER	6	−9	−1
Maeda et al.	1981	[130]	5	TCM	1–4	DIL	12– 15	−27	
Hallin et al.	1983	[94]	30	BFZ	24	NIF	6	−3	+8
Wigler et al.	1984	[107]	8	D	Chronic	VER	104	−29	
Maeda et al.	1981	[130]	5	DIL	1–2	TCM	14– 15	−8	
Hallin et al.	1983	[94]	30	NIF	24	BFZ	6	−4	+2
Marone et al.	1984	[27]	10	NIF	6–8	CHLOR	6– 8	−6	NC
Ca-antagonist and beta-blocker									
Pedersen et al.	1980	[75]	9	PROP/ATEN/TIM/MET	4	NIF	4	−13	+6
Husted et al.	1982	[124]	10	PROP/TIM/MET	8	NIF	52–132	−21	0
Orö and Ryman	1984	[131]	12	MET	3	NIT	4	−23	NC
Tammen et al.	1984	[132]	8	MET/PROP	2–3	NIT	3	−14	+8
Yagil et al.	1983	[133]	22	PROP	4	NIF	14– 30	−26	NC
de Diviitis et al.	1984	[83]	15	ACEBUT	4	NIF	4	−9	+8
Wigler et al.	1984	[107]	5	PROP/OXPREN	Chronic	VER	104	−29	
Aoki and Sato	1982	[134]	7	NIL	8	PROP	8	0	−14
Eggertsen and Hansson	1982	[135]	13	NIF	12	MET	12	−5	
Ekelund et al.	1982	[25]	12	NIF	4	MET	12	−7	−26
de Diviitis et al.	1984	[83]	15	NIF	4	ACEBUT	4	−9	−16

Ca-antagonist and thiazide-type diuretic + beta-blocker									
Brennan and Blake	1982	[136]	18	BFZ + MET	?	NIF	8– 24	−18	
Dean and Kendall	1983	[137]	20	D + B	2	NIF	12	−13	−2
Murphy et al.	1983	[138]	15	ATEN + BFZ	Chronic	NIF	2	−7 to −16	+3 to +5
Gonzales-Gomez et al.	1983	[139]	16	PROP + CPZ	3	VER	3– 9	−15 to −27	+19 to −3
Ca-antagonist and sympatholytic									
Leary and Asmal	1979	[140]	40	RES	6	VER	6	−6	−4
Guazzi et al.	1980	[142]	12	MD	1.5	NIF	1.5	−25	
Leary and Asmal	1979	[140]	40	VER	6	RES	6	−5	−14
Guazzi et al.	1980	[142]	11	NIF	1.5	MD	1.5	−14	
Ca-antagonist and vasodilator									
Ueda and Musakami	1983	[141]	68	HYDR	2	NIF	6	−19	−1
Ueda and Musakami	1983	[141]	16	NIF	2	HYDR	6	+2	−2
Ca-antagonist and converting enzyme inhibitor									
Stornello et al.	1983	[88]	9	CAPT	1	NIF	1	−8	+5
Guazzi et al.	1984	[81]	14	CAPT	1	NIF	1	−9	
Stornello et al.	1983	[88]	9	NIF	1	CAPT	1	−9	−17
Guazzi et al.	1984	[81]	14	NIF	1	CAPT	1	−10	

[a] Compared to values of preceding treatment, combined with sedative agent

ACEBUT, acebutolol; ATEN, atenolol; B, beta-blocker, not specified or different types; BFZ, bendrofluazide; CAPT, captopril; CHLOR, chlorthalidone; CLON, clonidine; CPZ, cyclopenthiazide; D, diuretic, not specified or different types; DIL, diltiazem; HYDR, hydralazine; MD, alpha-methyl-dopa; MET, metoprolol; NC, no statistically significant change; NIF, nifedipine; NIL, niludipine; NIT, nitrendipine; OXPREN, oxprenolol; PROP, propranolol; RES, reserpine; TCM, trichlormethiazide; TIM, timolol; VER, verapamil and 10), no close correlation of average percentage BP reductions with the mean drugs dosages is apparent. This does not exclude a particular dose-BP-response relationship in individual hypertensive patients receiving stepwise increasing doses of CCB [126, 127]. The level of BP before treatment seems to be an important correlate of their effect. Considering the published reports on patients with benign essential hypertension and normal subjects, a significant relationship between basal mean BP and absolute or percentage BP responses to NIF or VER is apparent under conditions of both acute single dose or chronic monotherapy (Figs. 12 and 13). The existence of this relationship following an acute single dose or short-term therapy has already been noted by others [18, 26, 75, 128, 129] and also applies to hypertensive emergencies [78, 130] and to various CCB other than NIF or VER. It follows that the BP-lowering effect of CCB is minimal in normotensive subjects and tends to increase with the severity of essential hypertension. However, the dependence of responses on pretreatment BP is by no means specific for CCB, but is similarly characteristic at least for the thiazide diuretics [70], beta-blockers [72], and other sympatholytic agents [71]. It is probable that additional factors, such as the interactions with the sympathetic and renin-angiotensin systems and other BP-regulating components may also modulate the BP effects of CCB.

Certain others have postulated that the antihypertensive efficacy of both CCB and beta-blockers depends upon the age of the patients [105]. Based on a still-limited number of observations, they envisioned age-related treatment strategies. There are presently not enough data available to support or refute an increasing antihypertensive effect of CCB with increasing age. However, the Swiss bopindolol study [72] provided an opportunity to finally test the age-hypothesis for beta-blockers. No correlation existed between beta-blocker-induced decreases in BP and age (which in the 561 patients with moderate essential hypertension ranged from 22 to 82 years). We may have to tell physicians to disregard age as a determinant of the potency of at least this beta-blocker and to be cautious before accepting similar claims for CCB.

The potential value of a monotherapy with CCB in essential hypertension requires further assessment of the efficacy and benefit/risk ratio by long-term studies. At the present time, diuretics and beta-blockers are accepted step 1 drugs for the treatment of essential hypertension. With regard to the antihypertensive effect, it is evident that certain CCB are at least as potent as thiazide-type diuretics or beta-blockers in the first 6 months or even 2 years of treatment. Thus, all three drug classes given as monotherapy may lower BP in essential hypertension by an average of about 12% to 15% [13].

Combination therapy

Compared to monotherapy, an additional BP-lowering effect can be obtained in essential hypertension when CCB are combined with a thiazide-type diuretic, beta-blocker, sympatholytic such as alpha-methyldopa or reserpine, a previous two-drug regime with a beta-blocker and diuretic [25, 27, 29, 32, 75, 81, 84, 88, 94, 107, 124, 130–142], or angiotensin converting enzyme (ACE) inhibitors [81, 88] (Table 2, Fig. 14). NIF added to a pre-existing therapy with the post-synaptic alpha$_1$-blocker prazosin produced excessive symptomatic decreases in BP in a few patients [143]. It is evident that the complementary potencies of various combinations deserve further clarification, particularly regarding long-term conditions.

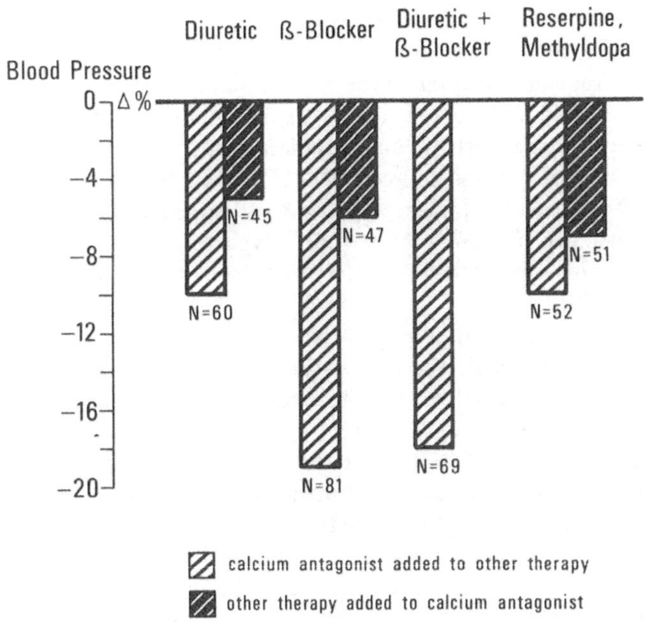

Fig. 14. Additional BP-lowering effects of some drug combinations as compared to monotherapy, in essential hypertension. Values represent means of reports in different treatment categories as further specified in Table 2

Other Forms of Hypertension

A paucity of controlled data on the effect of CCB monotherapy in various secondary forms of hypertension at present prevents definite conclusions. Acute BP reductions were noted following single doses of NIF or other CCB in sporadic cases with pheochromocytoma, primary hyperaldosteronism, renal artery stenosis or parenchymal disease, and in terminal renal failure [5, 39, 110, 144, 145].

While a certain antihypertensive effect was obtained following short-term monotherapy with DIL in some patients with mild to moderate renal failure of various origin or chronic nephritis [146, 147], some combination studies with other agents are difficult to evaluate as regards specificity of patient groups.

Hypertension accompanying diabetes mellitus deserves particular consideration, since the second phase of insulin secretion depends upon the influx of Ca into the beta cells. An ongoing study in our institution suggests that a monotherapy with nitrendipine may be an effective and well-tolerated treatment of mild to moderate hypertension associated with diabetes type II [53]. Thus, a dose of 20–40 mg once daily provided satisfactory BP control in 10 patients observed from 6 weeks up to 1 year. Moreover, no adverse effect of CCB therapy on parameters of carbohydrate metabolism such as blood HbA_1 and basal and stimulated levels of plasma glucose and insulin were noted. In fact, CCB given in usual clinical doses had no relevant influence on glucose homeostasis in many non-diabetic or diabetic subjects [148–150], although the development of hyperglycemia was sporadically described [151].

Hypertensive Emergencies

NIF is now established as an important alternative for the treatment of certain hypertensive emergencies. A single dose of 5–20 mg, applied sublingually or sometimes orally, acutely and effectively reduced BP in many patients with life-threatening states complicating hypertension of various etiology [77, 152–154]. In patients with severe hypertension and left ventricular failure, concomitant improvement of BP and pulmonary congestion usually occurred [152, 153]. Hypertensive encephalopathy was influenced favorably in some cases [154, 155]. BP also responded in cases with pheochromocytoma [77, 156].

An important consideration of any antihypertensive emergency therapy is its effect on cerebral circulation. With NIF, the interesting constellation of an unchanged or even increased cerebral blood flow, despite a concomitant marked fall in BP, was reported [77]. However, this average tendency does not preclude a compromised perfusion in certain cases [157, 158]. The relative efficacy and safety of NIF in different types of hypertensive emergencies needs further clarification.

Following sublingual application of NIF, the reduction in BP is maximal at 15 to 30 min, and improvement may last for up to 4 h. This response is only slightly delayed after oral administration [13]. Furthermore, the induced individual decreases in BP correlate strongly with pre-treatment BP [77, 159], as also noted in benign essential hypertension. An exaggerated fall to hypotensive levels was not encountered upon NIF monotherapy, but sometimes may occur with the application of higher doses (15–20 mg) in patients already on diuretics, prazosin [143], or other potent antihypertensive therapy.

Other CCB, such as VER [160] or DIL [161] given i.v., or certain newer agents also were found to be effective in some patients with hypertensive crises.

Side Effects

CCB therapy is well tolerated by the majority of patients. Nevertheless, side effects may occur which differ in part between individual substances and sometimes lead to disruption of treatment. Table 3 gives merely an impression from the available literature ([13, 162], and references cited above), since the relative tolerance and frequency of side effects of the various CCB, particularly when used for treatment of hypertension, have not been clarified by comparative assessment. Certain symptoms, such as facial flushing, burning sensations, palpitations, and dizziness may be more pronounced in the initial stages and tend to diminish with progressive treatment. Intravenous administration of VER to patients with diseased hearts or already receiving another cardiodepressant with negative chronotropic and inotropic action, such as beta-blockers, digitalis, or quinidine (which, as VER, also blocks alpha-receptors) [55], has occasionally provoked serious episodes with bradycardia, heart block, and/or hypotension. Therefore, i.v. administration of VER or DIL to such patients is contraindicated; while oral prescription of VER or DIL in combination with other cardiodepressants warrants particular precaution even in patients without apparant cardiac disease [162–164], and should be avoided in patients with conduction disorders or left ventricular dysfunction. Pitting ankle edema which appears follow-

Table 3. Side effects of calcium channel blockers occurring during chronic administration

	NIF	VER	DIL
Cardiovascular			
Headache	++	+	+
Facial flushing, burning of face or legs; palpitations	++	+	+
Orthostatic hypotension	+	+	+
Bradycardia	–	++	+
AV-block	–	+	+
Ankle or leg edema	++	+	+
Gastrointestinal			
Anorexia, nausea or vomiting	+	+	+
Constipation	–	++	+
Diarrhea	+	–	–
Heartburn	(+)	–	(+)
Liver function disturbances			(+)
Gingival hyperplasia	(+)		
Skin rash, itching	(+)	(+)	(+)
Neurological			
Dizziness, vertigo	+	+	+
Weakness, asthenia	+		+
Renal, urogenital			
Aggravation of preexisting renal functional impairment	(+)		
Acute renal failure			(+)
Impotence	(+)		

Reported occurrence of side effects range from more common ++ to rare (+) and none –

ing initiation and also may improve with progressive CCB therapy often reflects a local, harmless hemodynamic alteration (probably increased capillary pressure due to arteriolar dilatation without venular dilatation), rather than congestive heart failure or marked body sodium fluid volume retention. In a few cases, gingival hyperplasia during NIF treatment [165], or acute impairment of renal function following initiation of therapy with NIF [166] or DIL [167], were reported.

For the still-limited periods evaluated so far, CCB therapy has been remarkably free of relevant metabolic side effects. Plasma potassium was generally unchanged except for a mild decrease on NIF in some patients [7, 168]. Serum total and high-density lipoprotein cholesterol, total or very low-density lipoprotein triglycerides, glucose and insulin, when measured, also were usually not affected adversely by

NIF, VER, or DIL [13, 57, 148–150, 169–174]; the same conclusion applies for the use of nitrendipine in a group of patients with diabetes mellitus type II [53]. Nevertheless, the long-term situation still remains to be assessed.

In patients on digoxin therapy, serum digoxin levels are increased by VER, DIL, or some other CCB, due to decreased renal and extrarenal digoxin clearance [162, 175, 176]. Serum digoxin concentrations should be maintained within therapeutic limits when such combinations are used.

Practical Antihypertensive Therapy

What is the place of CCB, particularly as compared with diuretics and beta-blockers, in practical antihypertensive pharmacotherapy in 1985? Since they are comparatively equivalent in antihypertensive potency (at least 6 months to 1 year) to monotherapy, and because of their acceptable subjective tolerance and relative metabolic "neutrality," CCB clearly deserve consideration as an alternative to beta-blockers, low-dose diuretics, and probably also angiotensin converting enzyme (ACE) inhibitors, either as initial or second drugs (Fig. 15). Beta-blockers, CCB, and ACE inhibitors are more expensive, but they (and the two latter in particular) have less biochemical side effects than diuretics. Recently, some suspicion has arisen that thiazide-type diuretics used in high dosage may possibly have an adverse influence on coronary heart disease in certain individuals with mild hypertension [177, 178] and contribute to excess cardiac death in elderly hypertensive males [179]. Hypokalemia may undoubtedly favor the appearance of cardiac arrhythmias in susceptible, often elderly individuals. Therefore, the possibility to prescribe a CCB instead of a thiazide-type diuretic may be of particular interest in those patients in whom diuretic-induced symptomatic hypokalemia, associated cardiac arrhythmias, attacks of gout, or an aggravation of a hyperglycemia have already developed or where they should whenever possible be avoided. CCB have also been found to be effective in some patients with hypertension poorly responding to conventional drug combinations [137, 180, 181], and it may be worthwhile to try these agents in hypertensive patients with diabetes mellitus in whom diuretics and $beta_2$-blockers tend to have undesirable metabolic effects.

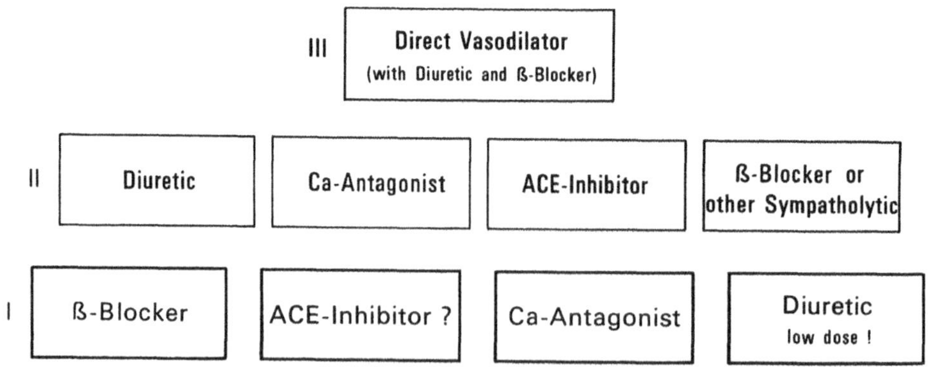

Fig. 15. Antihypertensive pharmacotherapy 1985: A general plan of alternatives which may be useful for treating hypertension

Table 4. Calcium antagonist therapy in essential hypertension

Precautions

Avoid abrupt discontinuation in coronary artery disease

Concerning VER and DIL:

- AV-block I
- Combined *oral* administration with beta-blocker

Contraindications

Congestive heart failure[a]

Pregnancy (except VER)

Digitalis toxicity

Concerning VER and DIL:

- Sick-sinus-syndrome
- AV-block II or III
- Bradycardia
- Parenteral use in presence of beta-blocker or quinidine

Dosage	mg/day	doses/day
NIF retard	20– 80	2
VER retard, sustained release	240–480	1–2
DIL	90–360	3
Nitrendipine	20– 60	1–2

[a] Nifedipine useful for hypertensive emergencies with acute left ventricular failure

Table 5. Emergency treatment upon hospitalization for severe or malignant hypertension with acute left ventricular failure or encephalopathy, or for malignant hypertension without these complications but unresponsive to gentle drug therapy

Consider a single dose of the following alternative agents[a]:

Agent	Means	Dose
Nifedipine	orally	5–20 mg
Labetalol	i.v. bolus or i.v. infusion	60–100 mg 2 mg/min
Clonidine	i.v.	0.15 mg over 5–10 min
Nitroprusside	i.v. infusion titration in regard to blood pressure reduction	no constant dosage
Diazoxide	i.v. bolus	(150)–300 mg

[a] Repeat if necessary; complement with early build-up of usual oral drug combinations

Practical dosages, precautions, and contraindications regarding the use of NIF, VER, and DIL are summarized in Table 4. A relatively short duration of antihypertensive action, necessitating two to three applications per day [8, 13], has represented a certain disadvantage of the earlier commercially available CCB. However, newer developments such as the longer-acting nitrendipine [182] or a sustained release oral dosage from of VER [183] may possibly allow once-daily dosage.

Considering emergency treatment, severe or malignant hypertension complicated by severe congestive heart failure, simultaneous anticoagulant therapy, or hypertensive encephalopathy, or malignant hypertension without these complications, but resistant to more gently acting drug therapy within the first 24h, are life-threatening conditions which require rapid lowering of BP. Among the possible emergency drugs for this indication (Table 5), NIF applied sublingually or orally is now considered to have particular value because of its easy and safe application as well as its possible lack of an adverse effect on cerebral blood flow in many patients. The potential value of a CCB in the other types of hypertensive emergencies such as pheochromocytoma crisis or hypertension with stroke or dissecting aortic aneurysm needs to be clarified.

References

1. Weidmann P (1983) Essential, renal and endocrine hypertension. In: Massry SG, Glassock RJ (eds) Textbook of nephrology, vol 2. Williams and Wilkins, Baltimore, pp 6.38–7.382
2. Weidmann P, Massry SG, Coburn JW, Maxwell MH, Atleson J, Kleeman CR (1972) Blood pressure effects of acute hypercalcemia. Studies in patients with chronic renal failure. Ann Intern Med 76:741–745
3. Marone C, Beretta-Piccoli C, Weidmann P (1980) Acute hypercalcemic hypertension in man: role of hemodynamics, catecholamines and renin. Kidney Int 20:92–96
4. Llach F, Weidmann P, Reinhart R, Maxwell MH, Coburn JW, Massry SG (1974) Effect of acute and long-standing hypocalcemia on blood pressure and plasma renin activity in man. J Clin Endocrinol Metab 38:841–847
5. Aoki K, Yoshida T, Kato S, Tazumi K, Sato I, Takikawa K, Hotta K (1976) Hypotensive action and increased plasma renin activity by Ca^{2+}-antagonist (nifedipine) in hypertensive patients. Jpn Heart J 17:479–484
6. Lewis GRJ, Morley KD, Lewis BM, Bones PJ (1978) The treatment of hypertension with verapamil. NZ Med J 87:351–354
7. Pedersen OL, Mikkelsen E, Christensen NJ, Kornerup HJ, Pedersen EB (1979) Effect of nifedipine on plasma renin, aldosterone and catecholamines in arterial hypertension. Eur J Clin Pharmacol 15:235–240
8. Olivari MT, Bartorelli C, Polese A, Fiorentini C, Moruzzi P, Guazzi MD (1979) Treatment of hypertension with nifedipine, a calcium antagonistic agent. Circulation 59:1056–1062
9. Fleckenstein A (1983) Calcium antagonism in heart and smooth muscle. Experimental facts and therapeutic prospects. Wiley, New York
10. Katz AM, Reuter H (1979) Cellular calcium and cardiac cell death. Am J Cardiol 44:188–190
11. Katz AM, Hager WD, Messineo FC, Pappano AJ (1984) Cellular actions and pharmacology of the calcium channel blocking drugs. Am J Med 77:2–10
12. Antman EM, Stone PH, Mueller JE, Braunwald E (1980) Calcium channel blocking agents in the treatment of cardiovascular disorders: I. Basic and clinical electrophysiologic effects. Ann Intern Med 93:875–885
13. Weidmann P, Gerber A, Laederach K (1984) Calcium antagonists in the treatment of hypertension: a critical overview. In: Crosnier J, Maxwell MH (eds) Advances in nephrology. Year Book Medical Publishers, Chicago, pp 197–232

14. Bianchetti MG, Beretta-Piccoli C, Weidmann P, Link L, Boehringer K, Ferrier C, Morton JJ (1983) Calcium and blood pressure regulation in normal and hypertensive subjects. Hypertension [Suppl 2] 5: II-57–II-65
15. Park CS, Han DS, Fray JCS (1981) Calcium in the control of renin secretion: Ca^{++} influx as an inhibitory signal. Am J Physiol 240: F70–F74
16. Oehmar H, Kubo S, Masaoka S, Kanazawa I, Yuasa A, Tsuchioka Y, Matsuura H, Kurogane H, Kajiyama G (1983) Sympathetic nerve and hormonal responses to a single dose of nifedipine in patients with essential hypertension and normal subjects: comparison among renin subgroups. Hiroshima J Med Sci 32: 187–197
17. Leonetti G, Cuspidi C, Sampieri L, Terzoli L, Zanchetti A (1982) Comparison of cardiovascular, renal, and humoral effects of acute administration of two calcium channel blockers in normotensive and hypertensive subjects. J Cardiovasc Pharmacol [Suppl 3] 4: 319s–324s
18. Kiowski W, Bertel O, Erne P, Bolli P, Hulthen UL, Ritz R, Bühler F (1983) Hemodynamics and reflex response to acute and chronic antihypertensive therapy with the calcium entry blocker nifedipine. Hypertension [Suppl 1] 5: I-70–I-74
19. Corea L, Miele N, Bentivoglio E, Agabiti-Rosei E, Muiesan G (1979) Acute and chronic effects of nifedipine on plasma renin activity and plasma adrenaline and noradrenaline in controls and hypertensive patients. Clin Sci 57: 115s–117s
20. Corea L, Alunni G, Bentivoglio M, Boschetti E, Cosmi F, Giaimo MD, Miele N, Motolese M (1980) Acute and long-term effects of nifedipine on plasma renin activity and plasma catecholamines in controls and hypertensive patients before and after metoprolol. Acta Ther 6: 177–189
21. Muiesan G, Agabiti-Rosei E, Alicandri C, Beschi M, Castellano M, Corea L, Fariello R, Romanelli G, Pasini C, Platto L (1981) Influence of verapamil on catecholamines, renin and aldosterone in essential hypertension patients. In: Zanchetti A, Krikler D (eds) Proceedings of the international symposium on calcium antagonism in cardiovascular therapy. Excerpta Medica, Amsterdam, p 238
22. Muiesan G, Agabiti-Rosei E, Castellano M, Alicandri CL, Corea L, Fariello R, Beschi M, Romanelli G (1982) Antihypertensive and humoral effects of verapamil and nifedipine in essential hypertension. J Cardiovasc Pharmacol [Suppl 3] 4: s325–s329
23. Slike B, Ahuja RC, Okoli C, Nelson GIC, Taylor SH (1983) Blockade of slow calcium channels and regulation of circulatory pressor responses in uncomplicated hypertension. Isr J Med Sci 152: 364–372
24. Corea L, Bentivoglio M, Cosmi F, Alunni G, Carnovali M (1981) Nifedipine versus prazosin in essential hypertension: a double-blind study. Curr Ther Res 30: 708–717
25. Ekelund LG, Ekelund C, Roessner S (1982) Antihypertensive effects at rest and during exercise of a calcium blocker, nifedipine, alone and in combination with metoprolol. Acta Med Scand 212: 71–75
26. McGregor GA, Rotellar C, Markandu ND, Smith SJ, Sagnella GA (1982) Contrasting effects of nifedipine, captopril and propranolol in normotensive and hypertensive subjects. J Cardiovasc Pharmacol [Suppl 3] 4: S358–S362
27. Marone C, Luisoli S, Bomio F, Beretta-Piccoli C, Bianchetti MG, Weidmann P (1985) Body sodium-blood volume state, aldosterone, and cardiovascular responsiveness after calcium entry blockade with nifedipine. Kidney Int 28: 658–665
28. De Leeuw PW, Smout AJPM, Willemse PJ, Birkenhaeger WH (1981) Effects of verapamil in hypertensive patients. In: Zanchetti A, Krikler D (eds) Proceedings of the international symposium on calcium antagonism in cardiovascular therapy. Excerpta Medica, Amsterdam, pp 233–237
29. Leonetti G, Sala C, Bianchini C, Terzoli L, Zanchetti A (1980) Antihypertensive and renal effects of orally administered verapamil. Eur J Clin Pharmacol 18: 375–382
30. Schwietzer G, Distler A, Reeck S, Thiede HM, Philipp T (1983) Hypotensive action of calcium antagonists as related to plasma noradrenaline and reactivity to noradrenaline. J Hypertens [Suppl 2] 1: 102–104
31. Spies HF, Koch M, Appel E, Palm D, Kaltenbach MM (1978) Einfluß oraler Langzeittherapie mit Verapamil und Metoprolol auf arteriellen Blutdruck, Herzfrequenz und Plasmakatecholamine bei Hypertonikern (Abstr). Z Kardiol 67: 196

32. Anavekar SN, Christophidis N, Louis WJ, Boyle AE (1981) Verapamil in the treatment of hypertension. J Cardiovasc Pharmacol 3:287–292
33. Hiramatsu K, Yamagishi F, Kubota T, Yamada T (1982) Acute effects of the calcium antagonist nifedipine on blood pressure, pulse rate and the renin-angiotensin-aldosterone system in patients with essential hypertension. Am Heart J 104:1346–1350
34. Guthrie GP Jr, McAllister RG Jr, Kotchen TA (1983) Effects of intravenous and oral verapamil upon pressor and adrenal steroidogenic responses in normal man. J Clin Endocrinol Metab 57:339–343
35. Laederach K, Gerber A, Weidmann P (1984) Effect of calcium antagonist on blood pressure, catecholamines, renin, aldosterone, and cardiovascular pressor responsiveness in normal and hypertensive man. In: Althaus U, Burckhardt D, Vogt E (eds) Proceedings of the international symposium on calcium antagonism. PMI, Frankfurt, pp 93–115
36. Soto ME, Thibonnier M, Sire O, Menard J, Corvol P, Milliez P (1981) Antihypertensive and hormonal effects of single oral dose of captopril and nifedipine in essential hypertension. Eur J Clin Pharmacol 20:157–161
37. Thibonnier M, Bonnet F, Corvol P (1980) Antihypertensive effect of fractionated sublingual administration of nifedipine in moderate essential hypertension. Eur J Clin Pharmacol 17:161–164
38. Bianchetti MG, Beretta-Piccoli C, Weidmann P, Boehringer K, Link L, Morton JJ (1982) Studies on aldosterone responsiveness to angiotensin II during clinical variations in calcium metabolism in normal man. Clin Sci 63:325–328
39. Nadler JL, Horton R, Hauch V (1984) Therapeutic effect of calcium channel blockade in primary aldosteronism. Clin Res 32:21A
40. Millar JA, McLean K, Reid JL (1981) Calcium antagonists decrease adrenal and vascular responsiveness to angiotensin II in normal man. Clin Sci 61:65s–68s
41. Weidmann P, Horton R, Maxwell MH, Franklin SS, Fichman M (1973) Dynamic studies of aldosterone in anephric man. Kidney Int 4:289–298
42. Philipp T, Distler A, Cordes U (1978) Sympathetic nervous system and blood pressure control in essential hypertension. Lancet 2:959–963
43. Weidmann P, Keusch G, Flammer J, Ziegler WH, Reubi FC (1979) Increased ratio between changes in blood pressure and plasma norepinephrine in essential hypertension. J Clin Endocrinol Metab 48:727–731
44. Weidmann P, Grimm M, Meier A, Glück Z, Keusch G, Minder I, Beretta-Piccoli C (1980) Pathogenic and therapeutic significance of cardiovascular pressor reactivity as related to plasma catecholamines in borderline and established essential hypertension. Clin Exp Hypertens 2:427–449
45. Bianchetti MG, Weidmann P, Beretta-Piccoli C, Rupp U, Boehringer K, Link L, Ferrier C (1984) Disturbed noradrenergic blood pressure control in normotensive offspring of hypertensive families. Br Heart J 51:306–311
46. Meier A, Weidmann P, Grimm H, Keusch G, Glück Z, Minder I, Ziegler WH (1981) Pressor factors and cardiovascular pressor responsiveness in borderline hypertension. Hypertension 3:367–372
47. Weidmann P, Beretta-Piccoli C, Keusch G, Glück Z, Mujagic M, Meier A, Ziegler WH (1979) Sodium-volume factor, cardiovascular reactivity and hypotensive mechanisms of diuretic therapy in hypertension associated with diabetes mellitus. Am J Med 67:779–784
48. Beretta-Piccoli C, Weidmann P, Schiffl H, Cottier C, Reubi FC (1982) Enhanced cardiovascular pressor reactivity to norepinephrine in mild renal parenchymal disease. Kidney Int 22:297–303
49. Van Zwieten PA, van Meel JCA, Timmermanns P (1982) Calcium antagonists and alpha-2-adrenoceptors: Possible role of extracellular calcium ions in alpha-2-adrenoceptor-mediated vasoconstriction. J Cardiovasc Pharmacol [Suppl 3] 4:S273–S279
50. Vanhoutte PM, Timele TJ (1982) Calcium and alpha-adrenoceptors in activation of vascular smooth muscle. J Cardiovasc Pharmacol 4:S280–S286
51. Vierhapper H, Waldhäusl W (1982) Reduced pressor effect of angiotensin II and of noradrenaline in normal man following the oral administration of the calcium antagonist nifedipine. Eur J Clin Med 12:263–267

52. Simon G, Snyder DK (1984) Altered pressor responses in long-term nitrendipine treatment. Clin Pharmacol Ther 36:315–319
53. Trost BN, Weidmann P (1984) Hypertension accompanying diabetes mellitus: Antihypertensive and metabolic effects of calcium antagonism. Proceedings of the IXth International Congress of Nephrology, Los Angeles, June 11–16, p 228A
54. Brock TA, Lewis LJ, Smith JB (1982) Angiotensin increases Na^+ entry and Na^+/K^+ pump activity in cultures of smooth muscle from rat aorta. Proc Natl Acad Sci USA 79:1438–1442
55. Maisel AS, Motulsky HJ, Insel PA (1985) Hypotension after quinidine plus verapamil. N Engl J Med 312:167–170
56. Aoki K, Kawaguchi Y, Sato K, Kondo S, Yamamoto M (1982) Clinical and pharmacological properties of calcium antagonists in essential hypertension in humans and spontaneously hypertensive rats. J Cardiovasc Pharmacol [Suppl 3] 4:S298–S302
57. Aoki K, Sato K, Kondo S, Yamamoto M (1983) Hypotensive effects of diltiazem to normal and essential hypertensives. Eur J Clin Pharmacol 25:475–480
58. Guazzi MD, Polese A, Bartorelli A, Loaldi A, Fiorentini C (1982) Evidence of shared mechanism of vasoconstriction in pulmonary and systemic circulation in hypertension: a possible role of intracellular calcium. Circulation 66:881–886
59. Bonaduce D, Ferrara N, Petretta M, Romano E, Postiglione M, Rengo F, Condorelli M (1983) Hemodynamic study of nifedipine administration in hypertensive patients. Am Heart J 105: 865–867
60. Lund-Johansen P, Omvik P (1983) Hemodynamic effects of nifedipine in essential hypertension at rest and during exercise. J Hypertens 1:159–163
61. Fouad FM, Pedrinelli R, Bravo EL, Abi-Samra F, Textor SC, Tarazi RC (1984) Clinical and systemic hemodynamic effects of nitrendipine. Clin Pharmacol Ther 35:768–775
62. Kishi Y, Okumura F, Furuya A (1984) Hemodynamic effects of nicardipine hydrochloride. Br J Anaesth 56:1003–1007
63. Garay RP, Dagher G, Pernollet MG, Devynck MA, Meyer P (1980) Inherited defect in Na^+, K^+-co-transport system in erythrocytes from essential hypertensive patients. Nature 284:281–283
64. Dorst KG, Zidek W, Losse H, Zumkley H, Wollnik S, Vetter H (1981) Intrazelluläres Natrium und Calcium als genetische Marker der essentiellen Hypertonie. Schweiz Med Wochenschr 111:1964–1966
65. Robinson BF (1984) Altered calcium handling as a cause of primary hypertension. J Hypertens 2:453–460
66. Blaustein MP (1977) Sodium ions, calcium ions, blood pressure and hypertension: a reassessment and hypothesis. Am J Physiol 232:C615–C173
67. Hulthen UL, Bolli P, Amann FW, Kiowski W, Bühler FR (1982) Enhanced vasodilatation in essential hypertension by calcium channel blockade with verapamil. Hypertension [Suppl 2] 4: II-26–II-31
68. Robinson BF, Dobbs RJ, Bailey S (1982) Response of forearm resistance vessels to verapamil and sodium-nitroprusside in normotensive and hypertensive men: evidence for a functional abnormality of vascular smooth muscle in primary hypertension. Clin Sci 63:33–42
69. Erne P, Bolli P, Burgisse E, Bühler FR (1984) Correlation of platelet calcium with blood pressure: effect of antihypertensive therapy. N Engl J Med 310:1084–1088
70. Beretta-Piccoli C, Weidmann P, de Châtel R, Hirsch D, Reubi FC (1977) Beziehungen zwischen Blutdruck, Blutvolumen und Plasmarenin während Diuretikatherapie bei essentieller Hypertonie. Schweiz Med Wochenschr 107:104–115
71. Flammer J, Weidmann P, Glück Z, Ziegler WH, Reubi FC (1979) Cardiovascular and endocrine profile of adrenergic neurone blockade in normal and hypertensive man. Am J Med 66:34–42
72. Weidmann P, Bousquet JC, Swiss Practitioners Bopindolol Study Group (1986) Antihypertensive treatment with bopindolol alone or combined with a diuretic in general practice. J Cardiovasc Pharmacol
73. Beer N, Gallegos I, Cohen A, Klein N, Sonnenblick E, Frishman W (1981) Efficacy of sublingual nifedipine in the acute treatment of systemic hypertension. Chest 79:571–574
74. Palau LG, Minambres FB (1984) Modificaciones ecocardiograficas y de la tension arterial tras la administracion aguda y prolongada (tres meses) de nifedipina. Med Clin (Barc) 83:146–150

75. Pedersen OL, Christensen CK, Mikkelsen E, Rämsch KD (1980) Relationship between the antihypertensive effect and steady state plasma concentration of nifedipine given alone or in combination with a beta adrenoceptor blocking agent. Eur J Clin Pharmacol 18:287–293
76. Chia BL, Ee B, Tan A, Choo M (1982) The immediate hypotensive effect of oral nifedipine. Curr Med Res Opin 8:139–141
77. Bertel O, Conen D, Radü EW, Müller J, Lang C, Dubach UC (1983) Nifedipine in hypertensive emergencies. Br Med J 286:19–21
78. Conen D, Bertel O, Dubach UC (1982) An oral calcium antagonist for the treatment of hypertensive emergencies. J Cardiovasc Pharmacol 4:S378–S382
79. Aoki K, Kondo S, Mochizuki A, Yoshida T, Kato S, Kato K, Takikawa K (1978) Antihypertensive effect of cardiovascular Ca^{2+}-antagonist in hypertensive patients in the absence and presence of beta-adrenergic blockade. Am Heart J 96:218–226
80. Degenhardt S, Hummerich W, Lang R (1984) Akute hämodynamische und hormonelle Effekte einer sublingualen Einmaldosis von Nifedipin bei Hypertonikern. Nieren Hochdruckkr 13:494–499
81. Guazzi MD, de Cesare N, Galli C, Salvioni A, Tramontana C, Tamborini G, Bartorelli A (1984) Calcium-channel blockade with nifedipine and angiotensin converting-enzyme inhibiton with captopril in the therapy of patients with severe primary hypertension. Circulation 70:279–284
82. Aoki K, Kondo S, Sato K, Kato K, Kawaguchi Y, Mochizuki A, Yamamoto M (1981) Hypotensive action of nifedipine (Ca-antagonist) and propranolol in acute trials and its long-term therapy of hypertensive coronary heart disease patients. Jpn Heart J 22:575–584
83. De Divitiis O, Petitto M, di Somma S, Fazio M, Galderisi M, Villari B, Liguori V, Santomauro M (1984) Acebutolol and nifedipine in the treatment of arterial hypertension: efficacy and acceptability. Drug Res 34(1)/6:710–715
84. Levenson JA, Safar ME, Simon AC, Boutier JA, Griener L (1983) Systemic and arterial hemodynamic effects of nifedipine (20 mg) in mild-to-moderate hypertension. Hypertension [Suppl 5] 5:V-57–V-60
85. Maeda K, Tanaka C, Minamikawa H, Komatsu H, Kotsumi K, Inoue E (1982) Antihypertensive effects of the calcium antagonistic agent nifedipine. Drug Res 32(1):267–271
86. Imai Y, Abe K, Otsuka Y, Irokawa N, Yasujima M, Saito K, Sakurai Y, Chiba S, Ito T, Sato M, Haruyama T, Miura Y, Yoshinaga K (1980) Management of severe hypertension with nifedipine in combination with clonidine or propranolol. Drug Res 30(1):674–678
87. Masotti G, Poggesi L, Castellani S, Moretti A, Galanti G, Scarti L (1984) A study of the antihypertensive effect and some pharmacodynamic aspects of nifedipine in medium-term treatment. Int J Clin Pharmacol Res 4(1):71–79
88. Stornello M, di Rao G, Iachello M, Pisani R, Scapellato L, Pedrinelli R, Salvetti A (1983) Hemodynamic and humoral interactions between captopril and nifedipine. Hypertension [Suppl 3] 5:III-154–III-156
89. Pedersen OL, Mikkelsen E, Andersson KE (1978) Effects of extracellular calcium on potassium and noradrenaline induced contractions in the aorta of spontaneously hypertensive rats – increased sensitivity to nifedipine. Acta Pharmacol Toxicol (Copenh) 43:137–144
90. Douglas-Jones AP, Mitchell AD (1984) Comparison of nifedipine (retard formulation) and mefruside in the treatment of mild to moderate hypertension – a prospective randomized double-blind crossover study in general practice. Postgrad Med J 60:529–532
91. Klein W, Brandt D, Vrecko K, Haerringer M (1983) Role of calcium antagonists in the treatment of essential hypertension. Circ Res [Suppl 1] 52:174–181
92. Erne P, Bolli P, Bertel O, Hulthen UL, Kiowski W, Müller FB, Bühler FR (1983) Factors influencing the hypotensive effects of calcium antagonists. Hypertension [Suppl 2] 5:II-97–II-102
93. Valdes G, Montero J, Tobar M, Chacon C, Croxatto HR (1983) Effecto initial y cronico de nifedipina en pacientes hypertensos. Rev Med Chil 111:1237–1240
94. Hallin L, Andrén L, Hansson L (1983) Controlled trial of nifedipine and bendroflumethiazide in hypertension. J Cardiovasc Pharmacol 6:1083–1085
95. Lewis GRJ (1980) Verapamil in the management of chronic hypertension. Clin Invest Med 3:175–177
96. Loaldi A, Pepi M, Agostini PG, Fiorentini C. Gracio S, della Bella P, Guazzi MD (1983) Cardiac rhythm in hypertension assessed through 24 hour ambulatory electrocardiographic

monitoring: effects of load manipulation with atenolol, verapamil and nifedipine. Br Heart J 50:118–126
97. Terzoli L, Bianchini C, Sala C, Sernesi L, Leonetti G, Zanchetti A (1978) Effetto sulla pressione arteriosa e sul bilancio indrosalino della somministrazione cronica del verapamil in pazienti ipertesi. Boll Soc Ital Cardiol 13(10):1773–1778
98. De Leeuw PW, Birkenhäger WH (1984) Effects of verapamil in hypertensive patients. Acta Med Scand [Suppl] 681:125–128
99. Mitbø K, Hals O (1980) Verapamil in the treatment of hypertension. Curr Ther Res 27:830–837
100. Anavekar SN, Christophidis N, Louis WJ, Doyle AE (1981) Verapamil in the treatment of hypertension. J Cardiovasc Pharmacol 3:287–292
101. Doyle AE (1983) Comparison of beta-adrenoceptor blockers and calcium antagonists in hypertension. Hypertension [Suppl 2] 5:II-103–II-108
102. Mitbø K, Hals O, van der Meer J (1982) Verapamil compared with nifedipine in the treatment of essential hypertension. J Cardiovasc Pharmacol 4:S363–S368
103. Hornung RS, Jones RI, Gould BA, Sonecha T, Raftery EB (1984) Propranolol vs verapamil for the treatment of essential hypertension. Am Heart J 108:554–560
104. Gould BA, Mann S, Kieso H, Subramanian VB, Raftery EB (1981) The 24-h intraarterial ambulatory profile of blood pressure reduction with verapamil. In: Zanchetti A, Krikler DM (eds) International Symposium, Florence. Excerpta Medica, Amsterdam, pp 280–291
105. Bühler FR, Hulthen UL, Kiowski W, Bolli P (1982) Greater antihypertensive efficacy of the calcium channel inhibitor verapamil in older and low renin patients. Clin Sci 63:s439–s441
106. Lund-Johansen P (1984) Hemodynamic effects of verapamil in essential hypertension at rest and during exercise. Acta Med Scand [Suppl] 681:109–115
107. Wigler I, Peer G, Sofermann G, Blum M, Aviram A (1984) Long-term treatment of arterial hypertension with verapamil. Int J Clin Pharmacol Ther Toxicol 22:162–166
108. Lopez LM, Metha JL, Baz R, Aguila E (1984) Effects of nitrendipine and hydralazine on plasma catecholamines in essential hypertension. Clin Pharm 36(4):444–450
109. Kazda S, Garthoff B, Rämsch KD, Schlüter G (1983) Nisoldipine. In: Scriabine A (ed) New drugs annual: Cardiovascular drugs. Raven, New York, pp 243–258
110. Wambach G, Breuer G, Kaufmann W (1984) Hypotensive Eigenschaften von Nisoldipin. Drug Res 34(1):620–623
111. Leonetti G, Gradnik R, Terzoli L, Fruscio M, Rupoli L, Zanchetti A (1984) Felodipine, a new vasodilating drug: blood pressure, cardiac, renal, and humoral effects in hypertensive patients. J Cardiovasc Pharmacol 6:392–398
112. Andersson O, Bengtsson C, Elmfeldt D, Haglund K, Hedner T, Seideman P, Sjöberg KH, Strömgren E, Aberg H, Oestman J (1984) Short-term effects of felodipine, a new dihydropyridine in hypertension. Br J Clin Pharmacol 17:257–263
113. Rosatti F, Cella PL, Fici F, Rossi F, Chieppa S, Marmo E (1984) Diltiazem in the therapy of arterial hypertension: Polygraphic assessment of left ventricular performance. Curr Ther Res 36:701–711
114. Yamakado T, Oonishi N, Kondo S, Noziri A, Nakano T, Takezawa H (1983) Effects of diltiazem on cardiovascular responses during exercise in systemic hypertension and comparison with propranolol. Am J Cardiol 52:1023–1027
115. Inouye IK, Massie BK, Benowitz N, Simpson PM, Loge D (1984) Antihypertensive therapy with diltiazem and comparison with hydrochlorothiazide. Am J Cardiol 53:1588–1592
116. Trimarco B, de Lucia N, Ricciardelli B, Volpe M, Veniero A, Cuocolo A, Cicala M (1984) Diltiazem in the treatment of mild to moderate essential hypertension. Comparison with metoprolol in a crossover double-blind trial. J Clin Pharmacol 24:218–227
117. Gerold M, Eigenmann R, Haeusler G (1982) Cardiovascular effects of tiapamil (Ro 11–1781), a new calcium entry blocker. J Cardiovasc Pharmacol 4:419–429
118. Laederach K, Weidmann P, Lauener F, Gerber A, Ziegler WH (1986) Comparative acute effects of the calcium channel blockers tiapamil, nisoldipine and nifedipine on blood pressure and some regulatory factors in normal and hypertensive subjects. J Cardiovasc Pharmacol (in press)
119. Ventura HO, Messerli FH, Oigman W, Dunn FG, Reisin E, Fröhlich ED (1983) Immediate hemodynamic effects of a new calcium channel blocking agent (nitrendipine) in essential hypertension. Am J Cardiol 51:783–786

120. Van Schaik BAM, Vanniste AE, Geyskess GG (1984) Antihypertensive and renal effects of nicardipine. Br J Clin Pharmacol 18:57–63
121. Klütsch K, Schmidt P, Grosswendt J (1982) Der Einfluß von „Bay a 1040" auf die Nierenfunktion des Hypertonikers. Drug Res 22:377–380
122. Yokoyama S, Kaburagi T (1983) Clinical effects of intravenous nifedipine on renal function. J Cardiovasc Pharmacol 5:67–71
123. Thananopavarn C, Golub MS, Eggena P, Barret JD, Sambhi MP (1984) Renal effects of nitrendipine monotherapy in essential hypertension. J Cardiovasc Pharmacol 6:S1032–S1036
124. Husted SE, Nielsen HK, Christensen CK, Pedersen OL (1982) Long-term therapy of arterial hypertension with nifedipine given alone or in combination with a beta-adrenoceptor blocking agent. Eur J Clin Pharmacol 22:101–103
125. Zawar PB, Chawhan RN, Gosavi SV, Gokhale PD, Jadhav AB (1982) Verapamil in hypertension – a long-term study. Indian Heart J 34:38–41
126. Taburet AM, Singlas E, Colin JN, Banzet O, Thibonnier M, Corvol P (1983) Pharmacokinetic studies of nifedipine tablet. Correlation of antihypertensive effects. Hypertension 5(2):II-29–II-33
127. Taylor SH, Silke B, Ahuya C, Okoli R (1982) Influence of nicardipine on the blood pressure at rest and on the pressor responses to cold, isometric exertion and dynamic exercise in hypertensive patients. J Cardiovasc Pharmacol 4:803–807
128. Magometschnigg D (1983) Acute hypotensive response to nifedipine. Hypertension [Suppl 2] 5:II-80–II-84
129. Yoshimura M, Takashina R, Shikuma R, Takahashi H, Takeda K, Ashizawa H, Ochi Y, Ijchi H (1983) Antihypertensive effect of nifedipine and its relationship to severity of hypertension. Drug Res 3:254–257
130. Maeda K, Takasugi T, Tsukano Y, Tanaka Y, Shiota K (1981) Clinical study on the hypotensive effects of diltiazem hydrochloride. Int J Clin Pharmacol Ther Toxicol 19:47–55
131. Orö L, Ryman T (1984) Long-term study of the combined antihypertensive action of nitrendipine and metoprolol. In: Scriabin A, Vanov S, Deck K (eds) Nitrendipine. Urban and Schwarzenberg, Munich, pp 527–534
132. Tammen AT, Stoepel K, Vollmer G, Blümchen G (1984) Efficacy and safety in patients with essential hypertension and coronary heart disease. In: Scriabin A, Vanov S, Deck K (eds) Nitrendipine. Urban and Schwarzenberg, Munich, pp 469–476
133. Yagil Y, Kobrin I, Stessmann J, Ghanem J, Leibel B, Ben-Ishay D (1983) Effectiveness of combined nifedipine and propranolol treatment in hypertension. Hypertension [Suppl 2] 5:II-113–II-117
134. Aoki K, Sato K (1982) Acute hypotensive, hemodynamic effects of long-term treatment with niludipine, a Ca^{2+}-antagonist, in patients with essential hypertension. Drug Res 32(2) 9:1141–1145
135. Eggertsen R, Hansson L (1982) Effects of treatment with nifedipine and metoprolol in essential hypertension. Eur J Clin Pharmacol 21:389–390
136. Brennan FN, Blake S (1982) The use of nifedipine as a third-step agent in the treatment of refractory hypertension. Ir Med J 75:29–30
137. Dean S, Kendall MJ (1983) Nifedipine in treatment of difficult hypertensives. Eur J Clin Pharmacol 24:1–5
138. Murphy MB, Scriven AJI, Dollery CT (1983) Efficacy of nifedipine as a step 3 antihypertensive drug. Hypertension [Suppl 2] 5:II-118–II-121
139. Gonzalez-Gomez A, Gamio-Capestany F, Garcia-Barreto D (1983) Hypotensive action of verapamil in a group of hydralazine-dependent hypertensive patients. Arch Intern Med 261: 268–277
140. Leary WP, Asmal AC (1979) Treatment of hypertension with verapamil. Curr Ther Res 25: 747–751
141. Ueda K, Musakami M (1983) A controlled comparative multicenter study on the clinical efficacy of nifedipine in the treatment of severe hypertension. In: Kaltenbach M, Neufeld HN (eds) 5th International Adalat Symposium. Excerpta Medica, Amsterdam, p 146
142. Guazzi MD, Fiorentini C, Olivari MT, Bartorelli A, Necchi G, Polese A (1980) Short- and long-term efficacy of a calcium-antagonistic agent (nifedipine) combined with methyldopa in the treatment of severe hypertension. Circulation 61:913–919

143. Jee LD, Opie LH (1983) Acute hypotensive response to nifedipine added to prazosin in treatment of hypertension (case reports). Br Med J 287:1514
144. Kusano E, Asano Y, Takeda K, Matsumoto Y, Ebihara A, Hosoda S (1982) Hypotensive effect of nifedipine in hypertensive patients with chronic renal failure. Drug Res 32:1575–1580
145. Kubo K, Shiraishi K, Muto H, Suzuki T, Sugino N (1983) Treatment of hypertension in hemodialysis patients with nifedipine. Hypertension [Suppl 2] 5:II–109–II–112
146. Yamakado M, Tagawa T (1978) Hypotensive effects of diltiazem HCl (Herbesser). Mod Clin Med 20:1877–1881
147. Sakurai T, Kurita T, Nagano S, Sonoda T (1972) Antihypertensive vasodilating and sodium diuretic actions of D-cis-isomer of benzothiazepine derivate (CRD–401). Acta Urolog Jpn 18:695
148. Trost BN, Weidmann P (1984) Effects of nitrendipine and other calcium antagonists on glucose metabolism in man. J Cardiovasc Pharmacol 6:S986–S995
149. Donelly T, Harrower ADP (1980) Effect of nifedipine on glucose tolerance and insulin secretion in diabetic and non-diabetic patients. Curr Med Res Opin 6:690–693
150. Abadie E, Passa PH (1984) Diabetogenic effects of nifedipine (Letter). Br Med J 289:438
151. Bhatnagar SK, Amin MAA, Al-Yusuf AR (1984) Diabetogenic effects of nifedipine. Br Med J 289:19
152. Guazzi MD, Olivari MT, Polese A, Fiorentini C, Magrini F, Moruzzi P (1977) Nifedipine, a new antihypertensive with rapid action. Clin Pharmacol Ther 22:528–532
153. Bartorelli C, Magrini F, Moruzzi P, Olivari MT, Polese A, Fiorentini C, Guazzi MD (1978) Hemodynamic effect of a calcium-antagonistic agent (nifedipine) in hypertension: therapeutic implications. Clin Sci Mol Med 55:291s–292s
154. Kuwajima I, Ueda K, Kamata C, Matsushita S, Kuramoto K, Murakami H, Hada Y (1978) A study on the effects of nifedipine in hypertensive crises and severe hypertension. Jpn Heart J 19:455–467
155. Huysmans FTM, Sluiter HE, Thien TA, Koene RAP (1983) Acute treatment of hypertensive crisis with nifedipine. Br J Clin Pharmacol 16:725–727
156. Magometschnigg D (1982) Zur Therapie bei hypertonen Krisen. Nifedipin per os. Dtsch Med Wochenschr 107:1423–1428
157. Anonymous (1983) Calcium antagonists and aneurysmal subarachnoid hemorrhage. Lancet I: 141–143
158. Nobile-Orazio E, Sterzi R (1981) Cerebral ischemia after nifedipine treatment. Br Med J 283:948
159. Polese A, Fiorentini C, Olivari MT, Guazzi MD (1979) Clinical use of a calcium antagonistic agent (nifedipine) in acute pulmonary edema. Am J Med 66:825–830
160. Bhat RP, Wasir HS (1982) Verapamil infusion in hypertension. Indian Heart J 34:228–231
161. Rosenthal J (1981) Die Behandlung der hypertensiven Krisen mit Diltiazem. In: Bender F, Greeff K (eds) 1. Diltiazem-Symposium. Excerpta Medica, Amsterdam, pp 227–248
162. Krebs R (1983) Adverse reactions with calcium antagonists. Hypertension [Suppl 2] 5:II-125–II-129
163. Eisenberg JNH, Oakley GDG (1984) Probable adverse interaction between oral metoprolol and verapamil. Postgrad Med 60:705–706
164. Hutchinson SJ, Lorimer AR (1984) Betablockers and verapamil: a cautionary tale. Br Med J 289:659–660
165. Ramon Y, Behar S, Kishon Y, Engelberg IS (1984) Gingival hyperplasia caused by nifedipine – a preliminary report. Int J Cardiol 5:195–204
166. Diamond JR, Cheung JY, Fang LST (1984) Nifedipine-induced renal dysfunction. Am J Med 77:905–909
167. Ter Wee PM, Rosman JB, van der Geest S (1984) Acute renal failure due to diltiazem. Lancet II:1337–1338
168. Murphy MB, Scriven AJI, Dollery CT (1983) Role of nifedipine in treatment of hypertension. Br Med J 287:257–259
169. Giesecke HJ, Guckenbiehl W, Hagemann I (1982) Ergebnisse einer Multicenterstudie mit Diltiazem bei Hypertonie. In: Bender F, Greeff K (eds) 1. Diltiazem-Symposium. Excerpta Medica, Amsterdam, pp 220–226
170. Schulte KL, Meyer WA, Distler A, Gotzen R (1983) Antihypertensive Langzeitbehandlung mit Diltiazem und Nifedipin bei essentieller Hypertonie. Therapiewoche 33:6011–6014

171. Röjdmark S, Andersson DEH (1984) Influence of verapamil on glucose tolerance. Acta Med Scand [Suppl] 681:37–48
172. Segrestaa JM, Caulin C, Dahan R, Houlbert D, Thiercelin JF, Herman P, Sauvanet JP, Larribaud J (1984) Effect of diltiazem on plasma glucose, insulin and glucagon during an oral glucose tolerance test in healthy volunteers. Eur J Clin Pharmacol 26:481–483
173. Walldius G (1984) Effect of verapamil on serum lipoproteins in patients with angina pectoris. Acta Med Scand [Suppl] 681:43–48
174. Weidmann P, Uehlinger DE, Gerber A (1985) Antihypertensive treatment and serum lipoproteins. J Hypertens 3:297–306
175. Lessem J, Bellinetto A (1983) Interaction between digoxin and the calcium antagonists nicardipine and tiapamil. Clin Ther 5:595–602
176. Pedersen KE (1984) The influence of calcium antagonists on plasma digoxin concentration. Acta Med Scand [Suppl] 681:31–36
177. Helgeland A (1980) Treatment of mild hypertension: a five-year controlled drug trial. The Oslo Study. Am J Med 69:725–732
178. Multiple risk factor intervention trial research group (MRFIT) (1982) Risk factor changes and mortality results. JAMA 248:1465–1477
179. Morgan TO, Adams WR, Hodgson M, Gibberd RW (1980) Failure of therapy to improve prognosis in elderly males with hypertension. Med J Aust 2:27–31
180. Evans MG, Olanoff LS, Hurwitz G, Cowart D, Conradi EC (1984) Use of nifedipine as an adjunct to current antihypertensive therapy. Arch Intern Med 144:985–987
181. Murphy MB, Bulpitt CJ, Dollery CT (1984) Role of nifedipine in the treatment of resistant hypertension. Am J Med 77(2B):16–21
182. Andren L, Hansson L, Oroe L, Ryman T (1982) Experience with nitrendipine – a new calcium antagonist – in hypertension. J Cardiovasc Pharmacol 4:S387–S391
183. Dunn JM, Groth PE (1984) Once daily verapamil. Lancet II:1338–1339

Converting Enzyme Inhibitors in the Treatment of Hypertension and of Cardiac Failure

J. I. S. Robertson[1]

In man the enzyme renin exists both in blood and the kidney partly in an active, and partly in an inactive form [1, 2,]. Active renin reacts with a circulating substrate, angiotensinogen, cleaving that substrate between a leucine and a valine residue to form the inactive decapeptide angiotensin I. Within the circulation, angiotensin I is in turn split by (angiotensin) converting enzyme (ACE), two amino acid residues are removed, and the principal active component of the renin system, the octapeptide angiotensin II, is formed. Angiotensin II has a wide range of physiological and pathophysiological actions: It raises blood pressure both by an immediate vasoconstrictor and a slower action; it stimulates the sympathetic nervous system at various sites; it inhibits vagal tone; at rather higher than physiological doses it stimulates vasopressin secretion; it has a wide range of direct renal effects; it can promote thirst; and it is an important regulator of aldosterone secretion. All of these actions are evidently concerned with the maintenance of arterial pressure and of the circulation. Not surprisingly, therefore, efforts have been made over the years to develop therapeutic agents which interfere with the renin-angiotensin system at various points.

Synthetic analogues of the octapeptide angiotensin II, which act as competitive antagonists to angiotensin II, have been available for many years. While these agents, of which the best known is saralasin, have provided a wealth of information on the physiological and pathophysiological effects of angiotensin II, they have had limited therapeutic application because of their need so far to be given intravenously.

More recently, various inhibitors of the enzyme renin have been developed. This approach is particularly attractive because renin is remarkably specific in its substrate requirements and a therapeutically effective renin inhibitor should have an action virtually restricted to the renin system proper.

The most important therapeutic agents so far developed to interfere with the renin system, however, have been inhibitors of ACE and especially the orally active converting enzyme inhibitors such as captopril, enalapril and lisinopril [3–8]. ACE is not specific for angiotensin I; this same enzyme provides one of the pathways of degradation of bradykinin. Nevertheless, the use of ACE inhibitors has been hitherto the most profitable means of abrogating the renin-angiotensin system clinically. Early ACE inhibitors were peptides isolated from the venom of a South American snake, bothrops jararaca. While very important in the evolution of therapeutically effective ACE inhibitors, these venom peptide analogues had limited clinical application because of their need to be given parenterally. The really major

[1] MRC Blood Pressure Unit, Western Infirmary, Glasgow G11 6NT, United Kingdom.

Primary Hypertension
Ed. by W. Kaufmann et al.

advance was with the development of captopril, the first orally active ACE inhibitor. The molecule of captopril contains a sulphydril group. This sulphydril group is important in two respects: It is necessary for the effectiveness of captopril as an inhibitor of ACE and it is also suspected – although there is not general agreement on this point – of being responsible for some of the adverse effects seen with that agent. The orally active ACE inhibitors of the second generation, typified by enalapril, do not contain the sulphydril group. The absence of this moiety will, it is hoped, minimise adverse reactions.

Enalapril is itself a largely inactive pro-drup which is converted in the liver to the active ACE inhibitor enalaprilat. Whereas captopril has a rapid onset of action, within 1 h of oral ingestion, the peak effect of enalapril is much slower, at around 4–6 h. Both captopril and enalapril are dependent mainly on the kidney for elimination from the body.

Following administration of an orally active ACE inhibitor such as captopril, enalapril or lisinopril, there is a fall in circulating angiotensin II with a converse rise in components of the renin-angiotensin system proximal to the site of enzymatic blockade. Thus, there is an increase in the concentrations of both active and total renin and in angiotensin I in the circulation. Blood pressure and plasma aldosterone, both in part dependent on angiotensin II, fall in parallel with the fall in circulating angiotensin II. The fall in plasma angiotensin II is maximal at around 2 h after captopril or 6 h after enalapril, and is closely correlated with the concurrent fall in arterial pressure. Interestingly, with continued administration of these drug over 2–3 weeks, there is a further fall in arterial pressure, possibly representing interference by ACE inhibitors with the slow pressor effect of angiotensin II [1]. Thus, with long-term treatment, there is a much less close correlation between the fall in arterial pressure and the fall in angiotensin II than is seen initially.

I propose to consider the use of ACE inhibitors in hypertension under three main headings: – (a) those used alone before operation in hypertension with renal artery stenosis; (b) those used in combination with a loop diuretic to treat previously intractable and usually severe hypertension; and most importantly, (c) those used in the treatment of mild to moderate hypertension both when given alone and in combination with a thiazide diuretic.

Hypertension with Renal Artery Stenosis

Although the situation is by no means straightforward, the balance of evidence now indicates very firmly that the renin-angiotensin system is fundamentally involved with the pathogenesis of hypertension due to unilateral renal artery stenosis [9]. One would expect, therefore, clear beneficial effects of ACE inhibitors in correcting the systemic hypertension in this disease. This was clearly demonstrated in a series of ten patients with hypertension associated with unilateral renal artery stenosis [10] in whom we were able to initiate enalapril therapy with the patients either untreated, or with any previous treatment withdrawn for a minimum period of 1 month. Enalapril in the dosage range 10–40 mg once daily was the only therapy employed in the first 3 months in this series. The patients ranged in age from 37 to 56; two were women. The diagnosis of unilateral renal artery stenosis was based on an arteriographic renal artery narrowing together with the characteristic appearances of unilateral renal artery stenosis on bilateral ureteric catheterisation. On isotope renography, there was diminution in renal plasma flow on the suspect side. At renal vein sampling, renin was elevated on the side with the arteriographic lesion. At 6 h from the first dose of active enalapril there were marked decreases in plasma ACE activity and in angiotensin II, with converse increases in blood levels of angiotensin I and in plasma active renin concentration. The small decrease in mean plasma aldosterone was not significant. A highly significant reduction in blood pressure accompanied the decrease in plasma angiotensin II, and these changes were significantly correlated ($r = +0.67$; $P < 0.05$); the decrease in blood pressure at 6 h also correlated with the plasma concentrations (before enalapril therapy) of active renin ($r = +0.76$; $P < 0.05$) and angiotensin II ($r = +0.70$; $P < 0.05$).

With continued enalapril therapy, suppression of plasma ACE activity and angiotensin II, similar to that observed on the first day, was seen at 6 days and at 3 months, 6 h after dosing. Active renin concentration increased progressively from the 1st to the 6th day and from the 6th day to the 3rd month of treatment. The mean blood concentration of angiotensin I also increased further from the 1st to the 6th day of enalapril treatment, but there was no further increase thereafter. The slight decrease in mean plasma aldosterone remained insignificant. Blood pressure remained controlled at 6 days and 3 months. However, during long-term treatment, the decrease in blood pressure was less closely related than on the 1st day to either the pretreatment plasma renin or angiotensin II concentrations, or to the long-term decrease in plasma angiotensin II (respective correlation coefficients 0.44, 0.42, and 0.56; none significant).

We were particularly interested to study the effect over 24 h of once daily enalapril therapy and measurements were made on the last day of placebo treatment and compared with those at the 3rd month of enalapril treatment, 24 h after the preceding dose, and again 6 h after the morning dose of the drug. It was evident that a continued enalapril effect was seen at the 3rd month, 24 h after the last dose of the drug. At this time there was a marked increase in circulating active renin and angiotensin I, and a converse reduction of ACE activity and angiotensin II. Blood pressure also remained significantly reduced 24 h after dosing in comparison with pretreatment values. Nevertheless, following the morning dose of enalapril, significant further reductions in plasma ACE activity and angiotensin II occurred, while mean values for active renin and angiotensin II were further increased. The small additional lowering of arterial pressure 6 h after dosing was not statistically significant.

It should be emphasised that while there had been a significant fall in arterial pressure by the 6 th day of enalapril treatment, this further decreased highly significantly by the 3rd month. Thus, the full antihypertensive effect of ACE inhibition may take some 3–4 weeks to be established. Possibly in part this represents antagonism of the slow pressor component of the action of angiotensin II. Enalapril treatment was not associated with postural hypotension and there was no significant elevation of heart rate in the group of patients as a whole.

While there were no systematic changes in total body potassium, total exchangeable sodium was reduced during therapy in nine patients and unchanged in the tenth, falling from a mean of 101% to 96% of predicted normal values. The mean lowering of exchangeable sodium was 140 mmol and was highly significant ($P < 0.001$).

It is thus evident that substantial clinical benefits accrue from treatment with an ACE inhibitor in hypertension associated with unilateral renal artery stenosis. However, some important theoretical disadvantages must be carefully considered. It is well established that in unilateral renal artery stenosis, the afflicted kidney is heavily dependent upon a raised intrarenal concentration of angiotensin II to help sustain glomerular filtration rate, urea excretion, and pressure in the renal artery distal to the stenosis [11]. It would be expected that these compensatory effects would be lost with ACE inhibition. In this series we found a small, but significant, overall reduction in creatinine clearance by the 3rd month of enalapril treatment and this was reflected in a modest, but distinct, increase both in serum creatinine and urea. There was also the expected small, but significant, increase in serum potassium, no doubt reflecting the fall in exchangeable sodium in the absence of an increase in aldosterone. Serum sodium concentration was unchanged. It will be recalled that one of the diagnostic criteria at entry was a reduced renal plasma flow, assessed isotopically, on the suspect side. Repeat isotope renography at the 3rd month of enalapril treatment showed opposing effects in the two kidneys. While effective renal plasma flow through the unaffected kidney was significantly increased by enalapril treatment, on the stenotic side, already with an impaired renal plasma flow, this fell further. In one man, who entered the trial with a tenuous renal artery supplying a small scarred kidney, this artery had occluded completely by the 3rd month, although there had been no symptoms and his increase in serum creatinine and urea was less than the average for the group as a whole. While there is an obvious suspicion that the use of enalapril may have hastened the renal artery occlusion in this man, this is a difficult point to establish, because many such patients progress to renal artery occlusion irrespective of the nature or effectiveness of treatment. Our current view is that in patients who are candidates for corrective renal artery surgery or transluminal balloon dilatation, treatment with ACE inhibitors should be given alone for no more than 1 month and the patient should then proceed to operation [11]. This should permit intervention under the most favourable circumstances with the full blood pressure lowering effect of ACE inhibition being achieved. At the same time, the duration of the risk to the kidney will be kept to a minimum. These considerations do not, it should be emphasised, mean that ACE inhibitors can not be used indefinitely in patients with hypertension and renal artery stenosis if the patients are unwilling to undergo operation or are otherwise considered unsuitable.

For similar reasons ACE inhibitors should be used with extreme caution with bilateral renal artery stenosis or with stenosis to an artery of the sole kidney. Diuretics are not usually required in combination with ACE inhibitors in renovascular hypertension. If they are to be employed they should be introduced with extreme caution.

Because the renin-angiotensin system is closely implicated in the pathogenesis of renovascular hypertension, there are theoretical reasons for supposing that the use of these agents before operation might permit prediction of the likely hypotensive response to be achieved by subsequent corrective renovascular surgery. In one series [12], we found that the immediate response to captopril correlated poorly with long-term surgical outcome. However, as mentioned above, the blood pressure reduction achieved by prolonged ACE inhibition is usually much greater than the immediate response. In the same series we found that the absolute levels of systolic and diastolic pressure attained by the 6th week of captopril treatment alone corresponded remarkably well with the values attained 3 months or more after surgical intervention with the patients remaining off therapy following operation. Similar results have since been reported by Staessen et al. [13]. While these results are encouraging, and have important theoretical implications, they do of course require to be confirmed in larger series.

Previously Intractable Hypertension

ACE inhibitors may be used in conjunction with loop diuretics, usually frusemide, in the treatment of severe, previously intractable, hypertension. The rationale of this approach in unresponsive hypertension is straight forward. The use of powerful diuretics, such as frusemide, in the treatment of hypertension will promote sodium excretion which will lead to an increased secretion of renin by the kidney. Thus there will be a reactive rise in circulating angiotensin II which, through various actions, will offset the hypotensive effect. If, however, in these circumstances, a loop diuretic is used in conjunction with an ACE inhibitor, the reactive increase in angiotensin II is prevented, and thus the blood pressure reduction will be more marked and sustained. In a series [14] of patients of this type we found the combination of frusemide with captopril, 150 mg 3 times daily, effective and well tolerated. In the series mean blood pressure values were around 220/120 mm Hg on previous therapy. By the 3rd month of the combination of captopril with frusemide, this had been reduced to mean values around 140/90 mm Hg. Despite often large doses of loop diuretics, captopril 450 mg daily produced sustained reduction in plasma angiotensin II throughout 24 h, with converse sustained increases in plasma active renin concentration and in blood angiotensin I. Again, despite the large doses of diuretic, plasma aldosterone was significantly depressed in parallel with the reduction in plasma angiotensin II. The sustained fall in plasma aldosterone in these circumstances deserves emphasis; because of this there was no tendency to hypokalaemia. Thus, neither potassium-conserving diuretics nor potassium supplements were required and indeed might have been dangerous particularly in those patients who had renal impairment. Caution was also necessary in those with renal impairment, since excessive diuretic dosage could provoke worsening uraemia. Several patients in this series had suffered crippling side effects on previous therapy and were much more tolerant of the combination of captopril with diuretic.

A further need for care in patients of this type occurred where complex antihypertensive drug regimens were previously being employed, often resulting in very high levels of circulating renin and angiotensin II. In these circumstances initiation of ACE inhibition can cause a very steep and dangerous fall in arterial pressure [15]. Thus, treatment should be begun under close supervision with facilities on hand for correction of hypotension, if necessary, by administration of angiotensin II. Because the action of captopril is very abrupt, such initial steep falls in pressure will occur often within 20–30 min of administration of that drug. With enalapril the onset of the hypotensive effect is slower, but at maximum its effect is equally severe. It should be emphasised that such steep and disturbing falls in arterial pressure are unlikely to be seen with the initiation of ACE inhibition in mild to moderate and previously untreated essential hypertension.

Essential Hypertension

I wish to turn now to what is numerically the most important area of treatment: essential hypertension. It has been known since the work of Chinn and Düsterdieck in 1972 [16], that in essential hypertension circulating levels of angiotensin II are within a range having a direct immediate effect on arterial pressure. Thus, one would expect and indeed does see, an initial fall in arterial pressure with ACE inhibition in proportion to the circulating level of angiotensin II [8]. However, in essential hypertension, as with renovascular hypertension, sustained ACE inhibition produces an additional fall in arterial pressure over 3–4 weeks of treatment beyond the initial response. Several controlled trials have now shown that both captopril and enalapril have an antihypertensive effect in essential hypertension comparable to that seen with thiazide diuretics and with beta-blockers when those agents are used as sole therapy [3–6]. Moreover, for the reasons discussed in detail above, the conjoint use of ACE inhibitors with thiazide diuretics is particularly effective in lowering arterial pressure. An especially attractive aspect recently reported is that enalapril has proved more effective than beta-blockade in lowering systolic pressure [17]. Even more encouraging, in one small pilot study (where atenolol and enalapril were compared separately against placebo in their effects on short-term memory), whereas atenolol produced minor but distinct memory impairment, no such effect was detectable with enalapril [17]. These observations clearly require confirmation, but, if substantiated, would be important attributes of enalapril treatment.

Cardiac Failure

In cardiac failure there are two main goals of treatment. First, we are attempting to improve exercise capacity. If this can be achieved, we should then like to improve prognosis. Present therapy for congestive cardiac failure is based firmly on the use of diuretics. These are usually combined with digitalis preparations although, 200 years after the introduction of digitalis by William Withering, there remains controversy as to the value of long-term digitalis therapy in cardiac failure with sinus rhythm. More recently vasodilator drugs such as hydralazine and prazosin have been introduced. Because the vasodilators are of more recent introduction, they have been subjected to more critical evaluation than has digitalis. Surveying the situation Cohn [18] concluded that vasodilators do, in cardiac failure, improve exercise capacity during chronic administration although there is no good evidence that they prolong life.

It is in the context particularly of vasodilator therapy that the ACE inhibitors have theoretical attractions in the treatment of cardiac failure. ACE inhibitors should have all of the benefits of vasodilating drugs, such as hydralazine or prazosin, in reducing "afterload" and probably "preload." In addition, however, the ACE inhibitors have a whole range of other actions which should reinforce the beneficial effects of vasodilation. We have already seen their capacity to lower aldosterone secretion; this effect should promote diuresis and also help to correct any potassium or magnesium deficiency that might have resulted from antecedent diuretic therapy. In turn it might be hoped that the ACE inhibitors might help to diminish arrhythmias. This last would be a particularly important point because the majority of patients with cardiac failure succumb suddenly and presumably from ventricular arrhythmia.

Furthermore, at rather higher than physiological levels, circulating angiotensin II can stimulate the secretion of vasopressin. Reduction of vasopressin secretion by lowering angiotensin II should again help to promote diuresis in cardiac failure.

However, the direct renal effects of ACE inhibitors in cardiac failure, as already noted in renovascular hypertension, might be less beneficial [8]. One of the earliest changes in cardiac failure is a marked reduction in renal blood flow. Nevertheless, despite this, both glomerular filtration rate and urea excretion are well maintained. In part, this maintenance of glomerular filtration and urea excretion is a compensatory effect of intrarenal angiotensin II [19]. In cardiac failure enhanced angiotensin II-mediated constriction at efferent glomerular arterioles helps to sustain glomerular filtration. Moreover, in cardiac failure the diminished blood flow is largely diverted through the large juxtamedullary glomeruli which give rise to long loops of Henle which descend deep into the medulla accompanied by vasa recta bundles. Normally poor in renin, the juxtamedullary glomeruli become renin-rich in cardiac failure. Angiotensin II-mediated increased tone in the vasa recta loops may improve counter-current exchange in the renal medulla and serve to sustain urea excretion. Thus, lowering of intrarenal angiotensin II with ACE inhibition would lead to loss of these compensatory effects and thus to a fall in glomerular filtration rate and elevation of serum urea. Only in very severe cardiac failure, with grossly excessive intrarenal angiotensin II, causing pre-glomerular arteriolar constriction, hyponatraemia and rapidly advancing azotaemia, are ACE inhibitors likely to improve renal function. Thus, theoretically ACE inhibitors should provide substantial benefits in cardiac failure, although their renal actions are delicately balanced [8].

In two double-blind trials of ACE inhibition in cardiac failure, one using captopril [20] and one using enalapril [21], we found sustained reduction of angiotensin II and aldosterone with converse elevation of renin and angiotensin I. Plasma aldosterone, vasopressin and noradrenaline were also decreased during active treatment. Both drugs significantly improved exercise time while diminishing dyspnoea. During placebo treatment, on a fixed background of diuretic and digitalis therapy, both total body and serum potassium were depressed; both were corrected during ACE inhibition. Twenty-four hour ECG monitoring showed with both drugs significant reduction in ventricular ectopic activity. Thus, in cardiac failure with ACE inhibition the expected benefits are clearly seen. Nevertheless, as had been feared, this was at the expense of modest deterioration in renal function. Although ACE inhibitors increased renal plasma flow, glomerular filtration rate was diminished and there were significant, although usually mild, increases in serum creatinine and urea.

The diminution in ventricular ectopic activity gives hope that these drugs may indeed improve prognosis in cardiac failure. If a similar effect were to be seen with the use of ACE inhibitors in hypertension, as indeed should very well be the case, the finding will have important implications for that disease also.

Conclusions

What is the likely future role of ACE inhibitors in the treatment of hypertension and of cardiac failure? It is self-evident that given the drugs are effective, their role eventually will be determined by their pattern of adverse effects [22]. It is further self-evident that a greater burden of side effects is acceptable in treating a severe disease with a poor prognosis, such as cardiac failure or intractable hypertension, than in fairly mild uncomplicated hypertension where the ideal drug would be effective without having adverse side effects and without impairing "quality of life." Of what is now a wide range of ACE inhibitors, only captopril and enalapril have been used sufficiently extensively clinically for evaluation of side effects to be made. The adverse effects recorded with captopril include morbilliform rash, proteinuria, occasional cases of nephrotic syndrome, leukopaenia (with occasional deaths from agranulocytosis), disturbances of taste, aphthous ulcers of the mouth, persistent unproductive cough, and Raynaud's phenomenon. The most commonly recorded side effect with enalapril is rash. Occasional cases of persistent cough have also been reported, as has Raynaud's phenomenon. Captopril was introduced into clinical medicine at a maximum dose of 450 mg daily which is presently reckoned by many workers to be probably excessive. The manufacturers now recommend that the maximum daily dose be 150 mg a day. Furthermore, captopril depends largely on the kidney for excretion; thus, in the presence of renal impairment dosage should be further reduced. The side effect burden of captopril is clearly dose-related, and since the dosage has been reduced with further downward adjustments made if there is renal function impairment, side effects have been substantially less common. Although diminution in white count is still seen at the lower doses [20], this is a good deal less frequent, as is proteinuria. However, disturbances of taste sensation and rash are still seen, not uncommonly, at present doses of captopril.

Enalapril also depends largely upon the kidney for excretion and with this drug, again, doses should be limited in the presence of renal impairment. With enalapril neutropenia, proteinuria and taste disturbance have rarely, if ever, been encountered, although it has to be said that generally enalapril has been used in less severe forms of hypertension than has captopril thus far. It appears hopeful, therefore, that with the second generation of ACE inhibitors, such as enalapril, the burden of side effects will be less than with captopril. However, proper evaluation can only be made with a prospective study in the same patient population using the two drugs side by side [22] and this, as far as I am aware, has not been done.

In my opinion, the ACE inhibitors will have a clear and increasingly important role in the treatment of congestive cardiac failure. In the severer grades of cardiac failure these drugs clearly improve symptoms and extend exercise capacity, while limiting arrhythmias. Their effect on prognosis is so far unassessed, but this looks a promising avenue for further exploration. The main price that has to be paid for these benefits is the expected impairment, fortunately usually modest, of renal function.

In hypertension the ACE inhibitors are clearly challenging the established pattern of therapy at various points. They are at least as effective as beta-blockers or thiazides as first-line therapy and they combine well with thiazides as second-step treatment. Although further information is urgently needed, early reports suggest that their side-effect burden and their impact on life-style compares favourably with those seen both with beta-blockers and with thiazides. Moreover, ACE inhibitors have an important role in combination with loop diuretics in treating previously intractable hypertension.

Although much more needs to be learned of this exciting group of drugs, the prospects for the future look remarkably good.

References

1. Brown JJ, Leckie BJ, Lever AF, McIntyre G, Morton JJ, Semple PF, and Robertson JIS (1983) The renin-angiotensin system and the regulation of the circulation. In: Robertson JIS (ed) Clinical aspects of essential hypertension. Elsevier, Amsterdam, pp 278–323 (Handbook of hypertension, vol 1)
2. Robertson JIS (1984 The renin-angiotensin system: its importance in physiology and medicine. In: Robertson JIS (ed) The renin-angiotensin system. Gower, London, pp 1.1–1.33
3. Zanchetti A, Tarazi RC (eds) (1982) Symposium on angiotensin converting enzyme inhibition: a developing concept. Am J Cardiol 49:1381–1579
4. Murphy MB (1983) Symposium on the renin-angiotensin-aldosterone system: treatment of hypertension and heart failure. J Hypertens [Suppl 1] 1:1–159
5. Laragh JH (ed) (1984) Converting enzyme inhibition for understanding and management of hypertensive disorders and congestive heart failure. Am J Med 77(2a):1–86
6. Svensson A, Hansson L (eds) (1984) Symposium on new approaches to the treatment of hypertension. J Hypertens [Suppl 2] 2:1–121
7. Hodsman GP, Zabludowski JR, Zoccali C, Fraser R, Morton JJ, Murray GD, Robertson JIS (1984) Enalapril (Mk421) and its lysine analogue (Mk521): a comparison of acute and chronic effects on blood pressure, renin-angiotensin system and sodium excretion in normal man. Br J Clin Pharmacol 17:233–241
8. Atkinson AB, Robertson JIS (1979) Captopril in the treatment of clinical hypertension and cardiac failure. Lancet 2:836–839
9. Mackay A, Brown JJ, Lever AF, Morton JJ, Robertson JIS (1983) Unilateral renal disease in hypertension. In: Robertson JIS (ed) Clinical aspects of secondary hypertension. Elsevier, Amsterdam, pp 33–79 (Handbook of hypertension, vol 2)
10. Hodsman GP, Brown JJ, Cumming AMM, Davies DL, East BW, Lever AF, Morton JJ, Murray GD, Robertson JIS (1983) Enalapril in the treatment of hypertension with renal artery stenosis. J Hypertens [Suppl 1] 1:109–117
11. Tillman DM, Malatino LS, Cumming AMM, Hodsman GP, Leckie BJ, Lever AF, Morton JJ, Webb DJ, Robertson JIS (1984) Enalapril in hypertension with renal artery stenosis: long-term follow-up and effects an renal function. J Hypertens [Suppl 2] 2:93–100
12. Atkinson AB, Brown JJ, Cumming AMM, Fraser R, Lever AF, Leckie BJ, Morton JJ, Robertson JIS, Davies DL (1982) Captopril in the management of hypertension with renal artery stenosis: its long-term effect as a predictor of surgical outcome. Am J Cardiol 49:1460–1466
13. Staessen J, Bulpitt C, Fagard R, Lignen P, Amery A (1983) Long-term converting-enzyme inhibition as a guide to surgical curability of hypertension associated with renovascular disease. Am J Cardiol 51:1317–1322
14. Atkinson AB, Brown JJ, Lever AF, Robertson JIS (1980) Combined treatment of severe intractable hypertension with captopril and diuretic. Lancet 2:105–108
15. Hodsman GP, Isles CG, Murray GB, Usherwood TP, Webb DJ, Robertson JIS (1983) Factors related to first dose hypotensive effect of captopril: prediction and treatment. Br Med J 286:832–834
16. Chinn RH, Düsterdieck G (1972) The response of blood pressure to infusion of angiotensin II: relation to plasma concentrations of renin and angiotensin II. Clin Sci 42:489–504
17. Lichter I, Richardson PJ, Wyke MA (1984) Differential effects of atenolol and enalapril on tests of memory during treatment for essential hypertension. J Hypertens 2:560
18. Cohn JN (1984) Unloading the heart in congestive heart failure. Am J Med 77 (2a):67–70
19. Brown JJ, Davies DL, Johnson VW, Lever AF, Robertson JIS (1970) Renin relationships in congestive cardiac failure, treated and untreated. Am Heart J 80:329–342
20. Cleland JGF, Dargie HJ, Hodsman GP, Ball SG, Robertson JIS, Morton JJ, East BW, Robertson I, Murray GD, Gillen G (1984) Captopril in heart failure: a double-blind controlled trial. Br Heart J 52:530–535
21. Cleland JGF, Dargie HG, Gillen G, Hodsman GP, Ball SG and Robertson JIS (1985) Effects of enalapril in heart failure: a double blind study on exercise performance, renal function, hormones and metabolic state. Br Heart J 54:305–312
22. Ball SG, Robertson JIS (1985) A need for new converting enzyme inhibitors? Br Med J 290: 180–181

Serotonin, Serotonergic Antagonists, and Hypertension

P. M. VANHOUTTE[1] and R. F. J. SHEPHERD

Whether the increased total systemic vascular resistance characteristic of chronic hypertension is a primary event or secondary to increased cardiac output is still debated. Whatever the initiating cause, the increased resistance must result from the narrowing of the small arteries and arterioles (Fig. 1). This may be due either to structural changes or to augmented contraction of the smooth muscle of these resistance vessels. The former probably reflects the adaptation of the blood vessel wall to the increase in distension pressure [24]. The latter may have many causes. One may be alterations of the neurogenic control of the circulation. Possibilities include changes in the activity of central nervous system (CNS) controlling centers, resetting of the control exerted by the arterial and cardiopulmonary mechanoreceptors, alterations in the many processes that can modulate transmitter release and disposition [24, 27, 31, 44, 45, 67, 68]. There may also be changes in the adrenoceptors and in the other receptors on the smooth muscle cells, or changes in the smooth muscles themselves, including abnormalities of membrane transport. Thus, the primary defect may be an increased permeability of the vascular smooth muscle cell mem-

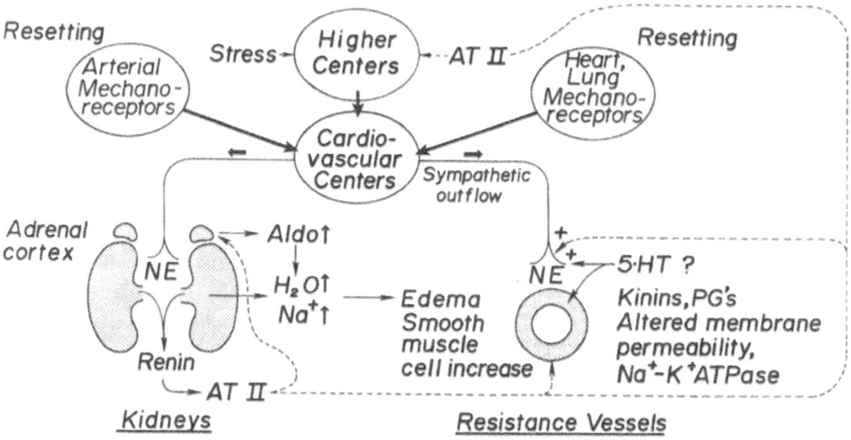

Fig. 1. Factors which may be involved in the genesis of essential hypertension. In addition, for each level of sympathetic nerve activity, the adrenergic nerve endings may liberate more norepinephrine than normal, and the α-adrenoceptors and S_2-serotonergic receptors of the vascular smooth muscle may be hyperresponsive. *ATII,* angiotensin II; *ATP,* adenosine triphosphate; *5-HT,* serotonin; *NE,* norepinephrine; *PG,* prostaglandin; ↑, increase; +, facilitation. (Vanhoutte [66])

[1] Department of Physiology and Biophysics and Division of Cardiovascular Medicine, Mayo Clinic, Rochester, MN 55905, USA.

Primary Hypertension
Ed. by W. Kaufmann et al.

brane to sodium. Other changes might involve increased activation of the renin-angiotensin-aldosterone system, or augmented secretion of a natriuretic hormone [20, 24, 30, 52, 66]. The role of vasopressin is debatable [12, 28, 49, 55, 80]. Likewise, whether or not 5-hydroxytryptamine (serotonin) plays a role in the maintenance of the increased peripheral resistance in chronic hypertension is still an unanswered question [66]; the concept of the putative role of this indole alkylamine has been revived by the observations that ketanserin, a drug whose primary action is to inhibit serotonergic receptors, can lower the blood pressure in primary hypertension [2, 18, 22, 51, 53, 65, 66, 69].

In this chapter, current knowledge of the acute and chronic actions of ketanserin in patients with primary hypertension will be reviewed. This will be preceded by an analysis of animal and human studies concerning the complex actions of exogenous serotonin on the cardiovascular system in normotension and hypertension, and an examination of whether or not serotonin is present in sufficient quantities to affect the systemic vascular resistance in hypertension.

Serotonin and Hypertension

Turnover of Serotonin

The major source of serotonin in the blood is the enterochromaffin cells of the gastrointestinal tract (see Fig. 2). Normally, the serotonin that they release is rapidly destroyed in its passage through the hepatic and pulmonary circulations [29, 63]. In hypertensive rats, the pulmonary clearance of serotonin is reduced [58].

The serotonin which reaches the blood is taken up and stored by the platelets which reach all parts of the cardiovascular system. The platelets release the serotonin they contain when they aggregate [35]. The released serotonin acts on S_2-serotonergic receptors on the platelets which amplifies the aggregation induced [14, 59]. In primary hypertension, although there is no evidence for an augmented concentration of serotonin in the plasma, the serotonin content of the platelets is reduced; they release serotonin more easily than in normal subjects and take it up again less avidly [1, 6, 7, 65, 66]. Beta-thromboglobulin levels are increased in the plasma of HT patients [48]; increased plasma levels of this platelet-specific protein reflect in vivo stimulation or destruction of circulating platelets [39]. These findings are compatible with an increased release and reduced disposition of serotonin at the level of the resistance vessels in hypertension, which could initiate constriction of these blood vessels. Subsequent metabolism by monoamine oxidase in the endothelium of the capillary and postcapillary vessels and recapture by platelets (albeit at a slower rate) would prevent the appearance of free serotonin in the blood of the large veins.

Vascular Effects of Serotonin

Vasoconstriction

Serotonin is a potent constrictor of blood vessels by its action on S_2-serotonergic receptors on the smooth muscle (see Fig. 3). When the amount of serotonin is too

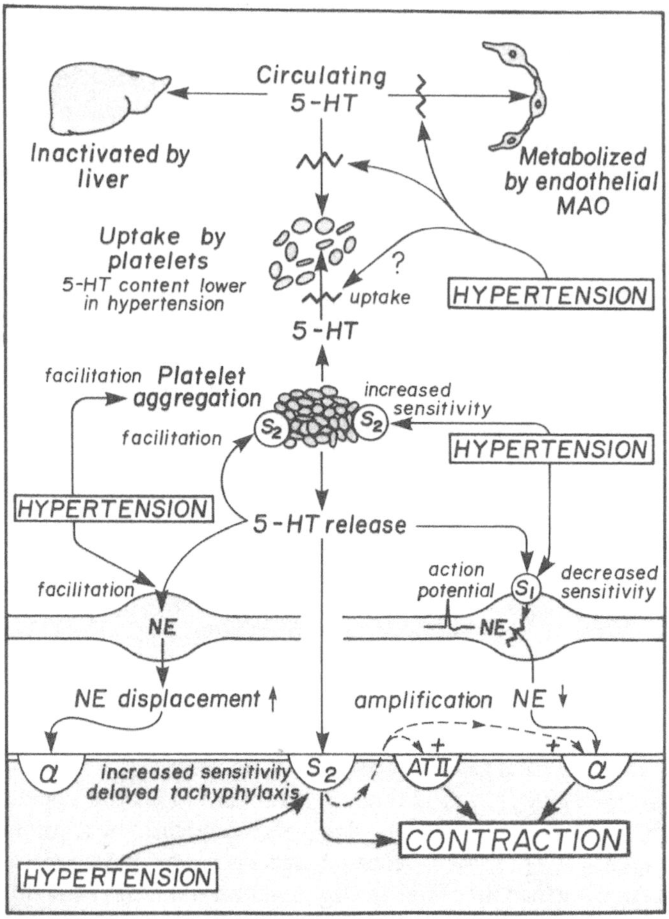

Fig. 2. Effects of high arterial blood pressure on the handling of serotonin *(5-HT)* by platelets and the blood vessel wall. α, α-adrenoceptor; *ATII,* angiotensin II; *MAO,* monoamine oxidase; *NE,* norepinephrine; S_2, serotonergic receptor. (Vanhoutte [66])

small to cause the vessels to constrict directly, the monoamine increases the sensitivity of the smooth muscle to norepinephrine (released from the sympathetic nerve endings) and angiotensin II. Alpha adrenoceptors may also be activated directly by serotonin. Thus, small amounts of serotonin may cause substantial contraction of the smooth muscle [64, 66, 70, 74, 75]. In addition, serotonin can cause the displacement of norepinephrine from adrenergic nerve terminals [68].

In adult hypertensive animals, the blood vessel wall is hypertensitive to the constrictor effect of serotonin. The augmentation of the vasoconstrictor response to serotonin is more pronounced than that to angiotensin II or norepinephrine. The rate of decay of the vasoconstrictor response to repeated exposure to high doses of serotonin (tachyphylaxis) is also reduced. This is not seen for the tachyphylaxis for angiotensin II. Thus, an augmented vascular responsiveness to serotonin, due to

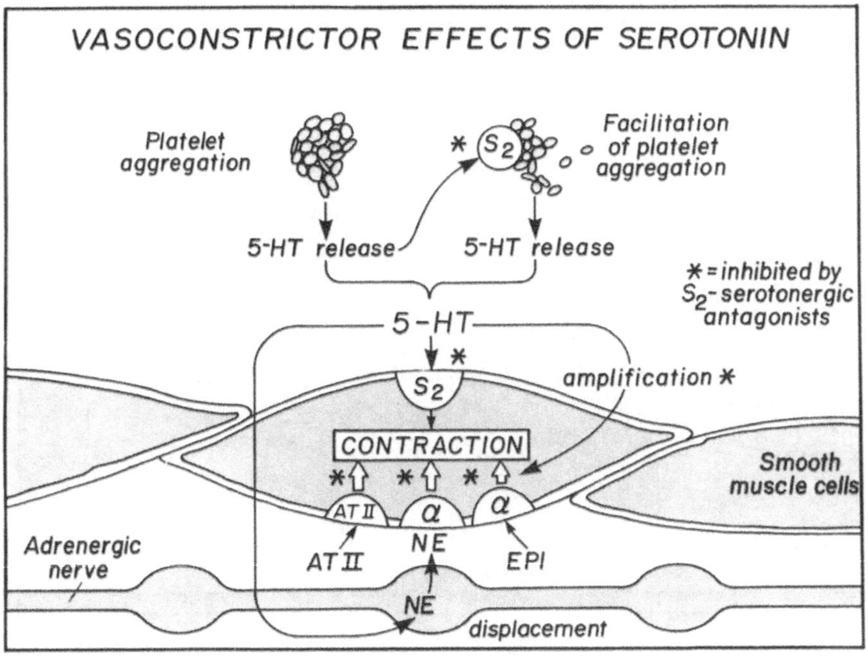

Fig. 3. Direct and indirect vasoconstrictor effects of serotonin. *α*, *α*-adrenoceptor; *ATII*, angiotensin II; *EPI*, epinephrine; *5-HT*, serotonin; *NE*, norepinephrine; S_2, S_2-serotonergic antagonist; ▽, receptors on vascular smooth muscle cells. (Vanhoutte [66])

both an increased sensitivity to and a prolonged effect of the monoamine, is an important characteristic of the hypertensive blood vessel wall [64, 75]. Augmented responsiveness and delayed tachyphylaxis to serotonin also occur progressively in aging, normotensive animals. Hence, the changes in sensitivity to serotonin observed in hypertension probably reflect the premature aging of the blood vessel wall, exposed to the chronic increase in distending pressure [64–66].

Vasodilatation

Serotonergic receptors are present on the sympathetic nerve endings (see Fig. 4). These prejunctional receptors, when activated by small amounts of serotonin reduce the amount of norepinephrine released during activation of the sympathetic nerves, leading to relaxation of the blood vessels [21, 43, 47]. In humans, intraarterial infusions of serotonin into the brachial artery can cause either constriction or dilatation of the forearm resistance vessels [57]. In the latter case, which is evident when the sympathetic nerves are active, the prejunctional action on the serotonergic receptors prevails over the direct constrictor action of the drug. The prejunctional effect of serotonin is reduced in spontaneously hypertensive rats (SHR) [40].

The endothelium forms vasodilator substances in response to various agonists (including serotonin) that can relax the underlying smooth muscle [9–11, 36] (Fig. 2). To judge from results obtained with acetylcholine and histamine, the ability of the

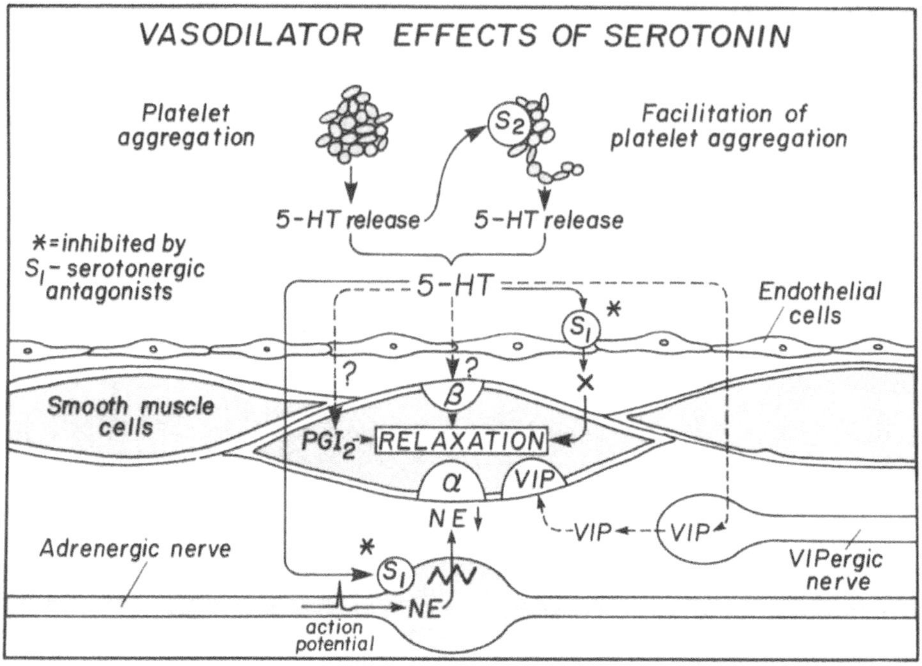

Fig. 4. Direct and indirect vasodilator effects of serotonin. *α*, *α*-adrenoceptor; *β*, *β*-adrenoceptor; *5-HT*, serotonin; *NE*, norepinephrine; *PGI*$_2$, prostacyclin-production; *VIP*, vasoactive interstitial peptide; *x*, unknown mediator; ?, uncertain; VV, inhibition of adrenergic neurotransmission. (Vanhoutte [66])

hypertensive blood vessel wall to relax upon stimulation of endothelial receptors is reduced [78].

Central Effects

Dahlstrom and Fuxe [13] demonstrated the existence of serotonin-containing neurons in the brain located near neural cardiovascular control sites. However, the role of these serotonergic neurons in cardiovascular regulation has still to be determined [41, 79].

Ketanserin and Primary Hypertension in Man

Ketanserin is a selective S_2-serotonergic antagonist in blood vessels, platelets, and bronchial smooth muscle. It differs from other serotonergic antagonists in that it has no agonistic actions. At concentrations higher than required to inhibit S_2-serotonergic receptors, the compound is a competitive $alpha_1$ adrenergic antagonist [42, 69, 71].

The presently available information on the effects of ketanserin in primary hypertension is summarized in Table 1.

Table 1. Action of ketanserin in primary hypertension

	Acute administration	Chronic administration
Systolic and diastolic blood pressure	[76, 77, 73, 81, 82, 19] ↓	[22, 53, 33, 2, 51] ↓
Heart rate	[76, 77, 82] ↑, [73, 81, 19] →	[22, 53, 33, 2, 51] ↓
Stroke volume	[77] ↓	[22] ↑, [51] →
Cardiac output	[76, 77] ↑ → ↓	[22] ↑, [51] ↓
Total systemic vascular resistance	[76, 77, 19] ↓	[22] ↓
Pulmonary artery pressure	[76, 77, 73, 19] ↓	[22] →
Pulmonary vascular resistance	[76, 77, 73] →, [19] ↓	[22] ↓
Renal vascular resistance	[76, 77] ↓	
Forearm vascular resistance	[76, 77] ↓	
Pulmonary capillary wedge pressure	[76, 77, 19] ↓	[22] →
Right atrial pressure	[76, 77, 19] ↓	[22] →
Renin/angiotensin II	[76, 77, 81, 82] ↑	[22, 2] ↓
Aldosterone	[76, 77, 81, 82] →	[22, 2] →
Norepinephrine	[76, 77, 81] ↑ →	[22] ↑ →
Epinephrine		[22] ↑

↑ increased; ↓ decreased; → no significant change

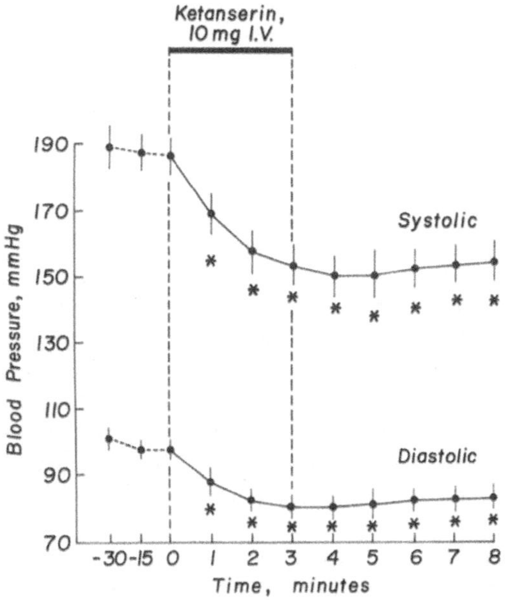

Fig. 5. In a group of elderly hypertensive patients, the intravenous (I.V.) injection of ketanserin causes a rapid and sustained reduction of both systolic and diastolic blood pressure. ∗, the effect of ketanserin is statistically significant. Data from De Crée et al. [16]. (Vanhoutte [66])

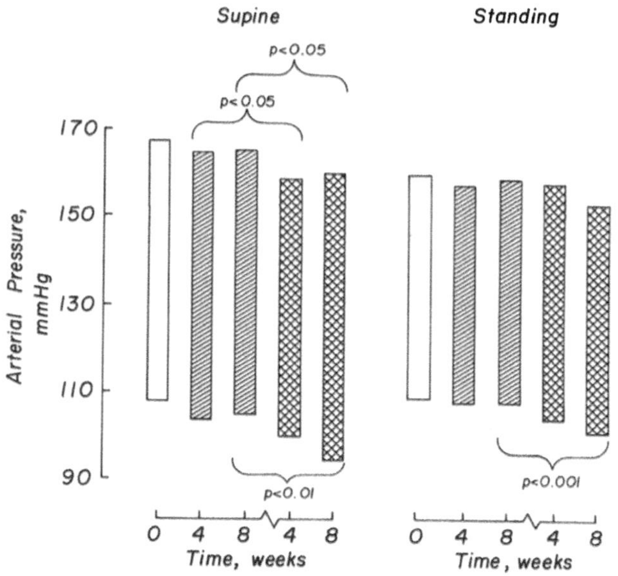

Fig. 6. Effects of ketanserin (40 mg; twice a day), on supine and standing systolic and diastolic arterial pressure. *Open bars,* run-in period; *hatched bars,* placebo period; *cross-hatched bars,* ketanserin period. (Schalekamp [60])

Antihypertensive Effects

Either acute (Fig. 5) [15, 16, 73, 76, 77, 81, 82] or chronic (Fig. 6) [3, 4, 22, 32, 33, 51, 53] administration of ketanserin lowers arterial blood pressure in primary hypertensive subjects. Although the number of trials and patients so far is limited, it appears that in the majority of subjects the efficacy of ketanserin as an antihypertensive agent is comparable to that of beta adrenergic blockers or diuretics [33]. Ketanserin appears to be more effective in elderly hypertensive patients [17].

Hemodynamic Effects

The hemodynamic effects that accompany the blood pressure reduction caused by ketanserin are complex with variable changes in heart rate and stroke volume. However, there appears to be uniform agreement that ketanserin given either acutely or chronically causes a decrease in calculated systemic vascular resistance which explains its antihypertensive effects.

When given intravenously, there may be a transient augmentation in cardiac output which is usually associated with an increase in heart rate; the heart rate then returns to the preinfusion value and stroke volume and cardiac output decrease. Throughout this entire cycle the arterial pressure and systemic vascular resistance remain significantly decreased (Fig. 7) [76, 77, 82]. Of the various vascular beds examined in humans, there is evidence for a decrease in renal and forearm vascular resistance which accounts in part for the decrease in total systemic vascular resistance [77].

Minor decreases in pulmonary arterial systolic and diastolic pressures have been reported with acute administration of the drug, without significant changes in pulmo-

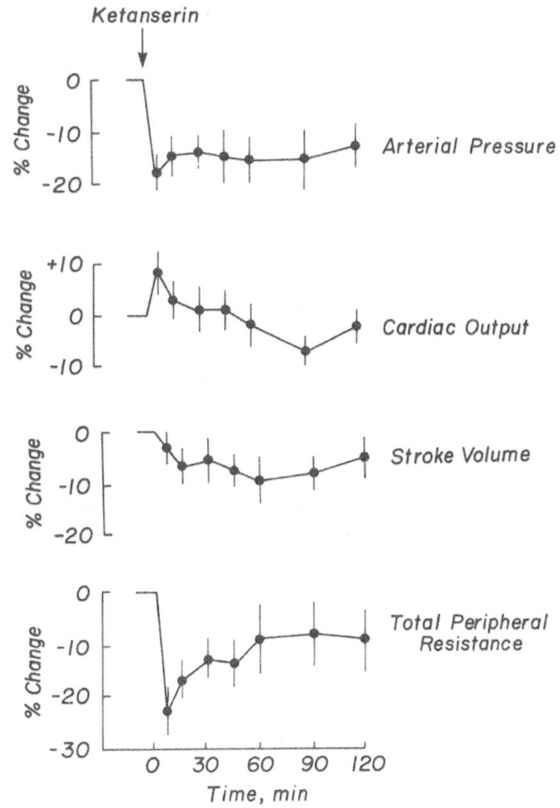

Fig. 7. Effects of ketanserin (10 mg i.v.) on systemic hemodynamics in 12 patients with essential hypertension. The decrease in arterial blood pressure *(upper)* was due to a decrease in total peripheral resistance *(lower)*. After 120 min, arterial pressure and total peripheral resistance were still below baseline. Data from Wenting et al. [77]. (Schalekamp [60])

nary vascular resistance [73, 76, 77]. Acute, but not chronic, administration of ketanserin decreases the right atrial pressure and the pulmonary capillary wedge pressure [19, 23, 76, 77]. This decrease in central venous pressure does not necessarily imply dilatation of systemic capacitance blood vessels, since many other factors can cause changes in right atrial pressure.

Ketanserin chronically decreases arterial blood pressure without a reflex increase in heart rate [34, 51, 53]. In fact, heart rate usually decreases. In one study, a significant decrease in pulmonary vascular resistance was reported [22]. Chronic administration of ketanserin either has little effect or lowers the increase in heart rate and arterial blood pressure during dynamic exercise [22, 53].

Hormonal Changes

Norepinephrine

In resting subjects, acute administration of ketanserin causes slight increases in the plasma level of norepinephrine [76, 77, 81, 82]. With chronic administration of the drug, the levels of norepinephrine may be unchanged [53] or increased [22].

Renin, Angiotensin II, and Aldosterone

With acute administration of ketanserin there is an increase in the plasma levels of renin and angiotensin II, but surprisingly no change in that of aldosterone [76, 77, 81, 82]. With chronic administration of the drug, the levels of renin and angiotensin II decrease, with again no change in that of aldosterone [2, 23].

Pharmacokinetics

Preliminary pharmacokinetic data indicate that the half-life of ketanserin is approximately 10 h, and that the drug should be administered twice a day to maintain the reduction in arterial blood pressure over a 24-h period [32, 34].

Side Effects

Intravenous administration of ketanserin may cause postural hypotension which is more marked in sodium-depleted subjects [82]. With chronic treatment (up to doses of 40 mg twice a day) postural hypotension does not occur [4]. When studied in double-blind trials, the occurrence of other side effects with ketanserin is not more pronounced than with other antihypertensive agents such as beta adrenergic blockers or diuretic agents (Symoens, personal communication). At higher doses (e.g., 60 mg t.i.d.), almost all patients withdraw from treatment due to dizziness and orthostatic hypotension; these symptoms correlated with the plasma levels of ketanserin [4].

Mechanism of Action

Of the different pharmacologic actions of ketanserin, the most likely to contribute to its antihypertensive effect would be the following.

Central Antihypertensive Effects

In the dog and rat, ketanserin, when given acutely, may cross the blood-brain barrier, and thus affect blood pressure by modulation of sympathetic outflow [26, 46, 50]. However, in the rat, central mechanisms probably do not contribute to the chronic hypotensive effect of ketanserin [54]. Likewise, in man, the changes in plasma levels of circulating catecholamines, and the absence of impairment of reflex control under treatment with ketanserin rule out that the drug causes hypotension mainly by a central nervous action.

Hormonal Effects

An action of serotonin on S_2-serotonergic receptors has been implicated in the production of corticosterone and aldosterone [26, 82]. However, ketanserin has no effect on the plasma level of aldosterone, and only a minimal effect on plasma renin activity and the level of angiotensin II. Thus, a major interference with the renin-angiotensin-aldosterone axis is not the likely explanation for the hypotensive effects of ketanserin.

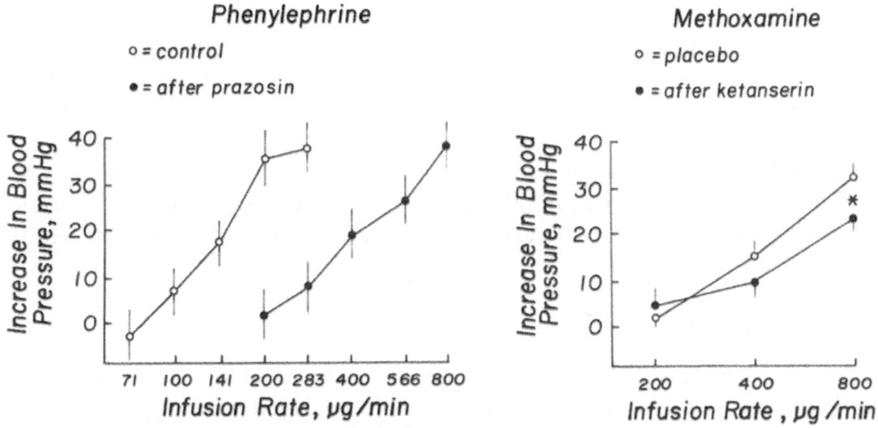

Fig. 8. In man, the selective α_1-adrenergic antagonist prazosin causes a parallel shift to the right of the dose-response curve to the pressor effect of the α_1-adrenoceptor agonist phenylephrine, which illustrates competitive inhibition (*left;* data from Singleton et al. [61]). By contrast, ketanserin causes a nonparallel depression of the dose-response curve to another α_1-adrenoceptor agonist, methoxamine (*right;* data from Fagard et al. [22])

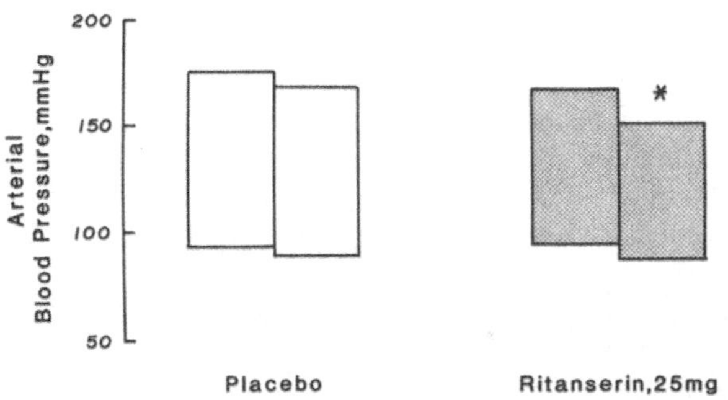

Fig. 9. Effect of chronic oral treatment with ritanserin (25 mg; *right*) as compared to placebo (*left*) in essential hypertensives. (Courtesy of Dr. J. Symoens)

Alpha Adrenergic Blockade

Discussion continues on whether or not the ability of ketanserin to antagonize alpha_1 adrenoceptors accounts, at least in part, for its ability to reduce systemic vascular resistance and thus lower arterial blood pressure in human hypertension.

The acute i.v. administration of ketanserin to normotensive subjects, with or without sodium depletion, and to patients with primary hypertension does not alter the pressor response to an infusion of phenylephrine. This implies that in man, unlike in the rat [8, 25, 38], ketanserin, if given acutely, has no adrenergic-blocking activity [5, 77, 81, 82]. By contrast, with a 3-h infusion of ketanserin, or chronic oral administration, there is a reduction in the pressor effects of alpha_1 adrenoceptor agonists (Fig. 8) [5, 22, 56]. However, unlike the selective alpha_1 adrenergic blocker prazosin, ketanserin does not shift the curves in a parallel manner, but depresses the response to higher concentrations of the alpha_1 adrenergic agonists more than that to lower doses (Fig. 8) [5, 22, 56]. In pharmacologic terms, this "non-competitive" behavior is difficult to reconcile with the available data indicating that ketanserin, albeit in higher concentrations than those required to antagonize S_2-serotonergic receptors, is a competitive antagonist at $alpha_1$ adrenoceptors [71]. The inhibitory effect of ketanserin on the response to $alpha_1$ adrenergic agonists could be explained by a nonspecific decrease in vascular responsiveness, resulting from the altered wall-to-lumen ratio following a reduction in arterial blood pressure (Fig. 9) [24]. Against this interpretation is the observation that, at least in normotensive subjects, chronic treatment with ketanserin does not seem to affect pressor responses to angiotensin II (S. Ball, personal communication).

Serotonergic Blockade

Ketanserin is a serotonergic inhibitor at concentrations which do not affect other autonomic receptors [71]. In normal volunteers, the increased aggregation of platelets caused by serotonin is inhibited by acute administration of ketanserin [2, 14]. This is in accord with the findings in vitro that ketanserin inhibits the reversible aggregation of human platelets caused by serotonin in human platelet-rich plasma as well as the amplification of platelet aggregation caused by other substances [14]. Ketanserin also increases the deformability of the red blood cells [16]. These two actions of the drug could contribute to the reduction of the total systemic vascular resistance. The vasoconstrictor effects of serotonin in normal individuals are also prevented by ketanserin [62]. Ritanserin, an S_2-serotonergic antagonist with much weaker alpha-adrenergic blocking properties than ketanserin [37], lowers arterial blood pressure in hypertensive, but not in normotensive people (Fig. 9; Symoens, personal communication). These findings all support the hypothesis that the anti-hypertensive effect of ketanserin may be related to its inhibitory effect on S_2-serotonergic receptors. If this is the case, it may be surprising that other available S_2-serotonergic antagonists (e.g., methysergide, cyproheptadine, pizotifen) do not appear to prossess overt antihypertensive properties. Among the possible explanations are the lack of agonistic properties of ketanserin and its high degree of selectivity for S_2-serotonergic receptors [66]. While no studies are available in man, judging from animal experiments, the fact that the action of ketanserin is specific for the S_2-serotonergic receptors on the smooth muscles would prevent the direct constrictor action of serotonin on vascular smooth muscle, and at the same time unmask the vasodilator properties of the monoamine [66].

References

1. Affolter H, Erne P, Buhler FR, Pletscher A (to be published) Increased sensitivity of blood platelets to 5-hydroxytryptamine in essential hypertension
2. Amery A, Fagard R, Fiocchi R, Lijnen P, Staessen J, Vermylen J (1984) Antihypertensive action and serotonin-induced platelet aggregation during long-term ketanserin treatment in hypertensive patients. J Cardiovasc Pharmacol 6: 182–185
3. Anderson A, Morgan T, Dumpys R (1983) The effect of ketanserin in essential hypertension. Clin Exp Pharmacol Physiol 10: 331–333
4. Andren L, Svensson A, Dahlof B, Eggertsen R, Hansson L (1983) Ketanserin in hypertension. Early clinical evaluation and dose finding study of a new 5-HT2 receptor antagonist. Acta Med Scand 214: 125–130

5. Ball SG, Zabludowski JR, Robertson JIS (1983) Mechanism of antihypertensive action of ketanserin in man. Br Med J 287:1065
6. Baudoin-Legros M, Le Quan-Bui KH, Guicheney P, Kamal LA, Meyer P (to be published) Platelet serotonin in essential hypertension and in mental depression. J Cardiovasc Pharmacol
7. Bhargava KP, Raina N, Misra N, Shanker K, Vrot S (1979) Uptake of serotonin by human platelets and its relevance to CNS involvement in hypertension. Life Sci 25:195–200
8. Cohen ML, Fuller RW, Kurz KD (1983) Evidence that blood pressure reduction by serotonin antagonists is related to alpha receptor blockade in spontaneously hypertensive rats. Hypertension 5:676–681
9. Cohen RA, Shepherd JT, Vanhoutte PM (1983) Inhibitory role of the endothelium in the response of isolated coronary arteries to platelets. Science 221:273–274
10. Cohen RA, Shepherd JT, Vanhoutte PM (1983) 5-Hydroxytryptamine can mediate endothelium-dependent relaxation of coronary arteries. Am J Physiol 245:H1077–H1080
11. Cohen RA, Shepherd JT, Vanhoutte PM (to be published) Endothelium and asymetrical responses of the coronary arterial wall. Am J Physiol
12. Crofton JT, Share L, Share RE, Lee-Kwon W-J, Manning M, Sawyer WH (1979) Importance of vasopressin in the development and maintenance of DOL-salt hypertension in the rat. Hypertension 1:31–38
13. Dahlstrom A, Fuxe K (1965) Evidence for the existence of monoamine neurons in the central nervous system. II. Experimentally induced changes in the intraneuronal amine levels of bulbospinal neurone systems. Acta Physiol Scand [Suppl 247] 64:1
14. De Clerck F, David JL, Jannsen PAJ (1982) Serotoninergic amplification mechanisms in blood platelets. In: De Clerck F, Vanhoutte PM (eds) 5-Hydroxytryptamine in peripheral reactions. Raven, New York, pp 83–94
15. De Cree J, Verhaegen H, Symoens J (1981) Acute blood pressure lowering effect of ketanserin. Lancet I:1161–1162
16. De Cree J, Leempoels J, Geukens H, de Cock W, Verhaegen H (1982) Are serotoninergic mechanisms involved in high blood pressure? In: De Clerck F, Vanhoutte PM (eds) 5-Hydroxytryptamine in peripheral reactions. Raven, New York, pp 183–192
17. De Cree J, Hoing M, de Ryck M, Symoens J (to be published) The acute antihypertensive effect of ketanserin increases with age. J Cardiovasc Pharmacol
18. De Leeuw PW, van Es Pn, van Soest GAW, Tchang PT, Birkenhager WH (1983) Effects of chronic oral treatment with katanserin, a new 5HT antagonist in essential hypertension. J Hypertens [Suppl] 2:379–380
19. Demoulin J-C, Bertholet M, Soumagne D, David J-L, Kulbertus HE (1981) 5-HT receptor blockade in the treatment of heart failure. Lancet I:1186–1188
20. De Wardener HE, MacGregor GA (1980) Dahl's hypothesis that a saluretic substance may be responsible for a sustained rise in arterial pressure: its possible role in essential hypertension. Kidney Int 18:1–9
21. Engel G, Gothert M, Muller-Schweinitzer E, Schlicker E, Sistonen L, Stadler PA (1983) Evidence for common pharmacological properties of [^{3}H] 5-hydroxytryptamine binding sites, presynaptic 5-hydroxytryptamine autoreceptors in CNS and inhibitory presynaptic 5-hydroxytryptamine receptors on sympathetic nerves. Naunyn-Schmiedeberg's Arch Pharmacol 324:116–124
22. Fagard R, Fiocchi R, Lijnen P, Staessen J, Moerman E, de Schaepdryver A, Amery A (1984) Hemodynamic and humoral responses to chronic ketanserin treatment in essential hypertension. Br Heart J 51:149–156
23. Fagard R, Cattaert A, Lijnen P, Staessen J, Vanhees L, Moerman E, Amery A (1984) Responses of the systemic circulation and of the renin-angiotensin-aldosterone system to ketanserin at rest and exercie in normal man. Clin Sci 66:17–25
24. Folkow B (1982) Physiological aspects of primary hypertension. Physiol Rev 62:347–504
25. Fozard JR (1982) Mechanism of the hypotensive effect of ketanserin. J Cardiovasc Pharmacol 4:829–838
26. Fuller RW, Snoddy HD (1984) Central serotonin antagonist activity of ketanserin. Res Commun Chem Pathol Pharmacol 46:151–154
27. Fuxe K, Bolme P, Agnati LF, Jonsson G, Andersson K, Kohler C, Hokfelt T (1980) On the role of central adrenaline neurons in central cardiovascular regulation. In: Fuxe K, Goldstein B,

Hokfelt B (eds) Central adrenaline neurons. Basic aspects and their role in cardiovascular function. Pergamon, Oxford, pp 161–182
28. Garvas H, Ribeiro AB, Kohlmann O, Saragoca M, Mulinari RA, Rames O, Gavras I (1984) Effects of a specific inhibitor of the vascular action of vasopressin in humans. Hypertension [Suppl 1] 6: I–156–I–160
29. Gillis CN (to be published) Peripheral metabolism of serotonin. In: Vanhoutte PM (ed) Serotonin and the cardiovascular system. Raven, New York
30. Haddy FJ (1983) Abnormalities of membrane transport in hypertension. Hypertension [Suppl 5] 5: V–66–V–72
31. Haeusler G (1976) Central adrenergic neurons in experimental hypertension. In: Onesti G, Fernandez M, Kim KE (eds) Regulation of blood pressure by the central nervous system. Grune and Stratton, New York, pp 53–64
32. Hedner T, Persson B, Berglund G (1983) Ketanserin, a novel 5-hydroxytryptamine antagonist; monotherapy in essential hypertension. Br J Clin Pharmacol 16: 121–125
33. Hedner T, Persson B, Berglund G (1984) Experience with ketanserin, a serotonin (S_2) agonist, in long-term treatment of essential hypertension. Clin Exp Hypertens [A] 6(3): 743–751
34. Hedner T, Persson B, Berglund G (to be published) A comparative and long-term evaluation of ketanserin in the treatment of essential hypertension. J Cardiovasc Pharmacol
35. Holmsen H (to be published) Platelet activation and serotonin. In: Vanhoutte PM (ed) Serotonin and the cardiovascular system. Raven, New York
36. Houston DS, Shepherd JT, Vanhoutte PM (1984) Platelets cause endothelium-dependent relaxation in some but not all isolated canine vessels. Fed Proc 43: 1084
37. Janssen PAJ (to be published) The pharmacology of potent and selective S_2-serotonergic antagonists. J Cardiovasc Pharmacol
38. Kalkman HO, Harms YM, van Gelderen EM, Batink HD, Timmermans PBMWM, van Zwieten PA (1983) Hypotensive activity of serotonin antagonists; correlation with α_1-adrenoceptor and serotonin receptor blockade. Life Sci 32: 1499–1505
39. Kaplan KL, Owen J (1981) Plasma levels of β-trhomboglobulin and platelet factor-4 as indices of platelet activation in vivo. Blood 47: 199–202
40. Kubo T, Su C (1983) Effects of serotonin and some other neurohumoral agents on adrenergic neurotransmission in spontaneously hypertensive rat vasculature. Clin Exp Hypertens [A] 5: 1501–1510
41. Kuhn DM, Wolf WA, Lovenberg W (1980) Review of the role of the central serotoninergic neuronal system in blood pressure regulation. Hypertension 2: 243–255
42. Leysen JE, Awouters F, Kennis L, Laduron PM, Vandenberk J, Janssen PAJ (1981) Receptor binding profile of R41 468, a novel antagonist at 5-HT_2 receptors. Life Sci 28: 1115–1122
43. Lorenz RR, Vanhoutte PM (1984) Aggregating platelets and adrenergic neurotransmission in isolated canine blood vessels. Fed Proc 43: 430
44. Mancia G, Farrari A, Gregorini L, Parati G, Ferarri MC, Pomidossi G, Zanchetti A (1979) Control of blood pressure by carotid sinus baroreceptors in human beings. Am J Cardiol 44: 895–911
45. McCall RB, Humphrey SJ (1982) Involvement of serotonin in the central regulation of blood pressure; evidence for a facilitating effect on sympathetic nerve activity. J Pharmacol Exp Ther 222: 94–102
46. McCall RB, Schuette MR (1984) Evidence for an alpha-1 receptor-mediated central sympatho-inhibitory action of ketanserin. J Pharmacol Exp Ther 228: 704–710
47. McGrath MA (1977) 5-Hydroxytryptamine and neurotransmitter release in canine blood vessels. Circ Res 42: 428–435
48. Mehta J, Mehta P (1981) Platelet function in hypertension and effect of therapy. Am J Cardiol 47: 331–334
49. Mohring J, Mohring B, Petri M, Haak D (1977) Vasopressor role of ADH in the pathogenesis of malignant DOC hypertension. Am J Physiol 232: F260–F269
50. Mylecharane EJ, Phillips CA, Markus JK, Shaw J (to be published) Evidence for a central component to the hypotensive action of ketanserin in the dog. J Cardiovasc Pharmacol
51. Omvik P, Lund-Johansen P (1983) Long-term effects on central haemodynamics and body fluid volumes of ketanserin in essential hypertension. J Hypertens 1: 405–412

52. Overbeck HW (1979) Commentary. The sodium pump in cardiovascular muscle in hypertension. Whose hypothesis? Clin Exp Hypertens 1:551–556
53. Persson B, Hedner T, Berglund G (1983) Ketanserin in essential hypertension: effects during rest and exercise. Eur J Pharmacol 25:307–312
54. Pettersson A, Persson B, Henning M, Hedner T (1984) Antihypertensive effects of chronic 5-hydroxytryptamine (5-HT_2) receptor blockade with ketanserin in the spontaneously hypertensive rat. Naunyn Schmiedebergs Arch Pharmacol 327:43–47
55. Rabito SF, Carretero OA, Scidi AG (1981) Evidence against a role of vasopressin in the maintenance of high blood pressure in mineralocorticortial and renovascular hypertension. Hypertension 3:34–38
56. Reimann IW, Frolich JC (1983) Mechanism of antihypertensive action of ketanserin in man. Br Med J 287:381–383
57. Roddie IC, Shepherd JT, Whelan RF (1955) The action of 5-hydroxytryptamine on the blood vessels of the human hand and forearm. Br J Pharmacol 10:445–450
58. Roth RA, Wallace KB (1980) Disposition of biogenic amines and angiotensin I by lungs of spontaneously hypertensive rats. Am J Physiol 239:H736–H761
59. Schachter M, Grahame-Smith DG (1982) 5-hydroxytryptamine and the platelet: Specific binding and active uptake. In: De Clerck F, Vanhoutte PM (eds) 5-Hydroxytryptamine in peripheral reactions. Raven, New York, pp 49–59
60. Schalekamp MADH (to be published) Serotonergic blockade and hypertension. In: Vanhoutte PM (ed) Serotonin and the cardiovascular system. Raven, New York
61. Singleton W, Saxton CAPD, Hernandez J, Prichard BNC (1982) Postjunctional selectivity of α-blockade with prazosin, trimazosin, and UK-33,274 in man. J Cardiovasc Pharmacol 4:S145–S151
62. Symoens J, Vanhoutte PM (to be published) Role of serotonin in blood pressure regulation. In: Smith JAR, Watkins J (eds) Care of the postoperative surgical patient. Butterworth, London
63. Thompson JH (1971) Serotonin and the alimentary tract. Res Commun Chem Pathol Pharmacol 1:687–781
64. Vanhoutte PM (1982) Does 5-hydroxytryptamine play a role in hypertension? Trends Pharmacol Sci 3:370–373
65. Vanhoutte PM (1983) 5-hydroxytryptamine and vascular disease. Fed Proc 42:233–237
66. Vanhoutte PM (to be published) Peripheral serotoninergic receptors and hypertension. In: Vanhoutte PM (ed) Serotonin and the cardiovascular system. Raven, New York
67. Vanhoutte PM, Webb RG, Collis MG (1980) Pre- and post-junctional adrenergic mechanisms and hypertension. State of the art review. Clin Sci 59:211s–223s
68. Vanhoutte PM, Verbeuren TJ, Webb RC (1981) Local modulation of the adrenergic neuroeffector interaction in the blood vessel wall. Physiol Rev 61:151–247
69. Vanhoutte PM, van Nueten JM, Symoens J, Janssen PAJ (1983) Antihypertensive properties of ketanserin (R41 468). Fed Proc 42:182–185
70. Van Nueten JM (1983) 5-Hydroxytryptamine and precapillary vessels. Fed Proc 42:223–277
71. Van Nueten JM, Janssen PAJ, van Beck J, Xhonneu R, Verbeuren TJ, Vanhoutte RM (1981) Vascular effects of katanserin (L41 468), a novel antagonist of 5HT_2 serotoninergic receptors. J Pharmacol Exp Ther 218:217–230
72. Vermylen J, Fiocchi R, Fagard R, Lijnen P, Staessen J, Amery A (1983) $Alpha_1$ antagonistic and antiserotoninergic action during administration of serotonin. Br Med J 287:1551–1552
73. Walker JM, Wilmhurst PT, Juul SM, Coltari DI (1984) Acute effects of ketanserin on left ventricular function, metabolism and coronary blood flow. Br J Clin Pharmacol 17:301–307
74. Webb RC (1982) Increased vascular sensitivity to serotonin and methysergide in hypertension in rats. Clin Sci 63:S73–S75
75. Webb RC, Vanhoutte PM (to be published) Responsiveness of the hypertensive blood vessel wall to serotonergic stimuli. In: Vanhoutte PM (ed) Serotonin and the cardiovascular system. Raven, New York
76. Wenting GJ, Man in'T Veld AJ, Woittiez AJ, Boomsma F, Schalemkamp MADH (1982) Treatment of hypertension with ketanserin, a new selective 5HT_2 receptor antagonist. Br Med J 284:537–539
77. Wenting GJ, Woittiez AJJ, Man in'T Veld AJ, Schalekamp MADH (1984) 5-HT, alpha-adrenoceptors, and blood pressure. Effects of ketanserin in essential hypertension and autonomic insufficiency. Hypertension 6:100–109

78. Winquist RJ, Bunting PB, Baskin EP, Wallace AA (1984) Decreased endothelium-dependent relaxation in New Zealand genetic hypertensive rats. J Hypertens 2:541–545
79. Wolf WA, Kuhn DM, Lovenberg W (to be published) Serotonin and central regulation of arterial blood pressure. In: Vanhoutte PM (ed) Serotonin and the cardiovascular system. Raven, New York
80. Yamamoto J, Yamane Y, Umeda Y, Yoshioka T, Nakai M, Ikeda M (1984) Cardiovascular hemodynamics and vasopressin blockade in DOCA-salt hypertensive rats. Hypertension 6:397–407
81. Zabludowski JR, Zocalli C, Isles GG, Murray GD, Robertson JIS, Inglis GC, Fraser R, Ball SG (1984) Effect of the 5-hydroxytryptamine type 2 receptor antagonist, ketanserin, on blood pressure, the renin angiotensin system and sympatho-adrenol function in patients with essential hypertension. Br J Clin Pharmacol 17:309–316
82. Zoccali C, Zabludowski JR, Isles CG, Murray GD, Inglis GC, Robertson JIS, Fraser R, Ball SG (1983) The effect of a 5-HT antagonist, ketanserin, on blood pressure, the renin-angiotensin system and sympatho-adrenal function in normal man. Br J Clin Pharmacol 16:305–311

Critical Evaluation of Antihypertensive Pharmacotherapy

W. KAUFMANN[1] and R. LANG[1]

Round-Table Discussion with:
M. ANLAUF, Essen, Federal Republic of Germany; F. R. BÜHLER, Basle, Switzerland; J. I. S. ROBERTSON, Glasgow, Great Britain; K. O. STUMPE, Bonn, Federal Republic of Germany; P. M. VANHOUTTE, Rochester, USA; W. VETTER, Zürich, Switzerland; P. WEIDMANN, Bern, Switzerland

Introduction

The second round table discussion was held to evaluate critically the significance of new drugs (calcium antagonists, angiotensin I-converting enzyme inhibitors, serotonin antagonists) presented during the preceding morning session. In view of the great number of drugs available on the market, the discussion was aimed at working out a rational treatment of hypertension. The following summary reviews the pharmacologic properties of these drugs and their place in the presently known rationale of antihypertensive therapy.

Calcium Antagonists

Calcium antagonists are agents that inhibit the cellular entry of calcium through a broad group of voltage-dependent, receptor-operated, and calcium-selective plasma membrane ion channels (Weidmann). The various calcium antagonists differ not only in their chemical structure and their exact mechanism of action at the calcium channel, but also have a certain degree of tissue selectivity. The dihydropyridine derivate nifedipine produces pronounced arteriolar vasodilation and has only a minimal influence on cardiac pacemakers, in contrast to the aralkylanine derivative verapamil. The negatively chronotropic and dromotropic effect of diltiazem seems to be intermediate to that of nifedipine and verapamil. Sympathetic cardiovascular reflexes attenuate the potential negatively chronotropic, dromotropic, and ionotropic actions of these drugs. The antihypertensive effect of calcium antagonists is related to a decrease in total peripheral resistance in the presence of unchanged cardiac output. Thus, calcium antagonists lower blood pressure through a direct reduction in basal cardiovascular muscle tone, although a number of additional factors may play a modulating role (Weidmann). These mainly include effects on catecholamines and renin as well as on cardiovascular responsiveness.

[1] Department of Internal Medicine II, Merheim Hospital and Policlinic of the University of Cologne, Ostmerheimer Str. 200, D-5000 Cologne 91.

Primary Hypertension
Ed. by W. Kaufmann et al.

Effects on Catecholamines, Renin, Aldosterone, Electrolytes, and Cardiovascular Responsiveness

It is well known that rising calcium concentrations increase the release of catecholamines from sympathetic nerve terminals and from adrenal medullary tissue, while increased entry of calcium into the juxtaglomerular cells of the kidney may inhibit renin release. However, the mechanisms by which treatment with calcium antagonists influences circulating renin and norepinephrine are not entirely clear. The analysis of published reports about the influence of monotherapy with nifedipine or verapamil on plasma catecholamines and renin showed differences between the humoral effects of these calcium antagonists (Weidmann). During chronic therapy with both agents, therefore, plasma norepinephrine tends to be slightly increased. However, in contrast to the acute administration of verapamil, a single dose of nifedipine increases plasma norepinephrine by an average of 25%. Furthermore, nifedipine given either acutely or chronically increases plasma renin by 60%, while after verapamil application renin is almost unchanged. The significant correlation between the induced changes in circulating renin and norepinephrine suggests that renin variations may closely reflect the effects of calcium antagonists on sympathetic activity (Weidmann). The degree of sympathetic stimulation appears to be determined by the degree of peripheral vasodilatation with consecutive activation on the baroreflex mechanism. This is mainly true for nifedipine. However, after acute administration of verapamil, plasma norepinephrine remains relatively unchanged, despite a distinct fall in blood pressure. This effect and the different chronotropic effects of acutely administered nifedipine or verapamil may represent different influences of these two calcium antagonists on the sympathetic nervous system (Weidmann). Verapamil probably interferes with norepinephrine release from nerve endings; thus, heart rate depends not only on the direct effects of verapamil on pacemaker and conduction (Weidmann).

Following acute administration, nifedipine tends – in contrast to verapamil – to decrease plasma aldosterone concentrations slightly. However, during chronic administration of nifedipine, basal and angiotensin II-stimulated plasma aldosterone levels are unchanged, and plasma potassium and plasma sodium levels are not consistently modified (Weidmann).

Calcium antagonists are found to reduce blood pressure responsiveness to norepinephrine in the experimental animal and in certain human conditions such as borderline hypertension, early renal failure, and diabetes mellitus, where exaggerated cardiovascular pressor responsiveness to norepinephrine exists. The underlying mechanism seems to be a regionally variable dependence of alpha-adrenoceptor-mediated vasoconstriction on transmembranous calcium entry. Thus, calcium antagonists lower not only basal vascular tone, but also the reactivity of certain blood vessels. Further, improvement of norepinephrine hyperreactivity in essential or diabetes-associated hypertension seems to provide a rational antihypertensive therapy in these situations (Weidmann).

It is well known that calcium is a common intracellular trigger for various pressor substances. However, the extent to which abnormalities in calcium metabolism play a primary pathogenetic role in hypertensive states is presently unclear. Some observations have been interpreted in favor of calcium-dependent dysregulation in essential hypertension. Thus, spontaneous hypertension in the rat and human essential hypertension both seem associated with an increase in free cytosolic calcium in vascular muscle cells. There is a good correlation of the blood pressure-lowering effect of calcium antagonists with pretreatment blood pressure values in hypertensive patients, while they have almost no effect on normotensive subjects. Furthermore, there seems to exist a close relationship between blood pressure and blood platelet calcium content before and after treatment with nifedipine or verapamil. Nevertheless, there is still the question of whether calcium antagonists correct an underlying abnormality in essential hypertension (Weidmann).

Besides nifedipine and verapamil, various other calcium antagonists have also been found to lower blood pressure. Despite the considerable pharmacologic differences between them, both the calcium antagonists nifedipine and verapamil given in appropriate dosage, exert a similar antihypertensive effect. Nifedipine (5–30 mg) and verapamil (160–480 mg) lower supine mean blood pressure by an average of 10%–20% during chronic oral treatment. Heart rate tends to be slightly decreased during the chronic treatment with verapamil, while after nifedipine administration, the increase in heart rate tends to dissipate during chronic therapy. In contrast to other direct arteriolar vasodilatators, significant body sodium-fluid retention during long-term treatment with calcium antagonists does not occur. In fact, renal sodium excretion may be increased acutely by various calcium antagonists (Weidmann).

It has been postulated that the antihypertensive efficiency of calcium antagonists and beta-blockers depends on the age of the patients (Bühler). However, there are not enough data available presently to support or refute the notion of increasing antihypertensive effects of calcium antagonists with increasing age (Weidmann).

Calcium antagonists have a potency similar to that of thiazide-type diuretics or beta-blockers. However, the potential value of monotherapy with calcium antagonists in essential hypertension requires further long-term studies (Weidmann). Also, the complementary potencies of calcium antagonists in combination with other antihypertensive drugs, i.e., diuretics, beta-blockers, sympatholytic drugs, converting enzyme inhibitors, postsynaptic $alpha_1$-blockers, etc., deserve further long-term investigation (Weidmann).

Acute blood pressure reductions were noted following single doses of calcium antagonists in secondary forms of hypertension, and nifedipine is now established as an important alternative for the treatment of certain hypertensive emergencies. A single dose of 20 mg nifedipine, applied sublingually, reduces blood pressure within minutes in many patients with life-threatening states and, despite a marked fall in blood pressure, leaves cerebral blood flow unchanged.

Antihypertensive therapy with calcium antagonists is well tolerated by the majority of patients. This therapy is remarkably free of significant metabolic side effects. Certain symptoms such as facial flushing, burning sensations, palpitations, and dizziness may be more pronounced in the initial stage and tend to diminish with progressive treatment (Weidmann). In contrast to nifedipine, caution is warranted when verapamil is administered to patients with conduction disorders and patients receiving another cardiodepressant with negatively chronotropic action.

Angiotensin I-Converting Enzyme Inhibitors

Converting enzyme (ACE) provides one of the pathways for the degradation of bradykinin and is therefore not specific for angiotensin I. Within the circulation, converting enzyme splits angiotensin I, removing two amino acids, to form the principal active component of the renin system, the octapeptide angiotensin II. Thus, inhibitors of ACE are the most important therapeutic agents to interfere with the renin-angiotensin system. A major advance was the development of captopril, the first orally active inhibitor of ACE. The second generation of this drug, typified by enalapril, does not contain a sulfhydril group, probably minimizing adverse reactions. Whereas captopril has a rapid onset of action, within 1 h of oral ingestion, the peak effect of enalapril is much slower, at around 5 h after ingestion. The full antihypertensive effect of both ACE inhibitors, given chronically, may take several weeks to be established (Robertson). Following administration of an ACE inhibitor, there is a fall in circulating angiotensin II and, subsequently, a fall in blood pressure and plasma aldosterone, which are both partly dependent on angiotensin II. Parallel with the fall in circulating angiotensin II, there is a converse rise in angiotensin I and renin.

Substantial clinical benefits accrue from the treatment of hypertension associated with unilateral renal artery stenosis by means of ACE inhibition. For instance, enalapril was used alone for 3 months before surgery on 10 patients with hypertension due to unilateral renal artery stenosis (Robertson). During this long-term treatment, the decrease in blood pressure was less closely related than on the 1st day to either the pretreatment plasma renin or angiotensin II concentrations or to the long-term decrease in plasma angiotensin II. Active renin and angiotensin I concentrations increased progressively from the 1st day to the 3rd month of treatment. Repeat isotope renography at the 3rd month of enalapril treatment showed contrary effects in the two kidneys (Robertson). While effective renal plasma flow through the unaffected kidney was significantly increased, in the stenotic kidney, which already had impaired renal plasma flow, this measure fell further. In unilateral renal artery stenosis, the afflicted kidney is heavily dependent on raised intrarenal concentrations of angiotensin II to help sustain the glomerular filtration rate. Thus, patients who are candidates for corrective renal artery surgery or transluminal balloon dilatation should be treated with ACE inhibitors for no more than 1 month before undergoing surgery (Robertson). Extreme caution should be used in the case of patients with bilateral renal artery stenosis.

Another indication for this drug is severe, previously intractable hypertension, where ACE inhibitors are used in conjunction with powerful loop diuretics such as furosemide. The diuretic promotes sodium excretion, which leads to increased secretion of renin. The reactive rise in circulating angiotensin II is prevented by the ACE inhibitor, so that blood pressure reduction will be more marked. Despite large doses of loop diuretics, plasma aldosterone in this situation is significantly depressed, and there is no tendency to hypokalemia (Robertson). Care is necessary when complex antihypertensive drug regimes have been previously employed, as they often result in high levels of circulating renin and angiotensin II. In these circumstances, ACE inhibitors can cause a dangerous fall in arterial pressure, which is not the case in moderate and previously untreated essential hypertension. Nevertheless, we know that even in moderate essential hypertension, circulating levels of angiotensin II are capable of having a direct immediate effect on arterial pressure. Several controlled trials have shown that both captopril and enalapril have an antihypertensive effect on essential hypertension comparable to that induced by monotherapy with thiazide diuretics or beta-blockers. Even more effective is the joint use of ACE inhibitors with thiazide diuretics.

Like other vasodilators, ACE inhibitors improve exercise capacity in cardiac failure by reducing afterload and probably preload. Their capacity to reduce aldosterone secretion and vasopressin secretion by lowering angiotensin II also helps to promote diuresis in cardiac failure. On the other hand, the direct renal effects of ACE inhibitors in cardiac failure are less beneficial. Lowering intrarenal angiotensin II means a loss of compensatory effects and may lead to a fall in the glomerular filtration rate. Thus, the renal actions of ACE inhibitors in cardiac failure are delicately balanced, and mild increases in serum creatinine occur (Robertson).

The most commonly recorded side effect of captopril and enalapril is rash. Other adverse effects observed with ACE inhibitors, especially with captopril, include proteinuria, occasional cases of nephrotic syndrome, leukopenia, taste disturbances, aphthous ulcers of the mouth, persistent unproductive cough, and Raynaud's phenomen.

The side effect burden of captopril is clearly dose-related. With the second generation of ACE inhibitors such as enalapril, the burden of side effects is less than with captopril. However, as both enalapril and captopril depend largely on the kidney for excretion, doses should be limited in the presence of renal impairment.

Serotonergic Antagonists

Whether or not serotonin (5-hydroxytryptamine) plays a role in the maintenance of increased peripheral resistance in chronic hypertension is still an unanswered question (Vanhoutte). Normally, serotonin, which is released from enterochromaffine cells of the gastrointestinal tract, is rapidly destroyed in its passage through the hepatic and pulmonary circulations. However, serotonin that reaches the blood ist taken up and stored by platelets, and the platelets release the serotonin they contain when they aggregate, thereby promoting aggregation.

In primary hypertension, although there is no augmented concentration of serotonin in the plasma, the platelets release serotonin more easily at the level of the resistance vessels than is the case in normal subjects (Vanhoutte). Serotonin is a potent constrictor of blood vessels by its action on S_2-serotonergic receptors in smooth muscle. However, alpha-adrenoceptors may be also activated directly by serotonin. Besides these direct actions, serotonin can cause vessels to constrict indirectly by releasing norepinephrine from sympathetic nerve terminals and by increasing the sensitivity of smooth muscle to norepinephrine and angiotensin II. On the other hand, by activating prejunctional receptors, small amounts of serotonin may reduce the amount of norepinephrine released during activation of the sympathetic nerves. Thus, when the sympathetic nerves are active, prejunctional action on the serotonergic receptors prevails over the direct constrictor action of the drug, leading to relaxation of the blood vessels. Furthermore, in response to serotonin, the endothelium forms vasodilatator substances that can relax the underlying smooth muscle.

In hypertensive animals, the blood vessel wall shows augmented vascular responsiveness to the constrictor effect of serotonin, owing to both an increased sensitivity to and a prolonged effect of the monoamine as well as a reduction of its prejunctional and endothelial vasodilating effects (Vanhoutte).

The concept of a putative role of serotonin in the pathogenesis of hypertension has been revived by the observation that ketanserin can lower blood pressure in primary hypertension. Ketanserin is a selective S_2-serotonergic antagonist that has no agonistic actions. At higher concentrations, ketanserin is a competitive alpha$_1$-adrenergic antagonist. The efficacy of ketanserin as an antihypertensive agent is comparable to that of beta-adrenergic blockers or diuretics, in that it decreases systemic vascular resistance. When given acutely, there may be a transient augmentation of heart rate, but chronically applied, it decreases blood pressure without a reflex increase in heart rate (Vanhoutte). With chronic administration of ketanserin, norepinephrine levels are unchanged, but levels of renin and angiotensin II decrease slightly, with no change in that of aldosterone. Thus, a major interference with the renin-angiotensin-aldosterone axis is not the likely explanation for the hypotensive effects of ketanserin. The drug should be administered twice a day because the half-life of ketanserin is approximately 10 h. At higher doses (e.g., 60 mg t.i.d.), patients have considerable dizziness and orthostatic hypotension, mainly owing to a central nervous action of the drug. In general, side effects with ketanserin are not more pronounced than with other antiyhpertensive agents such as beta-adrenergic blockers or diuretic agents (Vanhoutte).

There are still discussions about the real mechanism of action because chronic oral administration of ketanserin leads to a reduction in the pressor effects of alpha$_1$-adrenoceptor agonists. However, this inhibitory effect of ketanserin on the response to alpha$_1$-adrenergic agonists could be explained by a nonspecific decrease in vascular responsiveness, resulting from an altered wall-to-lumen ratio following a reduction in arterial blood pressure. The antihypertensive effect of ketanserin is mainly related to its inhibitory effect on S_2-serotonergic receptors (Vanhoutte). Thus, the increased aggregation of platelets caused by serotonin in vitro and in vivo is inhibited by acute administration of ketanserin, and the vasoconstrictor effect of serotonin in volunteers is also prevented by ketanserin. In contrast to other available serotonergic antagonists, which show no antihypertensive properties, ketanserin has a very high degree of selectivity for S_2-serotonergic receptors in smooth muscle, thus explaining the mechanism of action by which it lowers blood pressure. Ketanserin prevents the direct constrictor action of serotonin on vascular smooth muscle, unmasking at the same time the vasodilator properties of serotonin (Vanhoutte).

Rationale for Established Antihypertensive Treatment and Its Effects on Morbidity and Mortality

The crucial point of the round table discussion was the form our therapy should take in the future, especially for patients with mild hypertension. This includes the criteria for selecting initial antihypertensive agents, for determining the sequence of combining such drugs, and for implementing new drugs? The decision of a clinician to treat a particular hypertensive patient with hypertensive drugs should be based on the health situation of this patient and on data derived from epidemiologic and pharmacologic sources (Amery). However, the widespread idea, based on epidemiologic surveys, that hypertensive drug treatment should be started more readily in hypertensive patients with additional risk indicators is so far only speculative and needs confirmation from controlled trials (Amery). Patients with permanently elevated diastolic *and* systolic blood pressure should be treated, meaning not only patients with a systolic pressure of 190 mm Hg, but also patients with a systolic blood pressure of 160 and even 150 mm Hg, since the latter are also at greater risk than subjects with a systolic blood pressure of 120 mm Hg (Amery). However, it is not acceptable to treat a symptomless adult with a diastolic blood pressure of 90 mm Hg with drugs over many years (Robertson).

The German League against Hypertension, like other scientific medical organizations, has repeatedly drawn up recommendations for antihypertensive drug therapy. However, the criteria for this stepped care approach to antihypertensive therapy have never been precisely formulated (Holzgreve). There exist various bases for the classification of antihypertensives, including, for example, the claim that an antihypertensive drug interferes with the pathogenetic mechanism of hypertension, that blood pressure during exercise is reduced, that left ventricular hypertrophy regresses, that the hemodynamic profile is positively affected, and that the circadian rhythm of blood pressure is physiologically influenced, etc. Of all these criteria, only the following two are especially significant (Holzgreve): (a) demonstrated efficacy, that is, prevention of the typical long-term complications of hypertension; (b) good tolerance and an acceptable side effect rate. Several hypertension intervention studies (Holzgreve) have clearly shown that drug therapy in hypertensive individuals between 30 and 65 years with diastolic blood pressure values of between 95 and 110 mm Hg improves life expectancy and decreases morbidity. In these studies, the calculated mean reductions are 31% for total mortality, 40% for cardiovascular mortality, and 63% for cerebrovascular accidents (Holzgreve). Today, collective evaluation of all studies also justifies the statement that antihypertensive treatment prevents fatal and nonfatal myocardial infarction and sudden death to a small but clearly discernible extent (12%). However, this improvement in the reduction of coronary heart disease mortality through current antihypertensive treatment is far too small and still very unsatisfactory (Korner). The Japanese, who have extremely low cholesterol levels despite a high prevelance of hypertension, do not have any major problems with ischemic heart disease. Thus, if we could bring our physicians to agree to simultaneous treatment of even moderately elevated cholesterol levels, we might be much more successful in preventing coronary heart disease as a sequel of hypertension (Heyden). There was agreement during the discussion that the personal management of antihypertensive therapy by the physician is most important.

The hypertension detection and follow-up program compared two treatment procedures: treatment of hypertensive patients in regularly available medical practice, the normally administered referred care and treatment in specialized centers and clinics, where several measures were taken to increase compliance (stepped care). The 5-year mortality of the total number of randomized patients was 17% lower with stepped care than with referred care (Amery).

While several studies have shown a reduction in mortality for patients under 65 years, as yet none has proven this for patients over 65, and convincing data are still lacking for elderly patients (Amery). For stroke survivors over the age of 65, antihypertensive drug treatment was not able significantly to decrease the recurrence of stroke (Amery). Moreover, a decrease in cerebrovascular events is assumed only for treated male, but not for female patients (Amery). Thus, an overwhelming number of intervention studies find no explanation for the vast majority of patients, namely, white female subjects with uncomplicated essential hypertension (Amery). They do not prove that, through the use of hypertensive drugs in this group of patients, mortality in general, cardiovascular mortality only, or even the incidence of cardiovascular events can be decreased (Amery). In the female group of the Australian mild hypertensive study, which is a most relevant trial because of its methodology and the number of patients randomized, there were no significant differences between the actively treated and the control groups (Amery). Further, the Hypertension Detection and Follow-up Program study, where the largest number of patients were entered, does not indicate that we can prolong life expectancy in hypertensive white female subjects by means of antihypertensive drugs (Amery).

Based on long-term intervention studies, proof that hypertensive organ complications can be prevented is most thoroughly documented for diuretics, not quite as thoroughly for beta-blockers, reserpine, and alpha-methyldopa, and as yet not at all for calcium antagonists and ACE inhibitors (Holzgreve). The conclusion of the MRFIT study that diuretic treatment is harmful to hypertensive individuals with preexisting pathologic ECG changes is statistically unacceptable and stands in crass contradiction to the findings of all other studies (Holzgreve).

The second criterion for the selection of antihypertensives is the rate of side effects at equally effective doses. Since this is extremely difficult to determine, methodically sound therapeutic studies are mandatory (Holzgreve). The reported frequency and pattern of side effects differ not only between different hospitals in the same city, but between different investigators working at the same clinic, thus, showing clearly the influence of the investigator on the patients (Robertson). A valid study must compare the antihypertensive action, tolerance, and side effects of new drugs with those of standard therapy and must involve sufficiently large patients populations studied over a reasonably long period of time. Any new agent claiming a preferential status in antihypertensive treatment will have to be examined in the light of known large-scale therapeutic studies and will have to be compared with diuretics or beta-blockers (Holzgreve).

What is the Place of Calcium Antagonists, ACE Inhibitors, and Serotonin Antagonists?

Based on the argument that an ideal reduction of coronary morbidity has not yet been achieved, we must also give a chance to certain newer classes of antihypertensive drugs, which are of interest with regard to cardiovascular complications (Weidmann). These new drugs, especially the calcium antagonists and ACE inhibitors, are clearly challenging the established pattern of therapy in hypertension, although we certainly do not yet know what the long-term outcome will be (Weidmann).

In mild hypertension, therapy should normally be initiated with a beta-blocker and a thiazide diuretic. However, these drugs are not free from substantial deficiencies. They are unsuitable for patients with respiratory disease and diabetes mellitus. Furthermore, beta-blockers cause mental lassitude and deficiency in memory (Robertson). Thus, other drugs suitable for first-line treatment seem to be the calcium antagonists (Weidmann, Bühler) and the ACE inhibitors (Stumpe). Calcium antagonists deserve particular consideration as an alternative to beta-blockers, low-dose diuretics, and probably also ACE inhibitors, either as initial or second drugs. The overall tolerability is excellent (Bühler), and it seems important that calcium antagonists can be combined with all different antihypertensive varieties effectively (Weidmann). This is especially true of calcium antagonists combined with ACE inhibitors if two drugs are necessary to normalize blood pressure (Bühler). Concerning the combination of calcium antagonists with a higher cardiodepressant potential (i.e., verapamil) and beta-blockers given orally, there are only very few reports of bradycardia and heart block in the literature (Bühler). When long-term diuretic treatment is replaced by therapy with calcium antagonists, about 5% of patients have fluid retention (Bühler). However, if calcium antagonists are employed initially, the sodium-fluid retention problem is a minor one and occurs only in patients with chronic venous insufficiency. In the discussion, it was stressed that, for hypertensive patients with diabetes mellitus in whom diuretics and $beta_2$-blockers tend to have undesirable metabolic effects, calcium antagonists are worth trying (Weidmann).

ACE inhibitors are at least as effective as beta-blockers or thiazides as first-line therapy, and they combine well with thiazides as second-step treatment (Robertson). In combination with loop diuretics, they play an important role in the treatment of previously intractable hypertension. Moreover, ACE inhibitors will have an increasing part in the treatment of severe congestive heart failure (Robertson). In the treatment of mild hypertension, which affects almost 10% of the adult population, with specific drugs, the issue of well-being becomes increasingly important (Stumpe). Therefore, it was interesting to hear that a comparison of the effects on short-term memory of the ACE inhibitor enalapril and the beta-blocker atenolol showed a better outcome for enalapril (Robertson).

This still leaves the question of what the physician should do with elderly patients who have not had a complete work-up for renal artery stenosis (Rosenthal). Should he give an ACE inhibitor without knowing the condition of the renal artery and without having excluded the possibility of intrarenal artery lesion? The answer of the panel was yes, but serum creatinine levels should be carefully monitored at very short intervals in order to discover early effects on renal function (Robertson).

Besides effectiveness and tolerability, practicability was also mentioned (Vetter). Modern drugs should be taken only once a day to improve the compliance of the patient. New calcium antagonists (nitrendipine and a special form of verapamil) and a second generation of ACE inhibitors (enalapril) show satisfactory levels throughout the day with single dosing (Weidmann, Robertson).

In the generally accepted treatment of hypertension, the panel could come to no final conclusion concerning the place of a drug like ketanserin, which seems convincingly effective and reasonably safe, but for which only a limited amount of material is available as yet. In view of the great number of drugs for the treatment of hypertension recommendations for this new drug were differed somewhat, depending on personal experience. Ketanserin is a rather mild antihypertensive agent of the same order as beta-blockers and thiazide (Robertson). At the present time, one might predict from the pharmacology of ketanserin that, with established hypertension where there is an increased turnover of platelets and aging blood vessel walls, that is especially for elderly patients with artheriosclerosis, this drug should be more effective than others (Vanhoutte). In Sweden and Belgium at least several groups seem to achieve remarkable results with this drug when administered to patients with migraine and peripheral vascular disease (Vanhoutte). However, at the end of the round table discussion, disappointment was expressed (Holzgreve, Anlauf), as some participants of the panel had put the new substances on a par with beta-blockers and diuretics without having cited any long-term studies testing these new drugs. Thus, the long-term benefit-risk ratio of these drugs still has to be evaluated in the future.

References

Amery A, Fagard R, Fiocchi R, Lijnen P, Staessen J, Vermylen J (1984) Antihypertensive action and serotonin-induced platelet aggregation during long-term ketanserin treatment in hypertensive patients. J Cardiovasc Pharmacol 6: 182–185

Anonymous (1984) The international prospective primary prevention study in hypertension (IPPPSH): Objectives and methods. Eur J Clin Pharmacol 27: 379–391

Bühler FR, Halthern UC, Kiowski W, Bolli P (1982) Greater antihypertensive efficacy of the calcium channel inhibitor verapamil in older and low renin patients. Clin Sci 63: 439–441

Fleckenstein A (1983) Calcium antagonism in heart and smooth muscle: Experimental facts and therapeutic prospects. Wiley, New York

Folkow B (1982) Physiological aspects of primary hypertension. Physiol Rev 62: 347–504

Guazzi MD, de Cesare N, Galli C, Salvioni A, Tramontana C, Tamborini G, Bartorelli A (1984) Calcium-channel blockade with nifedipine and angiotensin converting-enzyme inhibition with captopril in the therapy of patients with severe primary hypertension. Circulation 70: 179–284

Hedner T, Persson B, Berglund G (1983) Ketanserin, a novel 5-hydroxytryptamine antagonist: Monotherapy in essential hypertension. Br J Clin Pharmacol 16: 121–125

Hypertension Detection and Follow-up Program Cooperative Group (1982) The effect of treatment on mortality in "mild" hypertension. New Engl J Med 307: 976–980

Joint National Committee on Detection, Evaluation and Treatment of High Blood Pressure (1984) Report. Arch Intern Med 144: 1045–1057

Laragh JH (ed) (1984) Converting enzyme inhibition for understanding and management of hypertensive disorders and congestive failure. Am J Med 77 (2a): 1–86

Multiple Risk Factor Intervention Trial (1982) Risk factor changes and mortality results. JAMA 248: 1465–1477

Robertson JIS (ed) (1984) The renin-angiotensin-system. Gower, London

Svensson A, Hansson L (ed) (1984) Symposium on new approaches to the treatment of hypertension. J Hypertens 2 [Suppl 2]: 1–121

Weidmann P, Gerber A, Laederach K (1984) Calcium antagonists in the treatment of hypertension: A critical overview. In: Crosnier J, Maxwell (eds) Advances in Nephrology. Year Book Medical, Chicago, pp 197–232

Vanhoutte PM (ed) (1985) Serotonin and the cardiovascular system. Raven, New York

Subject Index

GPSR Compliance

The European Union's (EU) General Product Safety Regulation (GPSR) is a set of rules that requires consumer products to be safe and our obligations to ensure this.

If you have any concerns about our products, you can contact us on ProductSafety@springernature.com

In case Publisher is established outside the EU, the EU authorized representative is:

Springer Nature Customer Service Center GmbH
Europaplatz 3
69115 Heidelberg, Germany

Batch number: 10704763

Printed by Printforce, the Netherlands